Wars in the 19th Century were accompanied by a very heavy loss of life from infectious diseases. Typhus fever, dysentery, malaria, typhoid fever and yellow fever caused many more deaths than wounds inflicted by enemy actions. During the Peninsular War, for example, for every soldier dying of a wound, four succumbed to disease. This book examines the development and evolution of surgical practice against this overwhelming risk of death due to disease. It reviews three major conflicts during this time: the Peninsular War, the Crimean War and the Second Boer War, besides considering many minor wars fought by the British Empire in the intervening years, and highlights significant medical and surgical developments during these conflicts.

War surgery in the first part of the 19th Century was brutal and it had to be carried out swiftly. It was performed at speed because there were no anaesthetics and the wounded often died during the procedure. Surgeons focused their attention on wounds of the arms and legs, because limbs were both easily accessible to the surgeon (unlike organs inside the abdomen and chest) and lent themselves well to amputation. This was commonly the operation of choice for many war wounds of arms and legs. Some surgeons performed more difficult surgical procedures to try to preserve the limbs and attempted to repair damaged tissues but these operations took longer and caused greater suffering to the patient. Abdominal and chest wounds were not treated since surgeons did not have the means, the ability, or the understanding, to cut into the abdomen and chest to repair the damaged organs successfully.

An important development which contributed to surgery moving forwards was the discovery of general anaesthesia, which became available in time for the Crimean War. However, whilst it certainly rendered operations pain-free, it was associated with significant numbers of deaths during surgery on wounded soldiers because of the poorly understood effects that anaesthetics had, particularly on the heart. As a result, operative surgery did not extend its scope a great deal, and military surgery remained focused on surgery of the limbs. However, fewer amputations were performed during the Boer War at the end of this period. Britain sent observers to several wars in which it was not involved to learn military lessons and to understand the medical and surgical aspects of war. The American Civil War and the Franco Prussian War were two such conflicts. The Russo Japanese War resulted in a very significant advance in surgery for abdominal wounds, but Western observers either failed to notice or ignored pioneering work performed by a Russian female surgeon called Vera Gedroits. As a result when the Great War began in 1914, lessons had to be re-learned by British surgeons, and many soldiers who suffered penetrating abdominal wounds lost their lives when they should have survived. Unfortunately one of the hallmarks of war surgery is that successive generations of surgeons make the same mistakes as their forebears and the same lessons have to be learned time and again.

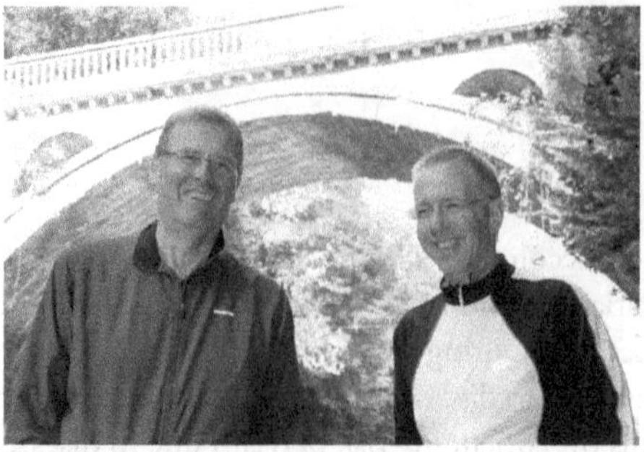

Tom Scotland (left) and Steve Heys (right)

Thomas R. Scotland

Born in St. Andrews and brought up in the East Neuk of Fife, Tom was educated at Waid Academy in Anstruther. He graduated in Medicine from the University of Edinburgh in 1971, becoming a Fellow of the Royal College of Surgeons of Edinburgh in 1975. He trained in orthopaedic surgery in Aberdeen, and after spending a year as a Fellow in the University of Toronto, returned to take up the position of Consultant Orthopaedic Surgeon with Grampian Health Board and Honorary Senior Lecturer at the University of Aberdeen. His particular interests were knee surgery, paediatric orthopaedics and tumour surgery, and for three years he was lead clinician for the Scottish Sarcoma Managed Clinical Network. He first developed his interest in the history of military surgery after many visits to the Great War battlefields of France and Flanders. He has co-edited a book, *War Surgery 1914-18*, with Steve Heys. Now he has joined forces with Steve again to publish this work on military medicine and surgery during the nineteenth century.

Steven D Heys

Born in Accrington in Lancashire and educated in England, Australia and Scotland, Steve graduated in Medicine from the University of Aberdeen in 1981 and undertook surgical training in the North-East of Scotland. He is a Fellow of the Royal Colleges of Surgeons of England, Edinburgh and Glasgow and underwent research training at the Rowet Research Institute in Aberdeen, obtaining a PhD in 1992. He specialised in general and breast cancer surgery for many years before latterly concentrating on breast cancer surgery. His research interests focus on the role of nutrition in the causation of cancer, and he has responsibilities for medical education both locally and nationally. He has published more than 200 scientific papers and written many book chapters on different aspects of surgery and played frequent national and international roles in surgery and the provision of surgical services. He spent time as a member of the 51st Highland Brigade RAMC (V) and is a keen bagpipe player. He formed a firm friendship with Tom on one of Tom's cycling expeditions to the battlefields of France and Flanders. *War Surgery 1914-18* was their first piece of work together. This is now their second publication on British military history.

WARS, PESTILENCE & THE SURGEON'S BLADE

The Evolution of British Military Medicine and Surgery during the Nineteenth Century

Thomas Scotland &
Steven Heys

Helion & Company Ltd

Helion & Company Limited
Unit 8 Amherst Business Centre
Budbrooke Road
Warwick
CV34 5WE
England
Tel. 01926 499 619
Fax 0121 711 4075
Email: info@helion.co.uk
Website: www.helion.co.uk
Twitter: @helionbooks
Visit our blog http://blog.helion.co.uk/

Published by Helion & Company 2013. Reprinted in paperback 2019
Designed and typeset by Farr out Publications, Wokingham, Berkshire
Cover designed by Farr out Publications, Wokingham, Berkshire
Printed by Lightning Source Limited, Milton Keynes, Buckinghamshire

Front cover: Watercolour by Charles Bell of a chest wound. This is a stab wound which has penetrated the chest wall. Patients with such wounds lived or died depending on whether any vital structure within the chest cavity had been significantly damaged. Surgeons were usually unable to intervene operatively. (Courtesy of the Royal College of Surgeons of Edinburgh). Rear cover: Statue of Sir James McGrigor in the library of Aberdeen Medico-Chirurgical Society. The full-sized version was located at the Royal Army Medical College at Millbank in London. (Courtesy of the Aberdeen Medico-Chirurgical Society).

ISBN 978-1-911628-33-0

British Library Cataloguing-in-Publication Data.
A catalogue record for this book is available from the British Library.

Dedication

This book is dedicated to our wives Lyn and Susan who proof read the chapters and endured bad tempers on many occasions. They also had to listen to the painful efforts of the elder author being taught the practice chanter for the bagpipes by the younger, a state of affairs which will continue and get worse long after this book has been submitted to the publisher.

Many women would have packed their bags and left for much less and much sooner! So thank you both very much.

Contents

List of Figures

List of Tables

About the Authors

Thomas R. Scotland

Born in St. Andrews and brought up in the East Neuk of Fife, Tom was educated at Waid Academy in Anstruther. He graduated in Medicine from the University of Edinburgh in 1971, becoming a Fellow of the Royal College of Surgeons of Edinburgh in 1975. He trained in orthopaedic surgery in Aberdeen, and after spending a year as a Fellow in the University of Toronto, returned to take up the position of Consultant Orthopaedic Surgeon with Grampian Health Board and Honorary Senior Lecturer at the University of Aberdeen. His particular interests were knee surgery, paediatric orthopaedics and tumour surgery, and for three years he was lead clinician for the Scottish Sarcoma Managed Clinical Network. He first developed his interest in the history of military surgery after many visits to the Great War battlefields of France and Flanders. He has co-edited a book "War Surgery 1914-18" with Steve Heys. Now he has joined forces with Steve again to publish this work on military medicine and surgery during the nineteenth century.

Steven D Heys

Born in Accrington in Lancashire and educated in England, Australia and Scotland, Steve graduated in Medicine from the University of Aberdeen in 1981 and undertook surgical training in the North-East of Scotland. He is a Fellow of the Royal Colleges of Surgeons of England, Edinburgh and Glasgow and underwent research training at the Rowet Research Institute in Aberdeen, obtaining a PhD in 1992. He specialised in general and breast cancer surgery for many years before latterly concentrating on breast cancer surgery. His research interests focus on the role of nutrition in the causation of cancer, and he has responsibilities for medical education both locally and nationally. He has published more than 200 scientific papers and written many book chapters on different aspects of surgery and played frequent national and international roles in surgery and the provision of surgical services. He spent time as a member of the 51st Highland Brigade RAMC (V) and is a keen bagpipe player. He formed a firm friendship with Tom on one of Tom`s cycling expeditions to the battlefields of France and Flanders. *War Surgery 1914-18* was their first piece of work together. This is now their second publication on British military history.

Foreword

'There must be a beginning of any good matter, but the continuing to the end, until it be thoroughly finished yields the true glory'.
(Drake to Walsingham)

As a military surgeon who has followed the drum of the Royal Army Medical Corps (RAMC), I feel honoured to contribute a foreword to this book. The history of warfare and the history of medicine are closely intertwined. Yet, there is surprisingly little written on the historical development of military medicine. For any serious student of the subject, and every member and prospective member of the Army Medical Services, *Wars, Pestilence and the Surgeon's Blade* is, quite simply, required reading.

The wars of the twentieth century have driven advances in many aspects of military medical and surgical treatment, which have translated into civilian medical practice and helped to shape our healthcare today. The Military Medical Services keep our forces fit, prevent and treat disease, repair the injured, and return them to active duty, as quickly as possible. Our troops stand in harm's way because they have morale borne of confidence in the casualty evacuation chain and the quality of treatment they will receive when wounded or ill.

Two hundred years ago, things were very different. The misery of the sick and wounded in war at the beginning of the 19th Century is almost beyond comprehension. Soldiers, it seemed, were expendable commodities. Armies were crippled by diseases for which medicine had no answer, and which ran rampant because of ignorance or neglect of the principles of sanitation and hygiene. Surgery focused on wounds of the limbs, and had to be quick, as there was no anaesthesia. Amputation was the procedure of choice for most surgeons; and mortality was high from blood loss and general infection. The frequent failures in casualty evacuation and medical care stemmed from the resistance of military commanders to provide adequate medical transport and personnel. Army doctoring was unattractive, not only dangerous, but considered by many as "the lowest step of professional drudgery and degradation". In 1808, Sir William Fergusson, Inspector General of Hospitals in Portugal during the Peninsular War was moved to say: "A better organisation, whether it regards humanity, or the efficiency of our Army, it is to be hoped will be made for future wars."

Wars, Pestilence and the Surgeon's Blade traces the evolution of the British Army Medical Services from the Peninsular War to the beginning of the Great War. It considers the three major conflicts Britain fought during that period: The Peninsular War (1808–1814), the Crimean War (1853-56) and the Boer War (1899 – 1902); and three major foreign wars - The American Civil War (1861-1865), the Franco-Prussian War (1870–1871) and the Russo-Japanese War (1904-1905). It is the second collaboration by Tom Scotland and Steven Heys, distinguished surgeons from Aberdeen. It stands well as a companion to *War Surgery 1914–1918* with which they established their reputations as military medical historians. It is beautifully written in their engaging and flowing style that is easy to read, but which nevertheless provides considerable biographical, historical and medical detail.

They tell of the seminal work of the great military doctors of the period. Men such as Sir James McGrigor, Director General of the Army Medical Department from 1815 – 1851, 'Father' of the Army Medical Services, whose documentation on every aspect of health and disease paved the way for an understanding of the epidemiology of disease, and cross infection; George James Guthrie whose work on the control of arterial haemorrhage, limb sparing surgery of the upper limb, and the "incalculable difference" between gunshot and blast wounds of limbs, which we witness today among our wounded in Afghanistan, established him as the outstanding surgeon of his era; and Sir Alexander Ogston, Regius Professor of Surgery in Aberdeen, who campaigned in the 1870's for reform and improvements in the field of medical organisation for war, and the care of the sick and wounded. His determination and authority were crucial to the formation of the RAMC.

At times, it is difficult to read this book without an immense sense of frustration at the apparent inability to learn the medical lessons of previous wars. McGrigor made significant improvements to the health of Wellington's forces during the Peninsular War. However, the measures he put in place were forgotten by the time of the Crimean War when conditions for soldiers were appalling, and there was a high incidence of cholera, typhus and typhoid due to a total neglect of hygiene. Following the horrors of the Crimea, and the Indian Mutiny, Army Medical

Reform became an issue of national importance and sanitary conditions for troops, barracks and hospitals were greatly improved. Yet, 40 years later, General Wolseley, Commander-in-Chief of the Army took the view that the sanitary officer was '*a very useless functionary*' who could well be left behind at base. As a result, during the Second Boer War, 14,000 troops died from disease, mainly typhoid, compared to 7,000 who died at the hands of the Boers. His attitude illustrated two fundamental issues that greatly retarded the development of British military medicine during the 19th Century: The systematic failure at the highest level to insist that military commanders should bear a responsibility for elementary hygiene in their units; and an entrenched prejudice on the part of the War Office and senior military commanders about service doctors holding military rank and enjoying comparable professional and social standing with other officers.

In surgery, there was little advance made upon the work of Guthrie in the Peninsular War. The failure of British military medical observers during the Russo-Japanese War to recognise the pioneering work of Vera Gedroits, Chief Surgeon of a Russian Red Cross Hospital train is particularly poignant. She advocated laparotomy for abdominal wounds within 3 hours of wounding. When there was a delay in treatment, the results were significantly poorer. This would become an extremely important surgical principle, which was rediscovered and eventually applied by British military surgeons during the Great War, but only after many thousands of soldiers had died from expectant management. In the field of anaesthesia, had doctors in Paris during the Franco-Prussian War made use of the substantial amount of nitrous oxide available to them, they would probably have recognised its relative safety for use with badly wounded soldiers who might succumb if given chloroform or ether. Instead, it was not until the Great War when it came into its own, as the only safe agent, in wounded soldiers close to death from shock.

There were important advances made: Sir Almroth Wright developed a successful vaccine against typhoid. Unfortunately, questionable fears about its safety meant it failed to gain approval for use during the Boer War, where it would have saved thousands of lives. Nevertheless, Britain would be the sole combatant to enter the Great War with its troops immunized against typhoid fever, a factor instrumental in making it the first war in which fewer British soldiers died from disease than from missile wounds. The methods employed to evacuate and treat huge numbers of wounded during the American Civil War, the Franco- Prussian War and the Russo-Japanese war were duly noted and meant that an effective casualty evacuation pathway with adequate doctors would be put in place for the First World War. By then, after a century of warfare, politicians and military commanders understood the importance of proper sanitary arrangements, hygiene, and inoculation, which would save the loss of thousands of men through disease and sickness. The hallmark lesson from the darkness and confusion of these 19th Century conflicts was the need for institutional military medical memory and due regard for the Army Medical Services. This would begin with the birth of the RAMC in 1898, the founding of the Journal of the Royal Army Medical Corps in 1903, the creation of an Army School of Sanitation at Aldershot in 1906, and the new Army Medical College at Millbank in 1907.

Wars, Pestilence and the Surgeon's Blade is a major and timely contribution to our understanding of the evolution of British Military Medicine. It is fascinating not just for what it reveals of the past, but also, for the lessons it provides that have relevance today. I commend it to you.

Michael P M Stewart
Colonel (Rtd.), CBE, MBChB (Abdn), FRCSGlas, FRCS Tr & Orth, FRCSEd (Ad hominem), L/RAMC,
Lately, Honorary Surgeon to H M The Queen, and Defence Medical Services Consultant Advisor in Trauma and Orthopaedics
Consultant in Trauma & Orthopaedic Surgery

Preface

Two surgeons are standing in Duthie Park in Aberdeen and are looking towards an obelisk which was erected here in a prominent position in the southern part of the park in 1906.It is on a hill overlooking the River Dee from where it can be clearly seen from far and wide. One of the surgeons is a retired orthopaedic surgeon who for many years worked in Aberdeen Royal Infirmary and the Royal Aberdeen Children's Hospital. The younger of the two is Professor of Cancer Surgery at the University of Aberdeen who specialises in the treatment of breast cancer at Aberdeen Royal Infirmary.

The obelisk is surrounded by rows of flower beds, which in the summer create a spectacular bloom and provide a pleasing setting for passing visitors to the park. As the surgeons look thoughtfully towards the obelisk, young mothers pushing prams on their afternoon outing and cyclists on their training schedules pass the landmark. Few give the obelisk as much as a glance and nobody stops to read the writing found on its base.

It used to stand at Marischal College in the centre of Aberdeen and which is part of the University of Aberdeen. It was erected there in 1860 to commemorate one of Aberdeen's most famous sons, Sir James McGrigor, who died in 1858. It was moved to its present site when Marischal College was extended in the early part of the twentieth century.

McGrigor came from a small village called Cromdale, in Speyside in the north of Scotland, and was a distinguished pupil at Aberdeen Grammar School. He initially graduated as a Master of Arts from the University of Aberdeen before enrolling in the University's medical school. On the completion of his medical studies he was a co-founding member of the Aberdeen Medical Society in 1789, which subsequently was renamed the Aberdeen Medico-Chirurgical Society in 1811. McGrigor joined the army in 1794 as a regimental surgeon and had an eventful early career in Flanders, the West Indies, India and Egypt before becoming the Duke of Wellington's Chief Medical Officer during the Peninsular War in December 1811, where his organisational skills set him apart as an outstanding medical administrator. He became Director General of Army Medical Services in 1815 at the age of 44, a week before the Battle of Waterloo. After Napoleon Bonaparte was defeated and exiled to St Helena, Baron Larrey and Baron Percy, his two principal medical officers, with whom McGrigor had formed a close friendship based on mutual respect, were both made Honorary Members of the Aberdeen Medico-Chirurgical Society.

How different it all must have been in McGrigor's day, when for every soldier who was killed or died from wounds during the Peninsular War, four succumbed to diseases such as typhus fever, malaria and dysentery. McGrigor himself was fortunate to have survived to a ripe old age. Many of his military medical contemporaries did not. Medical officers were no more immune to diseases than the men they were responsible for.

The two surgeons have written this book about British military medicine and surgery during the nineteenth century in which amongst many interesting developments, they acknowledge McGrigor's major contribution to improving the health of soldiers in the first part of the century which led to him becoming known as the father of British Military Medicine.

They previously joined forces to co-edit a book War Surgery 1914-18 which discusses the development of surgical and allied specialties during the Great War and which, like this book, has strong links with the University of Aberdeen.

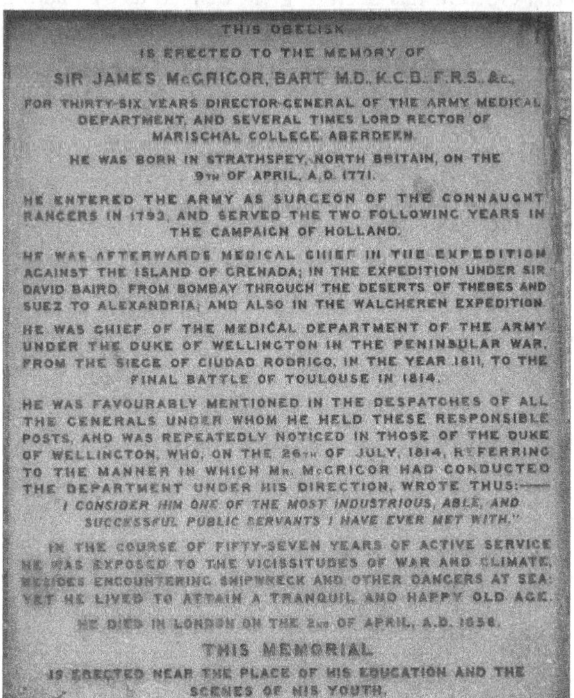

Acknowledgments

We are very grateful to Ann Robertson who wrote the chapter on the development of military anaesthesia during the nineteenth century. Ann graduated in Medicine from the University of Birmingham in 1975 and after training in anaesthesia became consultant in anaesthesia at Hairmyres Hospital, before moving to Aberdeen, where she worked with Tom Scotland for many years. She contributed a very important chapter to our previous publication *War Surgery 1914-18*. Now she has extended her interest in the history of anaesthesia to write a chapter on the evolution of military anaesthesia in the nineteenth century.

Mr. Gordon Stables of the Department of Medical Illustration, University of Aberdeen, has worked extensively with both authors on several occasions in the past on various medical projects. Gordon has been of great help to us by making the maps for this book. He also made a key contribution to our previous book *War Surgery 1914-18*, when he made many maps and illustrations. He has become an important member of our team and we are very grateful to him.

Colonel Mike Stewart, RAMC, very kindly agreed to write a foreword for this book. Mike is a graduate of the University of Aberdeen and is at the top of his profession in the British Army today. We could think of no one better placed and more appropriate to write the foreword.

We would also like to thank Robin Reid very much, who volunteered to proof read the text of the book with minimal persuasion. Robin also helped in many other ways.

We are also grateful to the many others who have given us permission to use illustrations in this book. We have endeavoured to obtain permission in every case where appropriate, although sometimes it has not been possible to trace the origin of every illustration or photograph. We sincerely hope we have not offended anyone by any inadvertent act of omission.

We hope this book will be read by anyone and everyone with an interest in military history. It has been written with a general readership in mind, although it should also appeal to health professionals. It is not a medical textbook, and it has been written to complement our previous work, *War Surgery 1914-18*.

1

Setting the Scene

This book sets out to examine the developments which took place in British military medicine and surgery between the early nineteenth century and the opening years of the twentieth century. It spans more than one hundred years of advances in both medicine and surgery and provides an in depth analysis of three major conflicts; the Peninsular War, the Crimean War and the Boer War. It charts how lessons that were learned from these wars were applied to subsequent conflicts.

THE THREE PRINCIPLE CONFLICTS

The Peninsular War (1808-1814) was notable because many more soldiers died as a result of disease than were either killed by the enemy or died from wounds. James McGrigor was appointed as Wellington's chief medical officer in the Peninsular campaign in 1812, with the title of Inspector of Hospitals. He introduced many important changes to improve the care of the sick and wounded which will be discussed in detail in Chapter 4. McGrigor subsequently became Director General of Army Medical Services in 1815 and he continued to exert his influence on army medicine for a further 36 years. Such was the importance of his contribution that he would rightly become recognised as the "father" of modern military medicine.

The Crimean War (1853-1856) occupied a half way military point between the Battle of Waterloo and the Second Boer War. It was a war where soldiers' uniforms had not changed significantly since the Napoleonic Wars and infantry still stood in a thin red line facing the enemy. It was also a war where combatants were equipped with improved weapons capable of inflicting more devastating wounds. It formed a link between the wars of the earlier part of the century and the American Civil War (1861-1865) that approached the scale of conflict which was destined to characterise the Great War (1914-1918). The Crimean War, discussed in Chapter

10, was associated with logistical and tactical errors on a grand scale with a resultant immense cost in terms of human tragedy. The majority of deaths were the result of disease, neglect and poor hygiene and major changes were introduced in its aftermath to prevent such events ever happening again. These will be discussed and analysed in Chapter 11.

The Second Boer War (1899-1902) came as a very unpleasant shock to the British Empire, as Chapter 15 explains. Boer farmers successfully took on the might of the British Empire after long-standing resentment fuelled by British administration and expansionism boiled over and led to a savage conflict. It came after the Boers realised that British activity would lead eventually to loss of ethnic Boer control over the South African Republic. Diseases once again caused more deaths amongst British troops than enemy action.

Great Britain was heavily criticised by other nations during the Boer War and Germany was particularly vocal in its condemnation of British actions. Great Britain's stance of "splendid isolation", which it had maintained for much of the nineteenth century, came to an end and it reached out for the support of allies. Firstly, Britain signed a treaty with Japan in 1902 aiming to thwart Russian expansion in the east, and then the "Entente Cordiale" with France was signed in 1904. This was necessary to counteract Germany's growing industrial and military might as the Triple Alliance, which comprised Germany, Austria-Hungary and Italy, loomed ever larger on the European stage as a threat to peace. Many of the young doctors who were involved in treating the wounded during the Second Boer War went on to become medical and surgical leaders in their fields during the Great War.

MINOR WARS

These three major conflicts form the backbone of this book and were the source of most of the medical and surgical development during the nineteenth century. The British Empire was also involved in many "minor wars". These necessitated the deployment of small numbers of British troops to fight as part of coalition armies, frequently alongside soldiers from the East India Company. Such wars were often fought in extremely unhealthy and dangerous places from the point of view of disease and were characterised by few battle casualties but very heavy losses from a variety of diseases. While these minor wars may not have been associated with significant advances in medical and surgical knowledge, or with notable developments in care of the sick and wounded, they have been grouped together in two strategically placed chapters (Chapters 8 & 14) to highlight and summarise any important medical issues pertaining to them.

OTHER WARS

There were wars in which Great Britain did not participate, but which were important because significant developments occurred to influence medical military thinking and care. The American Civil War (Chapter 12) and the Franco-Prussian War (Chapter 13) are considered important in this regard. Sometimes, when Britain sent observers to other wars, it could, and should, have learned lessons but yet did not. The Russo-Japanese War (Chapter 16) is an excellent example of this.

THE EAST INDIA COMPANY

For much of the nineteenth century, there were two armies playing their respective roles in the British Empire. The first was the British Army proper which had its headquarters in Horse Guards in London. Its regiments were partly stationed at home and partly overseas, located wherever they were needed in the Empire. In the early part of the nineteenth century, officers usually bought their commissions. Their rank often depended more on their financial status and social standing than on their own military skills or leadership capabilities. Tactics were based on the principle of the "thin red line" to withstand on-coming infantry attacks and the formation of "squares" to deal with cavalry charges. Rigid discipline was enforced and men were frequently punished by flogging for misdemeanours, many of which were of a minor nature.

The other Imperial Army was a very different force. The East India Company was established following a Charter granted in 1600 by Queen Elizabeth I of England to enable a group of London merchants to trade with the Indies and to be in competition with the Dutch East India Company. The British East India Company had maintained its own army since the 17th century. There were three groups making up the overall army, which were raised by the three administrative divisions of British India, namely Bengal, Madras and Bombay.[1] Although the army was raised, and paid from the profits generated by the East India Company, it was effectively at the disposal of the British Crown, and formed a large mercenary force. In 1858 it came under direct control of the British Government following the Indian Mutiny.

There were some regiments of European soldiers in the ranks of the East India Company Army who were recruited mostly from Ireland. Most of the other ranks were Indians and were mainly Muslims and Hindus, although there were also Sikhs and Pathans. The commissioned officers were all British and were educated at the East India Company's own military academy in Addiscombe, Surrey. Commissions were not purchased, and promotion in the East India Company was generally on merit.[2] Addiscombe Military Academy was opened in 1809 and closed in 1861 when the East India Company ceased to exist after the Indian Mutiny in 1857.

There was often friction between these two armies, which had different values. Whilst British soldiers were described by Wellington as the "scum of the earth" because so many of them came from a squalid background of poverty, the sepoys in the East India Company regarded themselves as warriors. The sepoys were firmly committed to their religious faith, no matter whether they were Hindus or Muslims, and this led to conflict during the Indian Mutiny, which will be discussed in Chapter 14.

Medical personnel for the East India Company were generally recruited from civilian life, but that was not always the case. For example, Sir James McGrigor (1771-1858) was nearly recruited from the British Army at a relatively early stage of his career by the East India Company to become head of its medical department. The East India Company's gain would have been the British Army's loss, since McGrigor was destined to become responsible for many important improvements in army medical services. Fortunately, as things subsequently evolved, there was considerable opposition to his appointment. This was because many longstanding employees of the East India Company resented the appointment of an outsider to such a senior position and therefore McGrigor remained with the British Army. McGrigor's career will be discussed in Chapter 2.

Often, medical officers for the East India Company were recruited from doctors in the ships which traded between Britain and India[3] and they were taken on to look after Europeans who were employed by the company. One of their early medical officers was John Holwell who had survived the "Black Hole of Calcutta". This was a very small dungeon in the old Fort William where troops of the Nawab of Bengal (Siraj ud-Daulah), himself only 18 years of age, held British prisoners of war after the capture of the Fort on June 19 1756. It was so cramped, measuring only 14 x 18 feet, that men were starved of oxygen in the appalling heat and only 23 out of 146 prisoners are believed to have survived.[4]

When British regiments arrived, medical officers were interchangeable between the British and Indian units. As a general rule, when engaged in any activity with the East India Company, overall deployment of medical resources was under the direction of the East India Company. Just as there was friction between the two armies, so there was friction between the medical services of the two forces. On more than one occasion, the medical arrangements put in place by the Company were shown to be deficient, as will be discussed in Chapter 8. As a result, Sir James McGrigor, now Director General of Army Medical Services, decided that a senior Assistant Medical Director would have to be present to supervise the arrangements for any future operations which included British units.[5]

SURGERY

In the early years of the nineteenth century there were many pioneering and capable surgeons, who tackled the problems of severe wounds of the extremities. They had a sound anatomical knowledge which enabled them to plan operative procedures for different types of wounds. There were no anaesthetics in the earlier years of the century and consequently such procedures were necessarily short, and amputation was the solution in many cases. However, there were other operations developed and undertaken, and these will be discussed in the relevant chapters.

It is no coincidence that at first surgery focused on wounds involving the arms and legs, since limbs were both obvious and accessible. In contrast, wounds involving the thoracic and abdominal cavities were not and were outside the expertise of these surgeons. Such operative procedures would only become feasible in the fullness of time, when general anaesthesia became available allowing surgeons to develop procedures to deal with damage sustained by the vital organs within the chest and abdomen. Development of anaesthesia will be discussed in Chapter 9.

Soldiers who had sustained significant wounds of the chest or abdomen nearly always died, and surgical progress with such patients in the British Army was not made until the Great War when early surgical intervention for these types of wounds was shown to be lifesaving. As will be seen however, in Chapter 16, pioneering work on abdominal wounds was performed by a Russian surgeon, Vera Gedroits, during the Russo-Japanese War of 1904-5.

NON-SURGICAL TREATMENT AND DISEASE

Surgeons of today would certainly be able to understand and generally support the types of operations performed at the Battle of Waterloo or in the Crimean War. By contrast, the general supportive measures and non-operative treatments which were available, and which were used throughout much of the nineteenth century were, with few exceptions, without any scientific basis. At best they were ineffective, and at worst, they were positively harmful.

Bleeding (where blood was actually removed from a wounded soldier and discarded), with the intention of removing "bad blood", was a standard treatment which was used for just about any medical or surgical problem including wounds. The amount of blood withdrawn was directly proportional to the severity of the wound, and since the patient had often already lost a significant amount of the blood from his circulation, this could only make matters worse. The widespread application of leeches brought about a similar, although more gradual reduction in levels of haemoglobin in the blood, whilst "blistering" using heated cups was another useless remedy, employed in the belief that an illness could be burned out.

To the modern observer, whilst surgeons displayed considerable skill in performing difficult operations, based on scientific study and an understanding of human anatomy, they also employed remedies which were ineffective and commonly made the patient's clinical condition worse. This was a reflection of the very poor level of knowledge these practitioners had about disease.

To illustrate the point, here is a description of a man who had sustained a blunt abdominal injury. This case study is taken from a book written by John Hennen, one of the most outstanding military surgeons of the early nineteenth century. It concerns a man who was run over by a horse drawn wagon and the treatment this patient received must certainly have contributed to, or may even have caused, his death. [6]

> The wheel had passed over the iliac and hypogastric regions. He felt acute pain on pressure, but no other symptom of inflamed bowels; on the contrary, their functions remained natural and undisturbed. Next day he was bled to twenty-four ounces, which relieved the pain and reduced the pulse; but very shortly afterwards it rose to 140, full, and somewhat hard. Venesection was repeated the next day to twelve ounces. Pain still continued; and on attempting a repetition of the blood-letting, none could be procured from the arm. He died on the fourth day from the accident. On dissection, a quantity of dark-coloured blood was found effused under the peritoneum covering the abdominal muscles in the iliac and hypo gastric region and some in the pelvic region. The cellular membrane about the pubes was particularly injected with it. The peritoneal coat of the intestines was somewhat more vascular than common; but not the slightest symptom of inflammation or organic lesion could anywhere be traced.

It is clear from the autopsy that this man had sustained a major wound and was bleeding within his abdominal cavity, and this resulted in a reduction in his circulating blood volume. Yet his treatment involved the removal of even more blood, which must have accelerated the deterioration in his condition and was a causal factor in his death. He had 36 fluid ounces removed, which is just less than 2 pints!

Infectious diseases were very common in the nineteenth century, and far greater numbers of soldiers died from the effects of disease than were killed by enemy action or died from wounds. This will be discussed at length in the following chapters.

Diseases were attributed to a variety of causes including intemperance (alcohol abuse), exposure to heat or cold (with or without moisture), miasma (marsh vapour), and contagion. Painstaking documentation of data by James McGrigor, led to a subsequent groundbreaking piece of work by medical officer and statistician, Henry Marshall. In his work *Statistical Report on the Sickness, Mortality and Invaliding among the troops in the West Indies*, which was published in 1838,[7] Marshall provided evidence to refute many of the theories of causes of disease in the early to mid-nineteenth century and which were not based on scientific facts. Marshall's work will be discussed in full in Chapter 7.

Since the causes of diseases were unknown, it is perhaps not surprising that most remedies were completely ineffective. There was an occasional exception, and intermittent fever, which we know as malaria, was effectively treated using a Peruvian bark extract which had been brought to the European theatres of war from South America. Interestingly, Peruvian bark contains quinine, which is one of the most effective drugs still used in the treatment of malaria in the present day.

DEATHS FROM DISEASE AND DEATHS FROM WOUNDS

It is important to remember that disease wreaked havoc with all armies throughout the greatest part of the nineteenth century. During the Peninsular War of 1808-1814, for every British soldier dying as a result of enemy action, at least four died from disease. Indeed, the Franco-Prussian War (1870-1871) was the first conflict where deaths from enemy action exceeded deaths caused by disease. This development was not sustained, because in the Second Boer War British deaths from disease once again exceeded those caused by enemy action by almost two to one.

In some of the "minor wars", deaths from disease outnumbered deaths from enemy action by a much greater ratio. For example, during the first war in Burma, there were 2,716 British troops deployed with the East India Company. Sixty were killed in action and amongst those soldiers treated by the medical services, there were 1,311 deaths. 1,215 of the deaths were caused by various diseases, and only 36 died from wounds, meaning that for every soldier who died from a wound, approximately 33 died from disease.[8] This was, relatively speaking, one of the most costly wars ever fought by the Indian Government in terms of the high proportion of deaths from disease.

SCIENTIFIC DISCOVERIES WHICH TRANSFORMED MEDICINE IN THE NINETEENTH CENTURY

During the nineteenth century, there were many discoveries which gradually transformed medicine and improved knowledge and understanding. All these discoveries will be discussed, and their relevance to military surgery emphasised.

General anaesthesia was discovered, and the abolition of pain during surgical procedures opened the way for surgeons to undertake more extensive and complex procedures than was previously possible.

The work of Louis Pasteur in France during the 1850s resulted in the discovery of micro-organisms and this led to the introduction of the "Germ Theory" of disease. This work by Pasteur stimulated Joseph Lister, who was Professor of Surgery in Glasgow, to develop strategies to combat microorganisms and he published his work on the use of antiseptics (which destroy bacteria) in surgery in 1867. The introduction of aseptic surgery i.e. that performed in an environment so free from microorganisms that significant infection or suppuration does not supervene, was a logical progression from Lister's work. Ernst von Bergmann, a German surgeon, made a major breakthrough in asepsis when he successfully sterilized surgical instruments using steam in 1885. Further work by Robert Koch in Germany in the late 1870s and early 1880s led to the identification of specific bacterial causes of various diseases. Very importantly Sir Alexander Ogston, an Aberdeen surgeon, utilised the previous work to help him in his discovery of the micro-organism responsible for most wound infections and which causes abscess formation - staphylococcus pyogenes.

The role of the Anopheles mosquito in the transmission of malaria was discovered by Sir Ronald Ross in 1897. Ross was a medical officer who was born in India and who trained in London. He joined the Indian Medical Service as a young man, and was awarded a Nobel Prize in 1902 for his discovery.

The cause of yellow fever, responsible for killing thousands of British troops in the West Indies, and its transmission by the bite of a mosquito, was not discovered until 1900, by Major Walter Reid of the United States Army.

Blood transfusion was first used in the American Civil War and in the Franco Prussian War. Whilst there were many problems due to lack of knowledge about the existence of different blood groups (important for ensuring that the correct type of blood is used in a transfusion), at least it was realised that wounded soldiers who had lost blood required this to be replaced and not to be treated by removing even more blood.

An understanding of the epidemiology of disease brought logical methods of control and recognition of causative factors for specific diseases brought remedies in the form of vaccines. Edward Jenner introduced an effective vaccine against smallpox in the late eighteenth century by using the knowledge that milkmaids who had contracted mild cow pox were protected against the deadly smallpox. Jenner inoculated children, who were particularly susceptible to smallpox with cowpox, thus immunising them against the lethal disease. Critics ridiculed Jenner, and he was criticized by clergymen who claimed it was repulsive and sinful to inoculate someone using material from an infected pustule from a diseased animal. A satirical cartoon of 1802 showed people who had been inoculated sprouting cows' heads. Jenner had the resolve to overcome these prejudices and as a result of his work, the British Army started to immunise troops against smallpox in 1800. Thanks to the work of Jenner more than two hundred years ago, one of the most effective vaccines has finally eradicated smallpox from the surface of the earth.

SUMMARY

Over the course of the nineteenth century came a knowledge which transformed the understanding of disease. It was an "enlightenment" which began with James McGrigor in the early 1800s, who recorded every aspect of health and disease in the troops for whom he was responsible. It continued with the statistical work of Marshall in 1835. The discovery of general anaesthesia and its impact on surgical practice led eventually to the development of more major surgical procedures and while this brought abdominal surgery into the realm of possibility, it would take the massive numbers of casualties in the Great War and the demand that this made, to develop effective treatments leading to major advances in surgical practice. The discovery of micro-organisms and the germ theory of disease led directly to anti-sepsis, and the natural follow on from anti-septic surgery was aseptic surgery of the modern era. The discovery of individual bacteria led to identification of specific causative agents of disease, while the discovery of the life cycle of the Anopheles Mosquito by Sir Ronald Ross in 1897 was perhaps one of the most significant discoveries ever made.

ENDNOTES

1. Morris, J., *Heaven's Command. An Imperial Progress.* London: Faber and Faber, 1973, pp.88-89.
2. *Ibid.*
3. Cantlie, N., *A History of the Army Medical Department.* Edinburgh: Churchill Livingston, 1974, Volume 1, p.411.
4. *Ibid.*
5. *Ibid*, pp.483-485.
6. Hennen, J., *Principles of Military Surgery 3rd Edition.* London: John Wilson, 1829, p.103.
7. Marshall, H., *Statistical report on the sickness, mortality, and invaliding among the troops in the West Indies.* London: W. Clowes and Sons, 1838.
8. Cantlie, op. cit., p.459.

2

Sir James McGrigor - The Father of British Military Medicine

The essential purpose of this book is to examine the developments in military medicine and surgery which took place throughout the 19th century. Whilst there were many important physicians, surgeons and scientists who made important contributions in this field, arguably one of the most important was James McGrigor. His organisational skills and sheer commitment set him apart from his contemporaries, and he rightly became the most trusted medical officer in the Duke of Wellington's staff during the Peninsular War. His appointment to the position of Director General of Army Medical Services in 1815 firmly established McGrigor as the father of modern army medical services. He made changes which had far reaching consequences throughout the nineteenth century, and this included accurate data collection which paved the way for the statistical analysis of disease. He encouraged a scientific approach to solving some of the medical problems of the day.

James McGrigor was born in 1771 near the village of Cromdale in Strathspey, Invernesshire. He was the son of an Aberdeen merchant and he was educated at Aberdeen Grammar School, which was regarded at the time as one of the finest schools in Scotland. In his autobiography published after his death, McGrigor recalled that one of the most significant events of his life was when he was awarded the prize for best pupil after five years of study. He ran home to tell his father of his success:

> I ran to my father's house, at a quicker pace than I ever ran in the course of my life, to announce my success in having obtained the highest prize in the fifth or high class.[1]

He studied Greek at Marischal College in Aberdeen, taking the degree of A.M. (Master of Arts), and although his father would have liked him to have joined the family business McGrigor had other ideas. Many of his friends had enrolled to study medicine and McGrigor also decided to pursue this career. While his father was disappointed, he did not try to dissuade him. McGrigor began his studies under Dr French, Physician to the Infirmary in Aberdeen, which was situated outside the city boundary at Woolmanhill. This location had been chosen "because of the pureness of the air in that region". After spending three years at the Infirmary, McGrigor went to Edinburgh University, studying under the great Munro Secundus. Professor Alexander Munro was a Scottish anatomist, surgeon and medical educator. To distinguish him as the second of three generations of physicians of the same name, he was known as Secundus. McGrigor also studied under Dr James Gregory in the Practice of Physic.

Whilst studying in Edinburgh, McGrigor was very impressed by the learned discussions which took place amongst the various clinicians. When he returned to Aberdeen, he became a co-founder of the Aberdeen Medical Society in 1798, which was renamed the Aberdeen Medico-Chirurgical Society in 1811. The society was originally set up to help improve the education of undergraduate medical students in Aberdeen. There was a Professor of Medicine at Marischal College but this person also simultaneously held the Chair of Mathematics and McGrigor was keen for a real focus on medical education itself. Medical education was scanty as there were no regular classes or lectures. However it was common practice in those times to further one's education by travelling to Europe to what now would be regarded as centres of excellence in teaching, learning and clinical practice.

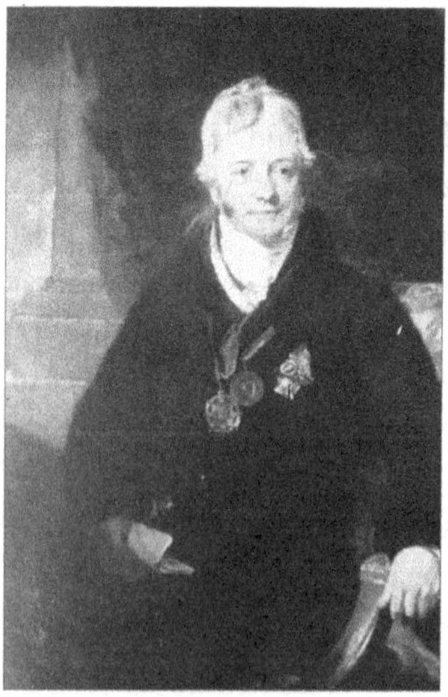

Figure 2.1. Portrait of Sir James McGrigor. (Courtesy of Aberdeen Medico-Chirurgical Society).

The Aberdeen Medico-Chirurgical Society flourishes to this day, and is extremely proud of its distinguished founder member. One of the society's most prized possessions is a collection of journals donated to the society by Sir James McGrigor in later life, and through his portrait McGrigor to this day looks down on proceedings in this society.

McGrigor maintained close ties with Aberdeen, and with the Aberdeen Medico-Chirurgical Society, throughout his long life.

A short time after returning to Aberdeen, McGrigor decided to join the army. He had apparently been influenced by a senior student friend of his who had exchanged his round bonnet for a smart cocked hat with a cockade:

> In this he strutted to the infirmary, where at 12 o'clock daily all the medical students usually attended to accompany the physicians and surgeons through the different wards.[2]

McGrigor set off by ship from Aberdeen to London in 1793 where he purchased a commission as assistant surgeon in the 88th Regiment (Connaught Rangers), and so began his long and illustrious career in the British Army.

Later in life, The Duke of Wellington, Wellington teased his old friend by saying of the Connaught Rangers:

> I hope from your long living with them you have not contracted any of their leading propensities. I hang and shoot more of your old friends for murders and robberies than I do of all the rest of the army.

Seeing that he had flustered McGrigor, he continued:

> One thing I will tell you, however, whenever anything very gallant, very desperate is to be done, there is no corps in the army I would sooner employ than your old friends –the Connaught Rangers.[3]

McGrigor went to Flanders during the years 1793-1794 where he had to deal with an outbreak of typhus fever affecting the troops under his care. Many of them died, and McGrigor himself contracted the disease. As with nearly all diseases at the time, the cause was unknown and it took until 1916 for a Brazilian doctor called Henrique da Rocha Lima to isolate the micro-organism responsible for typhus fever. He named it Rickettsia Prowazekii, after his colleague Stanislaus von Prowazekii, who had died of typhus in Hamburg in 1915. It was there that both men had been carrying out research at a prison hospital to investigate the cause of the disease.

Typhus fever is most likely to occur among people living in overcrowded, dirty conditions and where there are few opportunities to wash themselves or their clothing. As a result, typhus fever often occurs when cold weather, poverty, war and other disasters result in people living in squalid and overcrowded conditions where body lice can thrive and spread readily from one person to the next. Typhus fever is transmitted by body lice which become contagious by feeding on the blood of infected humans. The lice then defecate while feeding on another person and the faeces, which contain the typhus fever bacteria, can get rubbed into small wounds such as those caused by scratching lice-infected areas. It is the faeces, not the bite of the louse, that transmits the illness to humans. It is also possible to become infected through contact with the mucous membranes of the mouth and eyes, or by inhaling the dust of dried lice faeces. Typhus fever is not spread directly from person-to-person.

The illness usually starts suddenly with a headache, chills, fever, and generalized body aches. A rash appears in four to seven days, initially on the upper trunk, before spreading to the entire body, but usually sparing the face, palms, and soles. The rash starts as maculopapular, becomes petechial or hemorrhagic, and then develops into brownish-pigmented areas. The rash may be more concentrated in the axillae (armpits). Changes in mental status are common with delirium or coma and toxaemia is usually pronounced. Heart and kidney failure can occur when the disease is severe and this is usually quickly followed by death. Nowadays, prompt treatment with antibiotics can cure most cases, but antibiotics were of course not available in McGrigor's day and there was no effective treatment.

McGrigor was lucky to have survived, since disease in the early nineteenth century killed many more soldiers than did wounds inflicted by the enemy. Needless to say, medical officers who looked after the sick were no more immune to the various diseases than the patients whose lives they were attempting to save. This state of affairs continued throughout most of the 19th century, and it would not be until the Franco-Prussian War (1870-1871), that deaths from enemy action outnumbered those caused by disease. The very low percentage mortality from disease in the Great War, at 4.7% on the Western Front, reflects the good standard of medical care administered to the troops[4] and illustrates the tremendous improvement in the general health of soldiers which took place in the 100 years between McGrigor's time and the start of the Great War.

After returning to the United Kingdom following his time spent in Flanders, McGrigor then went to the Caribbean with Sir Ralph Abercromby's expedition. The intention was to capture the islands of St Lucia, Trinidad and Tobago and Grenada from the French. The West Indies was one of the unhealthiest places to be sent to, because there were many diseases which affected troops stationed there. Once again, there was an outbreak of typhus fever with an associated high mortality. McGrigor caught dysentery on this occasion which was also prevalent among the troops. He also survived being shipwrecked before a further severe attack of dysentery nearly resulted in his death. There was then an outbreak of the feared yellow fever, which was common in the West Indies and which was rightly regarded as one of the most deadly diseases. In his autobiography, McGrigor described the devastating effect of this outbreak:

> It presented itself with overwhelming force and with hideous mortality, being more fatal to the army by far than the enemy. The number that died of yellow fever was four times that of those who fell by the bullet and bayonet.[5]

McGrigor noted that there was serious overcrowding of the troops for the available accommodation, and he was convinced that:

> ...the disease was transmitted by contagion, although not in its origin a contagious disease.[6]

A contagious disease is one which is easily transmitted by physical contact with the person suffering the disease, by their secretions or objects touched by them. In fact, McGrigor was wrong. In 1881, a Cuban doctor by the name of Carlos Finlay (who was actually of French and Scottish descent) showed that the disease is carried by mosquitoes. We now know that yellow fever is caused by a virus, which is transmitted by the bite of female mosquitoes (the yellow fever mosquito, Aedes Aegypti and other species). It is found in tropical and subtropical areas in South America and Africa. The only known hosts of the virus are primates, including, of course, man, and several species of mosquito. The origin of the disease is most likely to be Africa, from where it was introduced to South America through the slave trade in the 16th century. In the 19th century yellow fever was one of the most dangerous diseases known to the British Army.

Yellow fever presents in most cases with fever, nausea and pain and it generally subsides after several days. In some patients, a toxic phase follows, in which liver damage with jaundice (giving the name of the disease) can occur and lead to death. Because of an increased bleeding tendency, yellow fever belongs to a group of diseases known as haemorrhagic fevers.

It is worth making the point that McGrigor had suffered from debilitating typhus fever and dysentery on consecutive postings. By good luck, he had also avoided getting yellow fever. Not all his fellow officers were so fortunate. As will be discussed in a later chapter, one of the outstanding surgeons of the era, an Irishman by the name of John Hennen, died of yellow fever in Gibraltar.

McGrigor's next posting with the Connaught Rangers was to India, and he set off in 1798. He first met Arthur Wellesley (later to become the Duke of Wellington) in India and he was present during the siege of Seringapatam.

McGrigor was appointed as Principal Medical Officer of an Anglo-Indian Army commanded by Sir David Baird and which embarked on an expedition from India to Egypt in 1801. At that time, Egypt was held by Napoleon Bonaparte. The aim of this expedition was to help to evict the French from Egypt, and thus to avert a French invasion of the East India Company territories in India.

It was planned that Baird's force would land at Suez, and attack Cairo from the south. As it happened, the Anglo Indian force ran into many problems. Bad weather prevented a landing at Suez, and the force disembarked at Cossier instead, before marching across a desert for 140 miles, and travelling down the Nile by boat to Ghiza.[7]

Once again, McGrigor was very sick, with what was known as remittent fever:

> I suffered an attack of fever which proved to be remittent, but which I first feared would prove to be the plague. The attack was a severe one, and followed by long and protracted debility.[8]

Remittent fever is not a disease entity, but is merely a descriptive term for a pattern of fever, and does not give an indication of the underlying cause. In the early part of the nineteenth century, no one knew of the existence of viruses, bacteria or parasites. Fevers were commonly divided into four basic types: typhus, intermittent, simple continued and remittent. Typhus is the disease we still know today; simple and remittent fevers were a mixture of infectious diseases including malaria, typhoid, relapsing fever and dysentery.[9]

It was a commonly held view that "miasmata", or vapours arising from putrefying organic matter, were the sources of disease. Whatever it was McGrigor was suffering from, he recovered once again.

As things turned out, the French garrison in Cairo surrendered to a Turkish force and the British sepoy force did not have to fire a shot. Having recovered, McGrigor took steps to deal with the imminent arrival of plague which was known to be coming. McGrigor made prudent arrangements by creating "pest" houses, houses of observation and quarantine areas. A pest house, or fever shed was a building used for persons affected by the disease. An observation house kept others exposed to the disease but as yet showing no manifestations of it under close review. Quarantine implies compulsory isolation, typically to contain the spread of the disease, where all those who had been in contact with a sufferer would remain until it was safe to release them. McGrigor set up a board of health and by so doing, he demonstrated the organisational skills for which he would become well known as an exceptionally gifted medical practitioner.

There was indeed an outbreak of fever. At first, there was typhus, which usually killed the patient and then there were cases of plague, with all the manifestations characteristic of the disease. Fungating infected groin lymph nodes or buboes were identified on men who quickly died and given his extensive contact with infected individuals, McGrigor was sure that he too would contract the disease. Thankfully the measures he had set in place helped to contain the disease and he was fortunate indeed that he did not contract plague himself. Once again, he had escaped death.

Bubonic plague is an infection of the lymphatic system usually resulting from the bite of an infected flea, Xenopsylla cheopis (the rat flea). The fleas are often found on rodents such as rats and mice and seek out other prey when their rodent hosts die. The bacteria form aggregates in the gut of infected fleas and this results in the flea regurgitating ingested blood, which is now infected, into the bite site of a rodent or human host. Once established, bacteria rapidly spread to the lymph nodes and multiply. Yersinia Pestis (formerly known as Pasteurella Pestis) bacilli can resist phagocytosis (which is the engulfing, ingestion and destruction of bacteria by the body's white blood cells) and even reproduce inside white blood cells whose function is to kill invading organisms.

As the disease progresses, the infected lymph nodes can bleed and become swollen and necrotic. Bubonic plague can progress to lethal septicaemic plague in some cases, meaning that it spreads through the blood stream. The plague is also known to spread to the lungs and become the disease known as the pneumonic plague. This form of the disease is highly communicable as the bacteria can be transmitted in droplets emitted when coughing or sneezing. Bubonic plague, along with the septicaemic plague and the pneumonic plague, which are the two other manifestations of Y. pestis, is generally believed to be the cause of the Black Death that swept through Europe in the 14th century and killed an estimated 75 million people, or 30-60% of the European population.[10]

In 1894, two bacteriologists, Alexandre Yersin of France and Kitasato Shibasaburō of Japan, independently isolated the bacterium responsible for plague in Hong Kong.

With the Peace of Amiens in 1802, war with France was over for a while. When still in Egypt McGrigor met Baron Larrey, Napoleon's Chief Medical Officer and he established a friendship that would last for the rest of their lives despite the fact that for much of the time they were on opposing sides in war.

In a letter to the National Library of Scotland dated 18 October 1826, McGrigor wrote:

> Sir James McGrigor presents his complements to Sir Walter Scott and has the honour to present a letter from Baron Larrey with his works in four volumes. Sir James McGrigor has known the Baron since the year 1800, when he left Egypt with the French Army, and he believes him to be a man of the greatest integrity.[11]

Such was the strength of their friendship, that McGrigor made Larrey an honorary member of the Aberdeen Medico-Chirurgical Society.[12,13]

After his return to India, he wrote an account of the expedition. *Medical Sketch on the Expedition to Egypt from India* is a detailed account of the diseases encountered by the expedition with particular reference to the outbreak of the plague.[14]

McGrigor's next posting was to the Royal Horse Guards (Blues) in November 1803, where he remained until 20 July 1805. During the time spent with the Horse Guards, McGrigor documented all admissions to hospital and the diagnoses of those admitted along with detailed notes of treatment given and progress. He documented the number of patients admitted in a month, the prevalence of different types of diseases, the number of soldiers discharged since the previous return, the number of deaths and if those still remaining were in hospital, barracks or billets, the numbers discharged on furlough or elsewhere were recorded.[15]

The sort of details he kept can best be illustrated by an example:

> Thomas Bingham, age 23, Captain Slingsby's troop. April 8th: has for last 3 days, in consequence of getting wet, had catarrhal symptoms, got last night sudorifics. He is now very hoarse, much pain of one side of head, dullness of hearing, little cough, no expectoration. Got last night a bolus of calomel and this morning a purgative powder, neither has operated.
>
> 14th: cough very loose, no dyspnoea, much hoarseness.
>
> 18th: had 9 motions from cathartic (an agent for purging the bowels), no syncope, cough loose; much hoarseness.
>
> 19th: only little cough, hoarseness less, no syncope.
>
> 29th: Dismissed cured.[16]

McGrigor made a practice of accurately documenting diseases which would continue for the remainder of his career.

During his time with the Horse Guards, there was an outbreak of typhus fever and hospital gangrene, which ran rapidly through most of the patients in the hospital. Hospital gangrene was relatively common at the time, and will be referred to again in subsequent chapters of this book. McGrigor was of the view that the hospital was too small and poorly ventilated for the number of cases admitted. After moving to a larger and better ventilated building cases of typhus disappeared and whilst cases of gangrene persisted he went on to say:

> By moving the men from one ward to another, changing the atmosphere, and destroying all the sponges used in dressing, together with other precautions, we finally got rid of the disease.[17]

Hospital gangrene will be discussed in the chapter dealing with surgery in the Peninsular War. Without any understanding of the bacteria which caused hospital gangrene, McGrigor worked out that overcrowding was a contributory factor and by "destroying all the sponges used in dressing", he helped to reduce the likelihood of transmitting the disease from one patient to the next.

McGrigor was nearly appointed Head of the Medical Department of the East India Company, on the invitation of his good friend Sir William Dundas. Fortunately (for the sake of the British Army), this change of direction in his career did not come to fruition. McGrigor remained with the British Army and was appointed to the promoted position of Deputy-Inspector of Hospitals in the North District which enabled him to fulfil a great ambition:

> My new appointment was one which was particularly congenial to my mind and habits. From my first entrance into the service I had some turn for statistical statements, for collecting medical facts and generalising upon them, and I made, for my own satisfaction, monthly, quarterly, and annual statements of the diseases which had come under my notice, both in the 88th Regiment and the Blues. I further extended them in various diseases to five and seven years, marking the proportional occurrence of the diseases and mortality. I now rejoiced to have a wider field before me for these researches and for the cooperation of others in whom I could confide, by which, either to correct any errors into which I might have fallen or to extend my deductions and have them confirmed.[18]

He went on to say that for far too long there had been detailed correspondences relating to unimportant matters such as the number of ounces of soap dispensed, or salt given to each patient. Now he was in a position to record, discuss and document matters of real importance relating to the health and well-being of the troops. There were many medical officers who were ignorant and whose medical education was sorely lacking. However, McGrigor used his new position to improve standards and to make sure that medical officers paid due attention to the health and well being of the troops under their care. He did so by discussion and encouragement and for the most part his words were met with an appropriate response. On some occasions, he had to have a word with the commanding officer concerned to ensure that his recommendations were acted upon. He encouraged the ongoing education of regimental surgeons which today would be known as continuing medical education:

> No man leaving the university or school of medicine in which he is brought up can conceive that he has finished his studies on leaving it.[19]

He encouraged experimentation with new treatments in the military setting, because he realised that military patients were under stricter control, allowing better observation and follow up. McGrigor recognised that it was more difficult for a regimental surgeon to continue his medical education than a doctor in civilian practice. Therefore he went to considerable trouble to draw this to their attention, and to remedy the deficiency by further study.

McGrigor was promoted to Deputy Director for the South-West District which included responsibility for Portsmouth. When he arrived at Winchester he found the hospitals in need of much reorganisation and being busy at work he had omitted to go to Sunday Worship. His absence was duly noted by the Duke of Cumberland, commander of South West District, who summoned him to Winchester Cathedral, holding back the service till McGrigor arrived. McGrigor was then given a public dressing down for his absence!

Many troops were concentrated in the south-west at the time, and there was a lot of sickness. All embarkations took place from Portsmouth, and McGrigor had to inspect every transport ship that arrived, and every vessel that set sail from Portsmouth, to assess the health of arriving and embarking troops. The scope for his statistical observations, for which he possessed the greatest zeal, was now complete.

Whilst at Portsmouth in 1808, almost the entire fleet from Sir John Moore's defeated army from the retreat from Corunna on the Peninsula arrived (see Chapter 3). Conditions were ideal for the spread of disease by contagion because healthy men were in immediate contact with sick individuals. The volume of work taxed McGrigor's organisational skills to the full, and he managed to obtain use of the naval hospital at Haslar to help deal with the many wounded and sick soldiers.

There was an outbreak of typhus fever and it took some time to clear Portsmouth of the many sick and wounded. His experience in Portsmouth would stand James McGrigor in good stead in times to come.

ENDNOTES

1. McGrigor, M., *The Scalpel and the Sword. The Autobiography of the Father of Army Medicine.* Dalkeith: Scottish Cultural Press, 2000, p.27.
2. *Ibid*, p.29.
3. *Ibid*, p.173.
4. Mitchell, T.J., G. M. Smith, *History of the Great War Medical Services Casualties and Medical Statistics.* London: His Majesty's Stationery Office, 1931, p.108.
5. McGrigor, M., *op. cit.*, p.64.
6. *Ibid.*
7. Milne, G.P., *Aberdeen Medico-Chirurgical Society A Bicentennial History.* Aberdeen: Aberdeen University Press, 1989, p.22.
8. McGrigor, M., *op. cit.*, p.91.
9. Howard, M.R., "Walcheren 1809: a medical catastrophe", *British Medical Journal,* 1999; 319: pp.1642-1645.
10. MacLeod, J., *Davidson's Principles and Practice of Medicine.* 13th Edition. Edinburgh: Churchill Livingstone, 1981, p.833.
11. McGrigor, M., *op. cit.*, p.243.
12. *Ibid,* p.244.
13. Riddel, J.S., *The Records of the Aberdeen Medico-Chirurgical Society from 1789 to 1922.* Aberdeen: W&W Lindsay, 1922, p.78.
14. McGrigor, J. *Medical Sketches of the Expedition to Egypt from India.* London: John Murray, 1804.
15. University of Aberdeen Collection GB 0817 Aberdeen Medico Chirurgical Society Ref No AMCS/4/1/4/28.
16. *Ibid.*
17. McGrigor, M., *op. cit.*, pp.114-115.
18. *Ibid*, p.127.
19. *Ibid*, p.13.

3

The Walcheren Campaign

On 30 July 1809, a British force of 40,000 men landed on the Dutch island of Walcheren. Its aim was to seize the port of Antwerp which was held by the French. Walcheren is now part of the reclaimed land mass of the Netherlands, but in 1808 it was an island in the province of Zeeland at the mouth of the Scheldt estuary. It lay between the Oosterschelde to the north and the Westerschelde to the south, and was roughly the shape of a rhombus.

The strategic aim of the expedition was to relieve Austria, Britain's ally in the Fifth Coalition. This was the smallest of a series of allied coalitions formed to take on the military might of Revolutionary and Napoleonic France. The Fifth Coalition effectively consisted of only Austria and Britain. Austrian troops were under severe pressure fighting Napoleon's forces on the River Danube. Therefore, by opening a second front in the north at Antwerp, Britain hoped to divert French reserves and

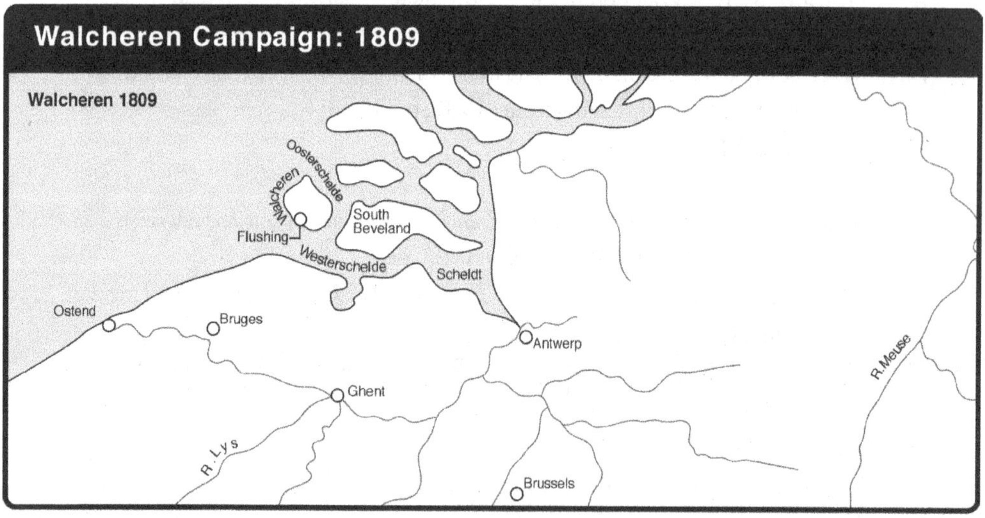

Figure 3.1. Map showing Walcheren in Holland.

thus prevent them from joining Napoleon's army in the south. Britain also planned to destroy the French fleet in Antwerp which at the time was a channel port of great strategic importance. The first aim of the campaign was to capture the port of Flushing and then to take Antwerp.[1]

This was one of the largest British forces ever assembled[2] but by the time it crossed the North Sea and landed at Walcheren on 30 July 1809, it was already too late to help its Austrian ally. It took far too long to make the necessary preparations and to set sail. Austria had been defeated at Wagram (on the Danube) by Napoleon on 5 and 6 July 1809. The two-day struggle at Wagram saw an Imperial French, German and Italian army, under the command of Napoleon Bonaparte, defeat an army of the Austrian Empire which was under the command of Archduke Charles of Austria-Teschen. The Battle of Wagram was the decisive military engagement of the War of the Fifth Coalition and the Walcheren Expedition was therefore "shutting the stable door, after the horse had bolted". Consequently, even if it had gone well, it would not have served any useful military purpose. As it was, it went disastrously wrong.

The British had landed too far from their immediate objective, the port of Flushing (see Figure 3. 1), giving the enemy plenty of time to dig in and block the way to Antwerp.[3] British forces were commanded by the Earl of Chatham, the elder brother of the late William Pitt the Younger. Chatham lacked the resolution to conduct an efficient military campaign and he brought his forces ashore in a leisurely fashion, giving the French ample time to make preparations to repel the invading army. Chatham had a reputation for being somewhat lazy and was known as "the late earl" because he took so long to get out of bed in the morning! This was a combined operation and needed close co-operation between the British Army and the Royal Navy, but Chatham was not on speaking terms with Admiral Strachan, his naval counterpart[4] and lack of cooperation between the two added to the delay. Following a naval bombardment of Flushing, the port was eventually captured with the loss of 700 casualties.

After a couple of weeks there was a serious outbreak of disease which began to take a heavy toll. Soon, out of a force of 40,000 men almost 4,000 died of disease, which was a mortality of 10% and many more suffered chronic ill health. Only 106 soldiers were killed in action or died from wounds sustained in battle.[5]

WALCHEREN FEVER

Nowadays, one does not associate the Netherlands with a high risk for developing virulent infectious diseases, but in the early part of the nineteenth century it was very different.

Writing in 1816, in his work entitled *History of the War against the French from the commencement of the French Revolution to the present time* Clark wrote:

> All the Dutch provinces are subject to marsh distempers, but Zealand in particular, is not only low and damp like the rest, but surrounded by the mouths of the Scheldt, whose oozy beaches unite with the marshy lands, so that except the sea breeze from the westward, every wind comes laden with the pestilential vapours. The bottom of every canal that communicates with the sea is thickly covered with ooze, which, when the tide is ebbed, disperses a most offensive and noxious effluvia. The sickly season begins with June and ends with October, continuing as long as the sun has power sufficient to draw up marsh miasmata.[6]

It was thought that the offensive smells or "miasmata" from estuaries such as the Scheldt were responsible for causing fever and it also so happened that the "sickly season" to which Clark was referring corresponded to the breeding season of the anopheline mosquito. The "marsh distemper" to which he alluded was malaria. It was a particularly severe outbreak which affected troops in Walcheren.

Malaria is caused by a group of parasites, Plasmodium falciparum, P. vivax, P.ovale and P. Malariae.[7] Infection occurs wherever there are human hosts with the parasite and there are enough mosquitoes to spread the disease after ingesting the parasites during a blood feed on a victim. Part of the life cycle of the parasite requires the mosquito for its development and part of the cycle requires a human host. Once in the human, the parasites go to the liver, where they multiply, before being released into the bloodstream to invade the red blood cells.

The parasites multiply within the red blood cells and then burst out, an event associated with fever. Each red blood cell cycle takes a definite period, depending on the specific causative parasite and it usually occurs every 48 or 72 hours, giving the fever an intermittent pattern. This is why physicians of the early nineteenth century called it "intermittent fever." Infection caused by P. falciparum is by far the most dangerous and may be associated with cerebral malaria, where the victim rapidly falls into a coma and dies. Between attacks the parasites may lie dormant within the liver so that there may be further attacks of intermittent fever many months after the original presentation. This was an important problem for survivors of the Walcheren Campaign, who suffered recurrent bouts of malaria when they were sent to the Peninsular War in Spain.

According to Howard, there is strong evidence to suggest that while malaria was implicated in Walcheren Fever, other diseases contributed to the high mortality. He maintains there was a lethal cocktail of disease which was a combination of malaria, typhus, typhoid and dysentery.[8] The soldiers would have been predisposed to these different diseases by overcrowding and poor sanitation coupled with an already existing high background level of morbidity resulting chiefly from poverty and drunkenness.

On the other hand, it has been suggested that whilst deaths from diseases such as typhus, typhoid, and dysentery occurred, contemporary accounts did not suggest there were large numbers of soldiers suffering from these diseases. Indeed, it is likely that many of the men were debilitated from a previous campaign. They were survivors from Corunna, one of the early battles in the Peninsular War and were in poor health from the outset. Consequently they suffered more severely from malaria than men in good health. Cantlie suggested that malaria was the principal disease and perhaps it was the malignant tertian variety, caused by P. falciparum, with cerebral complications, that was the main cause of death.[9]

The exact cause of Walcheren Fever will never be known for sure but whatever the aetiology, within a few weeks, the Walcheren force was reduced to a fraction of its initial strength and what was left of it would have to be evacuated. Many of those who survived to return home suffered ongoing morbidity and were never fit to serve again. The Walcheren Campaign provides a very clear example of how dangerous it was to send troops to an unhealthy location, where disease could so weaken a force as to render it helpless and unable to fight.

MEDICAL ORGANISATION AT THE TIME OF THE WALCHEREN CAMPAIGN

Army medical services were headed by a Physician General and a Surgeon General, who could be either senior regular army medical officers or be eminent members of the civilian medical profession. There was also an Inspector of Regimental Infirmaries who always came from a military background. These three men formed the Army Medical Board and those responsible at the time of the Walcheren Campaign were Sir Lucas Pepys, the Physician General, Sir Thomas Keate, the Surgeon General and Francis Knight, Inspector of Regimental Infirmaries.

Pepys was a civilian doctor with no military experience. In 1804, whilst holding the appointment of Physician General, he became President of the Royal College of Physicians of London. Keate had limited military experience and was responsible for providing medical staff, equipment and supplies for the expedition. There was an ongoing dispute between Pepys and Keate on one side, and Knight on the other. An army under the command of Sir John Moore had recently been evacuated from Corunna in January 1809 after fighting Napoleon on the Spanish Peninsula. Moore had fought a successful defensive battle although he himself had been killed, and the army arrived home in a dreadful state. 27,000 troops were evacuated. The disembarking soldiers were dressed in rags and approximately 6,000 of them were sick and wounded when they arrived back in Britain.

They were very capably dealt with by James McGrigor in Portsmouth, in his capacity as Deputy Director for the South-West District as explained in Chapter 2, but Knight had closed the general hospitals at Gosport, Plymouth and Deal on the grounds of economy, and there was not a single bed to receive them in these locations. This led to severe friction between Knight on the one hand and Keate and Pepys on the other. The dispute had not been resolved by the time of the Walcheren campaign, and Knight refused to have anything to do with the hospital arrangements in Great Britain. The members of the Army Medical Board were severely criticised by the Secretary of State for War and were instructed to work together and not to let personal animosities interfere with their duties. This did not auger well for the Walcheren expedition.

Surgeon General Keate, who was responsible for putting the medical arrangements in place, appointed Sir John Webb as Inspector of Hospitals. He had under his command a large staff of 80 personnel which included 3 Deputy Inspectors of Hospitals, 7 physicians, 22 staff surgeons, 2 apothecaries, 4 dispensers, 4 purveyors and more than 30 hospital assistants. He supplied enough stores to provide for 4,000 hospital beds, 10% of the force. In the event it was to prove hopelessly inadequate.[10]

Within three weeks of landing in Walcheren, it was reported that Sir John Webb had died of fever, and James McGrigor was sent to replace him. He hastily left Portsmouth on HMS *Venerable*, which unfortunately became grounded on a sandbank a short distance from its destination and nearly foundered when it started to ship water. Fortunately, all on board were safely evacuated when rescue boats set sail from Flushing and took them ashore on 3 October 1809.

McGrigor found that Webb was not dead, but he certainly was very ill. In the fullness of time Webb recovered his health, although he played no further part in the Walcheren campaign. McGrigor made the following assessment:

> The number of sick was immense, that of the wounded officers and men who could not be conveyed thither was considerable, and both together, most unhappily, nearly equalled that of the men in health. But the amount of sickness at Walcheren was great beyond all comparison with that which I had hitherto witnessed.[11]

There was very little that McGrigor could do, but he set to work and made the most of the facilities available to him. There were only 47 of the original 80 medical staff left, the others having fallen victim to disease. McGrigor inspected the hospitals and assessed his requirements. There was very little Peruvian bark available in store (necessary to treat intermittent fever) and McGrigor wrote repeatedly to Keate, requesting him to send a supply as quickly as possible since he was in danger of running out completely. He managed to purchase bark from an American merchant ship, "which just happened to arrive". Almost certainly those on board the American merchant man had heard of the acute shortage of bark being experienced by the British and seized the opportunity to make a quick profit selling it at inflated prices.[12]

On 1 September 1809, it was clear to Chatham that further successful operations were impossible and he re-embarked for England with half his force, leaving a garrison of 19,000 men on Walcheren under the command of Lieutenant General Sir Eyre Coote. By 17 September 1809, there were 8,600 men in hospital and by 1 October 1809 over 9,600 [13]

Table 3.1 shows the effective strength of rank and file together with numbers of sick and also those who died on specific dates.[14] Of those who survived, six months later there were still 11,000 men registered sick.[15]

Table 3.1. Strength of rank and file during Walcheren Campaign. Note - by 10th September, half the force had been sent home.

Date	Strength Rank & File	Sick	Died
25th August	37,737	2,702	114
10th September	17,870	7,491	221
17th September	17,410	8,660	277
24th September	16,400	9,196	287
1st October	16,156	9,680	354
8th October	14,927	8,942	217
21st October	14,927	9,800	-

From Cantlie, N., *A History of the Army Medical Department.* Edinburgh: Churchill Livingston; 1974, Volume 1, p. 402.

Figure 3.2 compares the morbidity and mortality from disease with losses sustained in battle and as can be seen the overwhelming majority of deaths were the result of disease.

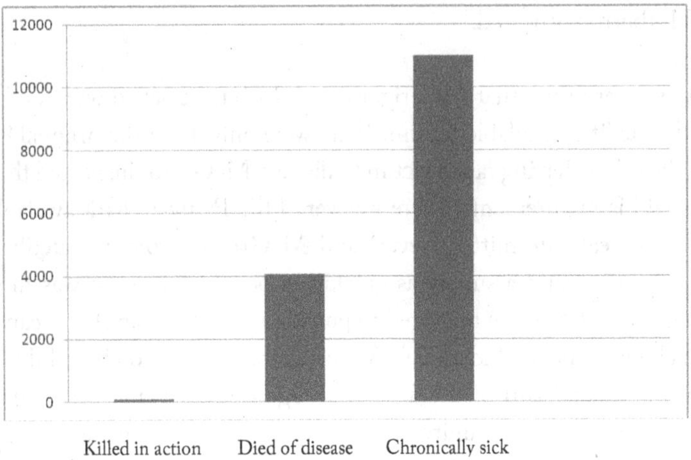

Figure 3.2. From Howard, M.R., "Walcheren 1809: a medical catastrophe", *British Medical Journal* 1999; 319: pp.1642-1645.

By the end of September 1809, there were 9,000 sick in hospital and the Commander-in Chief at Horse Guards pressed Sir Lucas Pepys to go to Walcheren to assess matters for himself. Pepys refused, saying he was not acquainted with active service conditions! The Secretary of State for War then wrote to Pepys and dismissed him. Neither Knight nor Keate offered to go to Walcheren but they did instruct two of the oldest medical officers to go instead of them. This abdication of responsibility resulted in the board being subjected to much ridicule and contempt. Keate at first tendered his resignation but later withdrew it.

Sir Eyre Coote was replaced as Commander in Chief by an experienced senior commander, Sir George Don, who immediately set about the business of evacuating the remaining troops. As the last men left on 9 December 1809, the dockyard at Flushing was set on fire, bringing down the curtain on a catalogue of mismanagement.

AFTERMATH OF THE WALCHEREN CAMPAIGN

A Commission of Inquiry was set up by the House of Commons and Pepys appeared before it. He was asked what acquaintance he had with army medical practice prior to his appointment as Physician General in 1794, to which he answered "None". He was then asked what acquaintance he had with army medical practice after his appointment, to which he also replied "None". He was asked if he had ever visited York Hospital at Chelsea (the military hospital at the time). He had never once visited it. He was rightly blamed for the shortage of medical supplies in Walcheren, which was one of his designated responsibilities.[16]

Surgeon General Keate put up a robust defence of his position. Dr Webb, the medical officer in charge at Walcheren, had put in a request for more Peruvian bark before he fell sick. However, because it had not been marked urgent there had been a delay in sending the request. Keate tried to switch blame from himself to Webb, but despite his protestations, the inescapable fact was that there had been a definite shortage of bark in Holland, either because it had never been shipped, or because there had been some administrative error in its distribution.

In the light of his involvement, McGrigor was summoned to appear as a witness before the Commission. This caused him considerable anxiety because he was not accustomed to appearing before such a gathering although he had absolutely nothing to reproach himself for. He went to the Speaker's chamber every day, growing increasingly anxious, until he was finally called to give evidence:

> I did this daily for upwards of a fortnight, being every day at the Speaker's chamber by four o'clock, the warrant being renewed and sent to me every day. At length my turn came and I was in some agitation, which the appearance of the witness cited immediately before me did not diminish.[17]

McGrigor went on to say:

> My examination by both sides of the house was a very long one. I kept fully possession of myself for a considerable time, but at last, from the extreme heat of the house, my position and the length of my examination, I became somewhat confused, and I completely stuck at one place relative to the supply of medicine to the sick.[18]

McGrigor went on:

> I had admitted at one time that our stores were nearly empty, and that little or no Peruvian bark remained. Reverting to my former replies that our sick did not suffer for want of medicine, he (his questioner) desired me to reconcile this apparent inconsistency. My reply was that I had given orders to the purveyor to purchase all the bark I could get. His next question was, "Where was a quantity of bark to be purchased in Walcheren? My reply was "From adventurers". He rejoined "What adventurers?" For the life of me, I could not remember the meaning of the word adventurer.[19]

As a result of the Commission of Enquiry, the old Army Medical Board was broken up. It was quite clear that although these men were eminent practitioners in London, they had no knowledge of military medicine and surgery and were most ill-suited to being responsible for an army in the field. It was decided that in future, members of the new Army Medical Department should be persons with first-hand knowledge of the service and who had served abroad with troops. The new board would be under the leadership of a Director General of Army Medical Services, assisted by two Principal Inspectors.

The Walcheren Campaign Commission of Enquiry ended and the final verdict was that no one was to blame. The campaign had been a disaster in military planning. McGrigor returned to his post as Deputy Director for the South-West District, where he remained until his next posting, when he was given orders to prepare for embarkation to the Peninsula, where he would become chief of the medical staff under Arthur Wellesley, later to become the Duke of Wellington.

ENDNOTES

1. Horne, A., *How far from Austerlitz?* London: Macmillan Publishers, 1996, pp.279-280.
2. Howard, M.R., "Walcheren 1809: a medical catastrophe", *British Medical Journal* 1999; 319: pp.1642-1645.
3. Horne, *op. cit.*, pp.279-280.
4. Cantlie, N., *A History of the Army Medical Department*. Edinburgh: Churchill Livingston, 1974, Volume 1, p.396.
5. *Ibid*, p.395.
6. Clark, H., *History of the War from the commencement of the French Revolution to the present time.* London: T. Kinnerty, 1816, p.170.

7. MacLeod, J., *Davidson's Principles and Practice of Medicine.* 13th Edition, Edinburgh: Churchill Livingstone, 1981, p.808.
8. Howard, *op.cit.* pp.1642-1645.
9. Cantlie, *op. cit.*, p.404.
10. *Ibid*, p.396.
11. McGrigor, M., *The Scalpel and the Sword. The Autobiography of the Father of Army Medicine.* Dalkeith: Scottish Cultural Press, 2000, p.158.
12. *Ibid.*
13. Cantlie, *op. cit.*, p.398
14. *Ibid*, p.402.
15. Howard, *op. cit.*, pp.1642-1645.
16. Cantlie, *op. cit.*, p.404.
17. McGrigor, M., *op. cit.*, p.162.
18. *Ibid.*
19. *Ibid*, p.162.

4

The Peninsular War

HISTORICAL BACKGROUND

War in the Spanish Peninsula began when Napoleon attempted to extend his Empire throughout the whole of Europe and beyond. Firstly, he joined in a convenient alliance with the Russians and Austrians to invade the Ottoman Empire, from where he hoped to invade India. Secondly, he would launch an offensive to attack Britain's naval base in Sicily and thirdly, he would attack the Iberian Peninsula with the strategic aim of using it as a launch pad for the invasion of North Africa.[1] The third goal was to be the one pursued most vigorously.

The whole of Northern Europe had already fallen under his controlling Continental System which was a systematic large-scale embargo against British trade. It began on 21 November 1806. Portugal, which was Britain's oldest ally, was the only remaining country in Europe which openly traded with Britain. Napoleon wanted to put a stop to this and to extend his Continental System throughout the whole of Europe. He aimed to remove Lisbon (which was under the protection of the Royal Navy) as Britain's last foothold on continental Europe. First, he had to send an army across Northern Spain to gain control there before he could move troops to Portugal. Besides, he considered that Spain needed to be "liberated" from the Bourbons.

In November 1807 Napoleon sent General Junot to invade Portugal. Junot crossed the Spanish border on 17 September 1807 and marched his army of 25,000 men through desolate countryside before occupying Lisbon on 1 December 1807. Of his original 25,000 troops, only 2,000 men remained and they were completely exhausted. This was a lesson in "scorched earth policy", where the farmers' crops were burned before the advancing French army, depriving them of food supplies. Such a policy would come to haunt Napoleon's armies in Spain over the ensuing years. Weakened by starvation, many men met their deaths through disease, or

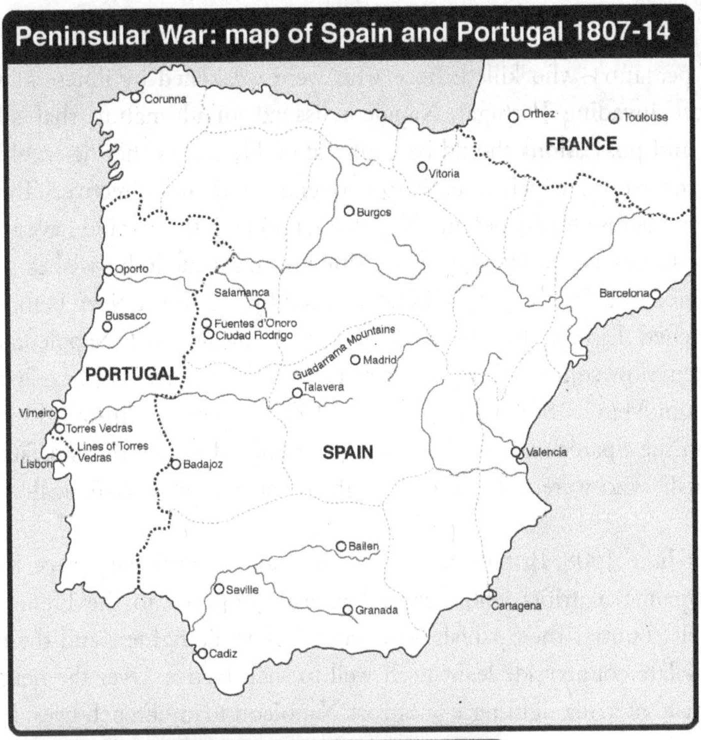

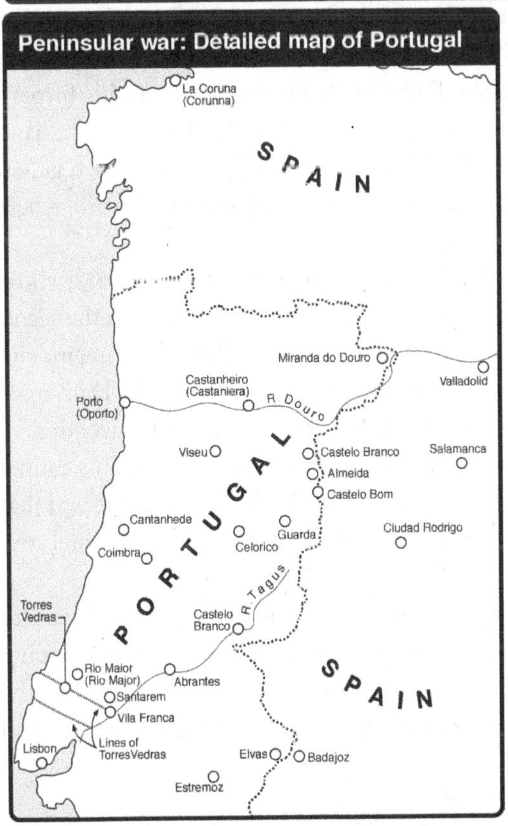

Figures 4.1 (a) and (b). Maps showing important locations in Spain and Portugal during the Peninsular War.

at the hands of peasantry who killed those who were weakened by illness and exhaustion. Before invading Portugal, Napoleon issued an ultimatum that all British property and possessions should be confiscated. He stated that he would declare war on any nation which refused to cooperate with his directive.[2] The Portuguese wavered before finally defying Napoleon, knowing they would have to take harsh consequences as a result of their decision not to accede to his wishes.

The Portuguese Royal family fled to Brazil, assisted by the Royal Navy, before Junot's army reached Lisbon. Britain's loss of Lisbon meant that Napoleon's Continental System now controlled the whole of Europe. Bonaparte sent Marshal Murat into Spain in March 1808 with an army of 100,000 men and installed his brother Joseph on the Spanish throne. He became embroiled in guerrilla warfare against the Spanish, who were not strong enough to wage open warfare against Napoleon.

By the end of June 1808, Britain decided to send an expeditionary force to Spain to assist Spanish patriots who were vehemently opposed to the French occupation of their country. The Spanish were natural guerrilla fighters and their primitive and desolate countryside leant itself well to such tactics. Over the next seven years, Spanish guerrilla fighting would cost Napoleon many French lives. It was very much in Britain's interest to harness the hatred of the Spanish guerrillas for their French oppressors. The British force was commanded temporarily by Sir Arthur Wellesley (later to become the Duke of Wellington), who in his fortieth year was the same age as Napoleon, and had made a name for himself in India at the Battle of Seringapatam in 1799. 9,000 British soldiers arrived in Portugal on 1 August 1808. Wellesley enjoyed initial success at the Battle of Vimeiro, where Junot and his remaining army were routed.

Unfortunately, Wellesley's superiors Hew Dalrymple and Harry Burrard, whose military, tactical and leadership skills were questionable, then arrived on the scene. Burrard prevented Wellesley from pursuing Junot after the Battle of Vimeiro and from following up on his success, whilst an equally cautious Sir Hew Dalrymple began peace negotiations with Junot. This led to the infamous Convention of Cintra, which allowed Junot's army to travel home in British ships. This caused outrage in Britain, and all three men were recalled. Wellesley must have feared that his career was over before it had properly begun and he retired to Dublin, bitter and angry at this turn of events.[3]

Meanwhile, Sir John Moore took command of British forces and began to forge closer associations with the Spanish forces. He advanced into Spain, hoping for help from the Spanish, but found he was facing the French by himself since the Spanish as already explained were neither prepared, nor capable, of waging open warfare. To make matters worse, Moore had to face Napoleon who had come to take personal command of the French forces.

Moore was forced into retreat, and Napoleon left, imagining the hard work in the Peninsula to be over. Bonaparte now had his attention fixed on waging war against his former ally, Austria and so left Marshal Soult to complete military operations against Moore. Moore made a stand at Corunna, defeating Soult on 16 January 1809, but was killed by a cannon-ball, which tore away his left arm at the shoulder and also his upper chest wall. He was buried in an unmarked grave and his adversary, Marshal Soult, subsequently erected a statue in his honour.[4] Moore's army escaped by sea, in a remarkable exploit bearing similarities to the evacuation of the British Expeditionary Force from Dunkirk in 1940. Despite severe gales, 27,000 men made it home to the United Kingdom, where they were attended to by James McGrigor when they reached Portsmouth, as described in Chapter 3.

Guerrilla resistance in the Peninsula continued and Lisbon still remained in British hands after the defeat of Junot. Wellesley used all his powers of persuasion to be given command of a second expedition to Portugal, and successfully re-launched his career. He returned to Portugal in the spring of 1809. General Beresford had already been sent to Portugal to organise Portuguese resistance and Marshal Soult crossed into Portugal to sustain French pressure. Soult was defeated by Wellesley at Oporto on 12 May, 1809.

Wellesley now advanced into Spain, taking the war to the French, although the Spanish remained unreliable allies and were still only fit for guerrilla warfare. Despite this, Wellesley beat the French at Talavera on 28 July 1809, before withdrawing into Portugal. He was given the title of "Viscount Wellington" after his victory at Talavera, although he would not become a Duke till 1814.He prepared a defensive position against a presumed French pursuit across the southern part of Portugal called the Lines of Torres Vedras, which extended across the southern end of Portugal from East to West and protected the port of Lisbon from the French.

The French storm gathered when two French armies, the Army of Portugal under Marshal Massena and the Army of Andalusia under Marshal Soult assembled on the border. Fortunately for Wellington, these two did not see eye to eye and there was no effective co-ordination of their activities. In July 1810, Massena advanced and was defeated by Wellington at Bussaco on 27 September 1810.[5] Despite his victory at Bussaco, Wellington remained behind his defences, and Massena spent a long and debilitating winter outside the British and Portuguese lines.

Wellington defeated Massena again in May 1811 at Fuentes de Oñoro, while the Portuguese allied army under Beresford attacked the fortress city of Badajoz with little success.

In January 1812, Wellington went on the offensive once again. He captured the border forts of Ciudad Rodrigo on 19 January 1812 and of Badajoz on 19 April. James McGrigor landed in Lisbon on 10 January 1812 and joined Wellington during the Siege of Badajoz. Wellington went on to defeat Massena's replacement, Marshal Marmont, at Salamanca on 22 July 1812 and briefly liberated Madrid, but once again withdrew to Portugal, rather than risk being cut off by numerically superior French forces. This was a hard and strenuous withdrawal, which taxed his retreating and demoralised troops to the full, who by now were suffering greatly from a variety of diseases. James McGrigor was to play a very important role during the retreat and over the winter months of 1812/13, to ensure that Wellington's army was fit and well enough by the spring of 1813 to resume the offensive.

Wellington faced Joseph Bonaparte, Napoleon's brother who had been installed "King of Spain" in 1808, and smashed the French Army, this time at Vitoria on 21 June 1813. Marshal Suchet tried to hold the mountain passes between Spain and France, but after several engagements, Wellington's forces entered France, driving northwards, and defeated Soult at Orthez in February 1814 and then captured Bordeaux.

Wellington fought Soult again at Toulouse on 10 April 1814 and defeated him in a battle which proved to be an unnecessary waste of life because Napoleon had already abdicated on 6 April 1814 and would soon be sent in exile to Elba. Unfortunately the news of the abdication had not reached the combatants in the South. Toulouse marked the end of the Peninsular War.

A key to the medical support in this campaign was the innovative changes which were introduced by James McGrigor and these will be discussed in some detail.

ADMINISTRATION OF MEDICAL SERVICES IN THE PENINSULA

Following the disaster of the Walcheren Campaign (Chapter 3), the army medical services had acquired a very bad reputation. Furthermore, the inability to recruit high quality medical personnel resulted in a lowering of standards of medical care. Many individuals, who were not appropriately qualified, found their way into the medical services. Doctors were mostly held in low esteem by the troops and were regarded by all as neither officers nor gentlemen.

In the Peninsular War, walking wounded were removed from the battlefield as quickly as possible by bandsmen, who were often more concerned about removing themselves from danger, whilst severely wounded soldiers remained on the battlefield, lying in agony and unattended. Even those wounded men who were fortunate enough to be collected by the bandsmen faced the prospect of an extremely uncomfortable and energy sapping journey in an unsprung ox cart to a makeshift and inadequate base hospital. These hospitals were positioned many miles behind the front line area since little attention had been given to providing an effective regimental hospital system much closer to the front line. Often the wounded did not survive the long journey. There were many more absentee troops from sickness and disease than there were new recruits. As a result, it became very difficult at times to wage war due to a shortage of able-bodied men who could fight. There was a chronic shortage of doctors where they were needed and the regimental returns documenting strength and sickness rates were inaccurate. This was yet another reflection of the inefficiency in the medical services.[6]

Statistical returns from regiments relating to their strength and sickness suggested that French soldiers were better cared for. Indeed, before Napoleon left the Peninsula, he declared:

> The English cannot hold the Peninsula; half of their army is on the sick list.[7]

The available statistical evidence shows some truth in what Napoleon said. Figure 4.2 details the monthly losses as a result of sickness and is based on data published in the *Journal of the Statistical Society* in 1856.[8]

The highest monthly ratio of sickness per 1,000 men amongst the French in the Peninsula was 194 per 1,000 and the lowest 103 per 1,000, with an average of 130 per 1,000. For comparative purposes, the highest rate in Wellington's Peninsular Army was 330 per 1,000 (in October 1811) and the lowest rate 94 per 1,000 (in April 1809), with an average of 225 per 1,000 (all in relationship to ration strength).[9]

In absolute terms, the rate of 330 per 1,000 in October 1811 meant that out of a total force of 57,781 men, no fewer than 19,880 were sick in hospital.[10] Troops wintered in northern and central Portugal and the main hospital was in Celorico. The surrounding villages were all taken over to form a huge sick enclave, where facilities were very poor, sanitation was inadequate and there was great overcrowding. These were ideal conditions for the spread of disease. Typhus fever contributed to the high mortality in October 1811, although pre-existing morbidity amongst troops who had been on the Walcheren Campaign was also a significant factor. Many suffered from a relapse of intermittent fever and were certainly experiencing recurrent bouts of malaria.[11]

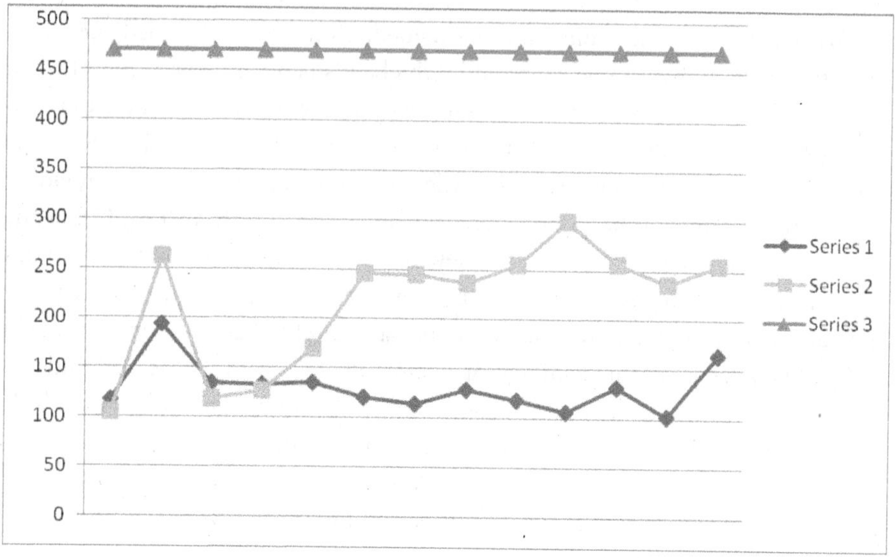

Figure 4.2. Monthly sickness rate per 1,000 for British and French troops on Peninsula, with comparative average figure for British losses on the Scheldt estuary.

Series 1 shows monthly French sickness returns per 1,000 ration strength, between October 1808 and December 1812;
Series 2 shows British returns during the same period;
Series 3 shows average figure for British losses on the Scheldt Estuary (Walcheren) in 1808, an action which began on 10 September, and lasted till 28 November 1808.
(From Hodge, W.B., "On the Mortality arising from Military Operations", *Journal of the Statistical Society* 1856:19; pp.219-271).

Wellington became very worried by the number of sick in hospital in Celorico. In the 77th Foot there were 287 men fit and 414 in hospital, which was 59% of their strength. The 40th Foot had 652 men in hospital out of 1,419 (46% of their strength).[12]

By November 1811, the sickness rate was less, but Wellington still maintained that his army was incapable of taking on any sizeable task. He needed a head of medical services who was dynamic and who could effectively reduce the incidence of sickness amongst the soldiers. He asked for "the most active and intelligent person that can be found" and he got James McGrigor.

Why was the sickness rate in the British Army apparently greater than the rate amongst French forces? It is clear that the single British Army was an army of "operation" constantly engaged in active service. In contrast, the French armies were, in general, armies of "occupation" and were regularly quartered in the country without necessarily being constantly engaged in fighting. There were more of them and they moved around like great chess pieces on a board the size of the Peninsula. The French only had to contend with Spanish guerrillas and feeble Spanish armies for the most part. So perhaps this was a factor.

However, the French Army in Portugal was more constantly engaged in fighting and its lowest ratio of sickness was 64 per 1,000 and maximum 235 per 1,000, with an average of 146. This is still significantly lower than the corresponding British figures.[13] One possible explanation was that the British Army was almost invariably successful in military operations against the French and therefore they lost very few wounded to the French. However, many French wounded were taken and treated by the British, thus lowering the numbers of French losses reported in French returns.

One of the principal tasks facing McGrigor when he set foot in Lisbon on 10 January 1812 as chief of Wellington's medical staff, was to assume the duties of Inspector General of Hospitals and to set about reducing the extremely high sickness rate. Wellington needed his army to be fit to enable it to sustain battle casualties over and above the attrition rate from sickness.

Losses sustained by the British Army from enemy action in various engagements are shown in Table 4.1. Three actions in the Peninsular Campaign at Salamanca, Vitoria and Toulouse are presented. For comparative purposes the table includes the Battle of New Orleans in the American War, and Waterloo, at which Wellington faced Napoleon himself, for the first and last time. The Waterloo figures include losses at Quatres Bras, which was a holding battle fought on 16 June 1815, two days before Waterloo and indicates British losses only.

The last two columns provide an estimate as to total numbers of deaths in each engagement.[14]

Table 4.1. Killed and wounded British soldiers in five battles. These figures are for British casualties only, and do not include figures for allies.

Date	Battle	Total strength	Casualties killed	Casualties wounded	Total	Per 1000 engaged	Estimated deaths total	Estimated deaths per 1000 engaged
22/7/12	Salamanca	30,500	388	2714	3,102	102	770	25.2
21/6/13	Vitoria	42,000	501	2,807	3,308	79	890	21.2
10/4/14	Toulouse	26,800	312	1,795	2,107	79	582	21.7
8/1/15	New Orleans	6,000	386	1,516	1,902	317	625	104.2
16/6/15	Quatres Bras	49,900	2,126	8,140	10,266	206	3,245	65.0
18/6/15	Waterloo							

From Hodge W.B., "On the Mortality arising from Military Operations". ***Journal of the Statistical Society of London***. 1856; 19; p.267.

Figure 4.3, further illustrates the numbers killed and wounded in each of the five battles at Salamanca, Vitoria, Toulouse, New Orleans and Waterloo.

When James McGrigor took over as Wellington's Chief Medical Officer, he kept accurate records of all diseases and the resultant deaths. Figure 4.4 details the ten commonest causes of death in the Peninsula between 1812 when he arrived in Portugal and the end of the Peninsular Campaign in June 1815. [15]

Wounds were the third commonest cause of death after dysentery and "febris continua" (persistent fever and this term actually covered a variety of febrile illnesses). As already explained, the causes of fevers were unknown and a descriptive term for the pattern of fever was employed.

Table 4.2 provides an annual breakdown of the figures relating to deaths from disease and deaths from enemy action amongst soldiers admitted to regimental and general hospitals. The figures do not include sick and wounded French prisoners of war.[16]

Table 4.2. Figures summarising deaths from disease and deaths from enemy action amongst soldiers admitted to regimental and general hospitals in 1812, 1813 and 1814. These figures do not include sick and wounded French prisoners of war. The great majority of deaths, almost 80%, were due to disease and the overall figures clearly illustrate that for every soldier who died from a wound, four died from disease.

Year	Total treated	Total deaths	Deaths from wounds	% Deaths from wounds	Deaths from disease	% Deaths from disease
1812	176,180	7,193	944	13.1	6,249	86.9
1813	123,019	6,866	1564	22.8	5,302	77.2
1814	53,073	2,909	845	29.0	2,064	71.0
Total	352,272	16,968	3,353	19.8	13,615	80.2

From McGrigor, J. Sketch of the Medical History of the British Armies in the Peninsula of Spain and Portugal during the late campaigns. *Medico-Chirurgical Transactions.* 1815; 6: pp.482-486

There was a significant reduction in the numbers of deaths from disease, from 6,249 in 1812 to 5,302 in 1813. There were only 2,064 deaths from disease in 1814, although the Peninsular campaign finished in June 1814 at the Battle of Toulouse. How was this reduction in deaths from disease achieved?

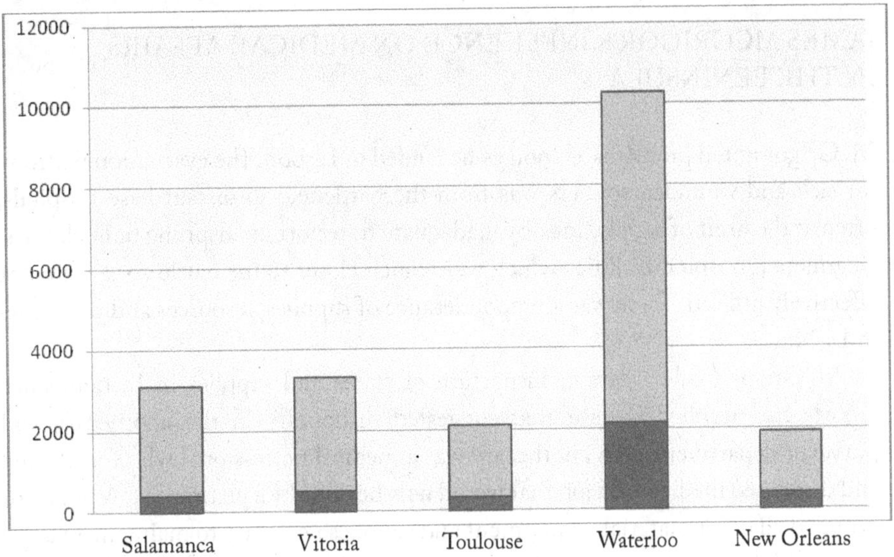

Figure 4.3. Numbers killed and wounded in five battles. Dark shade: killed, Light shade: wounded From Hodge, W.B., "On the Mortality arising from Military Operations", *Journal of the Statistical Society of London*.1856; 19; p.267.

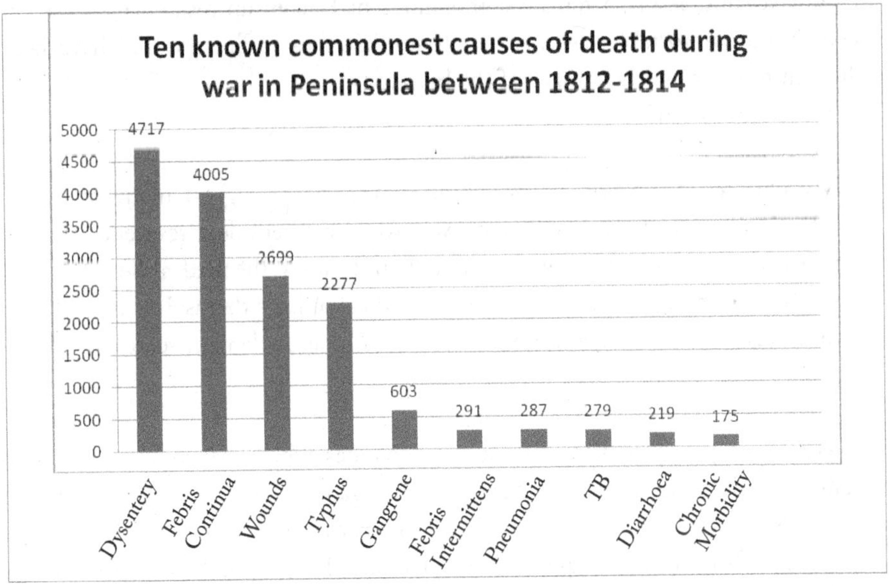

Figure 4.4. Ten commonest causes of death during Peninsular Campaign. From McGrigor, J., "Sketch of the Medical History of the British Armies in the Peninsula of Spain and Portugal during the late campaigns", *Medical and Chirurgical Transactions*. 1815; 6:p.381.

JAMES MCGRIGOR'S INFLUENCE ON MEDICAL AFFAIRS IN THE PENINSULA

McGrigor noted problems as soon as he landed in Lisbon. The evacuation pathway for sick and wounded soldiers was from the battlefield to distant base hospitals, often at the limit of supply lines, by inadequate transport in unsprung bullock carts. Regimental hospital facilities which were much closer to the battle zone were not effectively utilised. There was a preponderance of supplies, resources and personnel in Lisbon.

McGrigor made a careful inspection of stores and supplies in Lisbon, since reports had reached Britain that suggested dishonesty in the apothecary and purveyor departments. An apothecary was a medical professional who formulated and dispensed medicines, a job that would now be done by a pharmacist. A purveyor supplied all other materials, equipment and supplies necessary to maintain an army at war. McGrigor found no evidence of criminal activity, but did establish that there was stockpiling of every type of material. He set about putting this right.

There were many apparently sick officers resident in Lisbon, with a disproportionately high number of medical officers looking after them. A great many wives and assorted female companions had taken up residence in Lisbon, making it a comfortable oasis, so much so, that these officers would have been reluctant to return to the danger of the battle front.

McGrigor stated:

> My repeated inspection of all the hospitals, and of a great many of the officers, convinced me that Lisbon was so very agreeable a residence that many officers would be slow to resume their duties in the field, and that this was a much more attractive station for medical officers themselves than the divisions of the army about Ciudad Rodrigo in an inclement season of the year.[17]

McGrigor proposed three immediate changes which he communicated to Wellington by letter. Firstly, in future, with regard to other ranks, only special cases of wounded or sick would be sent to the rear to general hospitals at the base and only with McGrigor's approval. To facilitate this proposal, every army corps should have a temporary hospital where all minor conditions could be treated by regimental medical officers under the command of the Principal Medical Officer of the division. McGrigor proposed that minor cases should be treated as close to the front as possible, preventing them getting lost and forgotten in the base hospital areas. He proposed an expansion and better utilisation of the regimental hospital system.

Secondly, all sick and wounded officers would be treated in the same manner as the other men instead of being sent to Lisbon.

Thirdly, only the sick and wounded that were to be sent to Great Britain should go to Lisbon.

Most medical officers could be "freed up" from looking after those in Lisbon and should be ordered back to the forward area of Wellington's army, where their skills could be put to better use. Only a small number of designated personnel would remain in Lisbon to care for those wounded whose transfer to Lisbon from the battlefield or near the front had been authorised by himself.[18]

The numbers evacuated to general hospitals amounted to 90% of all admissions to hospitals.[19] There was a compelling argument to reduce the proportion of sick and wounded being sent all the way back to base hospitals, judging by the appalling condition of the wounded by the time they reached the general hospitals. They had endured long and arduous journeys in bullock carts. Many patients arrived so moribund that they died soon after. Even if their wounds or sickness were not serious, they were absent from their units for months since they were so far behind the fighting lines.

McGrigor had very definite ideas as to how sick and wounded should be managed to reduce this problem and to ensure that the maximum number of troops was available to take part in the fighting:

> The principal, if not the greatest means of preserving health in an army is the treating of every case when it can be done in the corps first and as long as it can be done. In acute disease everything depends upon active treatment being pursued at the very commencement.[20]

McGrigor directed his full attention to utilising regimental hospitals which were located near to the front more efficiently. Wellington requested that McGrigor should join him to discuss the proposals in his report and at the same time asked him to closely inspect various hospital stations on the way. McGrigor's first port of call was Coimbra (see Figure 1b), where he established a regulation which was subsequently applied to all hospitals – this was to segregate those who were sick from those who were wounded:

> I established at Coimbra a regulation which I subsequently found of the greatest service in all our hospitals - separate hospitals for care of continued fever, for dysentery, for wounds and ulcers, and for convalescents.[21]

He noted that many men with disease died from a relapse of the same disease after they were discharged from a warm hospital environment to a dreadfully cold army depot. McGrigor established a system of convalescent hospitals to take recovering sick for two to three weeks. Medical personnel were instructed to closely supervise these convalescent soldiers for any signs of relapse.

Base hospitals were at Lisbon, Santarem, Abrantes, Castelo Branco, Coimbra, Celorico and Castaniera (Castanheiro). McGrigor found men at Celorico and Castanheiro who were in a miserable and deplorable state who were suffering from tetanus, typhus and frost bite. They had been taken to these hospitals from Badajoz on bullock carts.[22] McGrigor was of the firm view that much better transport should have been provided for these men.

Base hospitals were too far away and McGrigor decided that as few as were absolutely necessary should be maintained. He considered that as many men as possible should be treated within the divisions of the army by their own surgeons in regimental hospitals each comprising 60 beds.

Wellington approved of many of McGrigor's suggestions, but would not sanction the use of vital transport to ferry the wounded to regimental hospitals. He believed that it should not be used for any purpose other than to move his army to engage the French in combat. His view was that using transport for the wounded would hamper his army's movements and would obstruct the roads which were needed to get men and supplies to the front.

Documentation of disease was poor, and from his past extensive experience McGrigor was able to rectify this. One of McGrigor's most important legacies was accurate recording of data, which would prove to be extremely useful in years to come. McGrigor provided Wellington with information about the numbers of sick and wounded in his army on a daily basis.

The siege of Badajoz in March/April 1812 was a costly affair, with 5,000 casualties who were killed or wounded. In May 1812 there were over 14,000 sick, the equivalent of 30% of the ration strength of each unit. Relapses of malaria, continued fevers, pneumonia and throat disorders were the major causes.[23]

Wellington was most impressed by McGrigor's diligence and organisational skills. Realising that morale was poor amongst medical personnel, McGrigor suggested that it would be beneficial if Wellington were to mention the medical services in dispatches. In his report from Badajoz, Wellington wrote:

> My Lord, It gives me great pleasure to inform your lordship that our numerous wounded officers and soldiers are doing well. I have great reason to be satisfied with the attention paid to these by Mr. McGrigor the Inspector General of Hospitals, and the Medical Gentlemen under his direction, and I trust that the loss to the Service upon this occasion will not eventually be great.[24]

While scarcely effusive in its praise, in a manner which was quite typical of Wellington, this nevertheless represented a major step in the recognition of the efforts of medical personnel.

There was no respite after Badajoz. Marshal Soult and his army were to the south, and they then marched north after hearing of the fall of Badajoz. However, they had to divert to protect Seville as a result of Spanish movements. To the east was Napoleon's brother Joseph, the recently declared "King of Spain". With only 20,000 men he was not a great threat. To the north, however, was Marshal Marmont with 70,000 men, and he posed a much greater threat. Wellington had to be very aware of the location of the different French armies.

Wellington was therefore very dependent on good intelligence to help him decide on his next move, and it is worth noting that his chief intelligence officer in the Peninsula was Colonel Colquhoun Grant, who was James McGrigor's brother-in-law. Grant was a master of many languages and could also speak different numerous dialects. He spent much of his time behind enemy lines and to the rear of the French armies, gathering information about troop movements. He frequently slept out in the fields, and had many narrow escapes where he almost fell into the hands of the French. He always felt himself to be safer in Spain, where he could depend on help from various Catholic priests or peasants. However, he could not count on the same help in Portugal and consequently he felt less secure. Word was sent to Marshal Marmont that Grant was nearby, and a force was sent to capture Grant, who was concealed in a house which was known to the French.

Grant jumped on his horse, and although many shots were fired after him by French infantry as he fled, he had managed to get away, at least initially. Unfortunately he was pursued and captured by a party of French cavalrymen. Grant was taken to Marmont's headquarters in Salamanca but even whilst he was a prisoner, he managed to get information out to Wellington via Spanish peasants. On the subject of Grant's capture, Wellington said:

> Sir, the loss of a brigade could scarcely have been more felt by me; I am quite in the dark about the movements of the enemy and as to the reinforcements which they expected.[25]

On one occasion Wellington received a crumpled piece of paper from a Spanish peasant and realised it was from Grant who was still managing to send information to Wellington whilst in captivity. Wellington declared:

> Grant is a very extraordinary fellow, a very remarkable character. What think you of him, at this moment, when a prisoner, sending me information? [26]

Grant was marched off towards Bayonne on the west coast of France with an escort of 300 men and six artillery pieces. The French clearly feared an attempt by Spanish guerrillas to rescue Grant. At Bayonne, Grant actually did escape and wondering where the French would be least likely to look for him, made for Paris under the assumed identity of an American citizen. Paris was certainly the last place on earth the French would search for him, and whilst pretending to be an American, Grant moved freely about Paris, and once again started to send information to Wellington.[27]

French secret police searched for him and eventually started to close in on Grant, who changed identity again. This time he assumed the role of a recently deceased American citizen. He changed his appearance and obtained a new passport. Despite this the net continued to close around him. He left Paris and made for the coast, where he learned that a British Man of War which was on blockade duty was stationed off the French coast. He engaged a French fisherman to take him out to the ship, but the fisherman lost his nerve and returned to the shore. Grant then learned that there was a French Marshal, who was of Scottish descent and who lived nearby. Interestingly, and by a complete coincidence, with another twist of fate the Marshal was a distant relative of Grant's mother.

Grant made for the Marshal's home, travelling by night and hiding in a ditch by day. The Marshal gave him money, but thought it unsafe for Grant to remain and was no doubt relieved to see him off his own premises. Grant returned to the coast, hired another fishing boat and prepared to embark to get to the British Man of War. He had to stand straight against the mast of the fishing boat and the lowered sail was coiled round him to hide him from French soldiers who came aboard to search the boat. Fortunately he was not found and he made it to the British ship. He contacted McGrigor from London and within a short time Grant was back in the Peninsula.

As a footnote to the story, Colquhoun Grant went to India after the final defeat of Napoleon, and served as a Brigadier-General in the First Burmese War where he contracted a fever (presumably malaria) and was sent home. He died as a result of this fever in 1829.

From Badajoz, Wellington moved north to Salamanca and after considerable manoeuvring fought the Battle of Salamanca, where he defeated Marshal Marmont on 22 July 1812. It was McGrigor's job to find accommodation for the wounded. 388 British soldiers were killed and 2,704 wounded. The French lost 14,000 men, including 7,000 prisoners.[28] McGrigor provided hospital accommodation for wounded British and French soldiers at Salamanca and further back at Ciudad Rodrigo.

There is an interesting story about surgeon James Guthrie, who was the senior surgeon at Salamanca where he treated many wounded French prisoners. Guthrie's Spanish allies were mistreating wounded French soldiers and would have killed them had Guthrie not threatened the Spanish with terrible retribution unless they dealt with the prisoners more humanely. Guthrie treated a particularly badly wounded French officer who eventually recovered from his wounds and was exchanged as a prisoner-of-war. The following year, Guthrie was captured by French cavalrymen and was taken prisoner, until that very same officer, who happened to be in the cavalry party, recognised his former surgeon and had him released.[29]

From Salamanca, Wellington advanced on Madrid and when McGrigor followed he found that many sick and wounded, who had accompanied their units on the march had been left behind because they were not physically able to keep up. Many were moribund. Determined to reduce their suffering as much as he could and otherwise helpless to render assistance, he ordered medical officers to come from Salamanca. He also demanded provisions to be sent to each of the places where the sick and wounded had managed to congregate by the wayside. He reported what he had done to Wellington who flew into a fit of rage and roared at McGrigor:

> I shall be glad to know who is to command the army, I or you. I establish one route, one line of communication for the army; you establish another, and order the commissariat and the supplies by that line. As long as you live, sir, never do so again; never do anything without my orders.[30]

In September 1812, the French withdrew to Burgos, and Wellington followed, but things went badly for him. He was short of engineers and artillery and after a month he had to withdraw, since he was now threatened by two French armies.

Soult and King Joseph were approaching from the south with 60,000 men and the defenders facing him in Burgos had been reinforced. Wellington was clearly troubled by the thought of having to abandon the sick and wounded, but McGrigor was able to inform his commander that he had already evacuated all those fit to be moved. By now it was late October, winter was coming, and Wellington's army faced a long retreat. The sickness rate had been steadily rising and there were difficult times ahead.

McGrigor had already evacuated the sick and wounded, much to Wellington's relief. He had moved them 80 miles to a general hospital in Valladolid by using every returning commissariat wagon and mule he could find.

The retreat continued from Valladolid to Salamanca but McGrigor found a great deal of drunkenness in the retreating and demoralised army. Alcohol abuse would have predisposed the soldiers to disease and it also suggested that soldiers were becoming difficult to control. McGrigor once again anticipated events by arranging to evacuate the wounded from Salamanca to the general hospitals in Celorico, Coimbra and Oporto. Eighty of the worst wounded had to be left behind at Salamanca. Wellington was delighted that McGrigor had been so efficient in evacuating the sick and wounded and made reference to it. McGrigor could not help reminding Wellington how he had blamed McGrigor for taking the initiative in Madrid, but Wellington simply shrugged off McGrigor's observation with the remark:

> It is alright as it has turned out, but I recommend you still to have my orders for what you do.[31]

The percentage sickness rate was 29.9% in May 1812 and 24% in July at the time of the Battle of Salamanca. After Salamanca, the situation started to deteriorate at the siege of Burgos, which lasted from Mid-September to late October. During the retreat which followed, the sick rate began to rise. The percentage sickness rate was 34.7% in August and 35% in September with 18,000 on the sick returns and over 16,000 in general hospitals. During the long retreat towards Portugal, the sickness rate was 37% in October and 36.4% in November.

Salamanca was the hardest pressed of all the hospitals during this time. The British retreat and the difficult conditions endured by the men are reflected in the sickness returns. Figure 4.5 shows the total numbers of sick admitted during the year 1812 while Figure 4.6 shows admissions as a percentage of ration strength.

Wellington spent the winter of 1812/13 in Portugal. When McGrigor made his statistical returns, many men were missing. McGrigor could not explain what had happened to them since many of them had not reached any hospital. Over

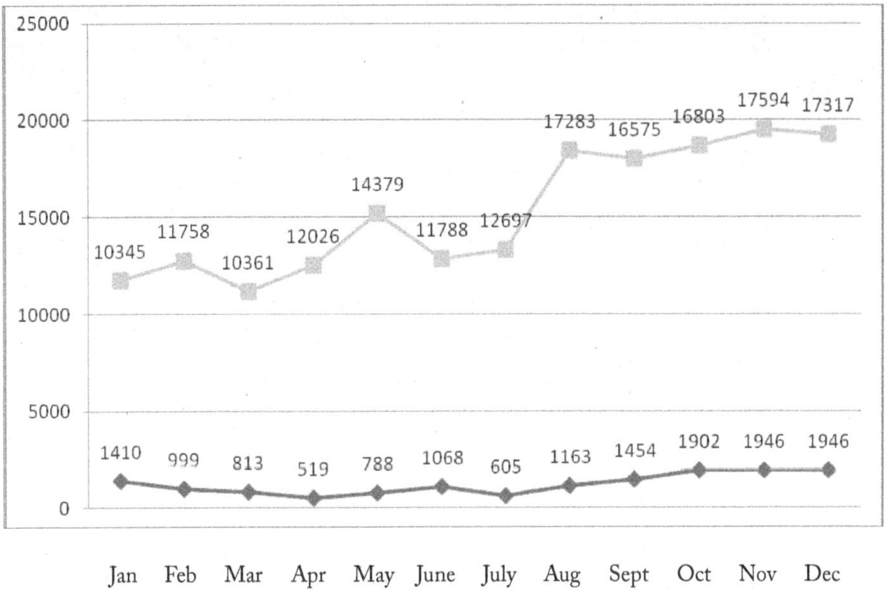

Figure 4.5. The total numbers of sick admitted to regimental and general hospitals each month during the year 1812. The bottom line is number of admissions to regimental hospitals, while the top line is number of admissions to general hospitals. From Cantlie, N., *A History of the Army Medical Department* Volume 1. Edinburgh: Churchill Livingston; 1974, p.505.

a few weeks, a significant number of men did turn up, but many had been left behind, too sick, or in some cases too drunk to go any further.

McGrigor was given the authority and responsibility to reorganise his medical facilities as he thought fit. Within a few months, he increased the total capacity of regimental hospitals from 2,000 to 5,000, to take the pressure off the general hospitals. He reduced evacuation over the longer distances to general hospitals to a trickle. Given the poor physical state of troops after the retreat, there was a fear that typhus fever might break out, which it duly did, and the Guards Division was worst affected. Typhus affected medical staff as well and 11 medical officers perished; [32] a timely reminder that medical officers were at high risk of contracting disease.

Dysentery also took its toll. Deaths from dysentery in 1812 numbered 2,340, while deaths from typhus fever totalled 999.[33] Soldiers also suffered from continued fever, which was mainly typhoid and many had relapses of malaria.

Unfortunately, medical treatments in the early nineteenth century were ineffective, with the exception of Peruvian bark which was used for intermittent fever (malaria). Various remedies including treatment with camphor, opium, leeches, blistering and cathartics were all employed without success. Better conditions with

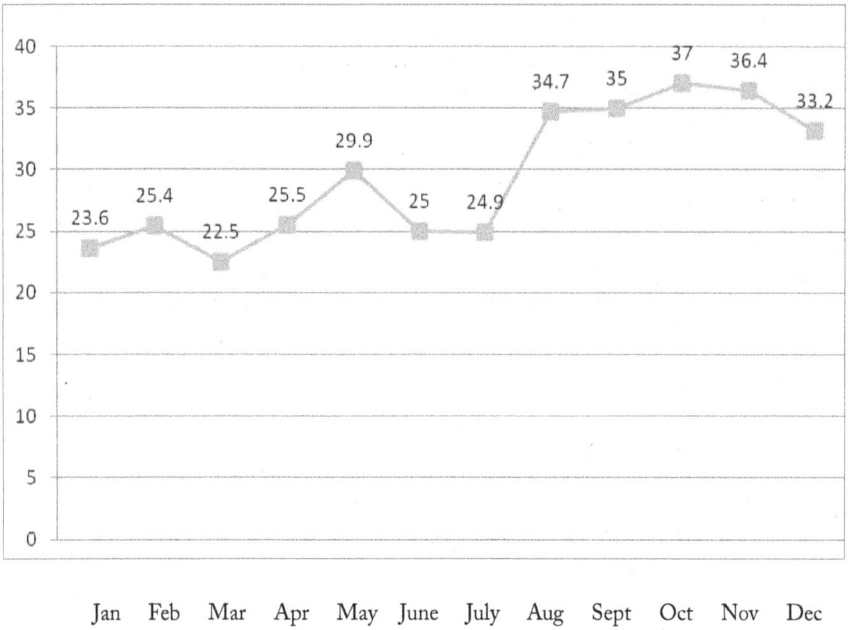

Figure 4.6. Showing total admissions in 1812 to regimental and general hospitals as a percentage of ration strength. From Cantlie, N., *A History of the Army Medical Department* Volume 1. Edinburgh: Churchill Livingston; 1974, p.505.

less overcrowding were the two key factors in limiting the morbidity and mortality of many diseases. McGrigor recorded:

> I may say of the whole of our hospitals in the Peninsula as well as of this station (Celorico) that at all times the utmost cleanliness of the wards and bedding and especially of the persons and linen of the patients have now been rigidly enforced. We regard cleanliness and ventilation not only as means of cure and of comfort but as essentially requisite to prevent contagion.[34]

Wherever there was the least suspicion of overcrowding, McGrigor insisted on redistribution of the sick to eliminate it. The entire Guards Brigade of over 2,000 men was badly affected by typhus fever and in an attempt to reduce the likelihood of contagion they were marched to Oporto. 700 remained in hospital, 700 marched to Oporto, and 700 remained in their graves.[35]

McGrigor asked for, and received, sectional wooden hutted hospitals to be sent from Britain to provide satisfactory accommodation for the sick and wounded. This helped to reduce overcrowding. Those divisions where overcrowding had been satisfactorily dealt with suffered much less from disease. The 4th Division, in good billets, did not have a single case of typhus.[36]

McGrigor's comprehensive returns enabled him to monitor the progress he was making. Once the soldiers were settled into winter quarters, fresh clothing and blankets were issued and good provisions improved the nutrition of the soldiers. At one stage, McGrigor stopped all energy-sapping journeys to base hospitals. In general hospitals, there were separate wards for sick and for wounded. All patients were provided with a bedstead, rather than straw on a cold and wet floor, which had been the case when McGrigor first arrived on the Peninsula.

As a result of these various measures, the sick rate fell by February 1813 to below 30%. By April, it was 20%. This fall can be attributed to better nutrition, good clothing and satisfactory accommodation, with less overcrowding.

McGrigor's efforts to improve the systems and delivery of medical care over the winter months of 1812 and 1813 were of great importance:

> By the extraordinary exertions of the medical officers, particularly at the large general hospitals in Lisbon, Coimbra, Oporto, Viseu and Celorico, a very large body of sick were sent out of the hospitals cured; and the weather being fine after their march, they joined their divisions of the army in firm health. Lord Wellington was highly pleased, as the number sent from the hospitals fit for duty was so much greater by some thousands than he had expected. Reinforcements having likewise joined from England, he determined on instantly commencing the campaign.[37]

MCGRIGOR'S SUCCESSES AND FAILURES IN THE PENINSULA

The successes that McGrigor achieved with his changes to medical care are summarised below. Whilst these were great achievements he did not complete all the improvements that he would have desired.

Successes

- Utilisation of the regimental hospital system; rapid treatment and reduction of the transport of debilitated patients to the rear with its associated high mortality;
- Restriction of the movement of large numbers of sick helped to reduce the spread of infection;
- McGrigor's efforts added the equivalent of a division of fighting troops at the Battle of Vitoria;[38]
- Segregation of cases of continued fever and dysentery from surgical patients, and provision of convalescent depots which reduced the probability of early relapse and death from disease;
- Institution of regular and accurate returns for sick and wounded; provision of accurate information for Wellington and institution of the database for future work on diseases affecting movements of troops in different environments;
- On appointment as Director General of Army Medical Services in 1815, McGrigor implemented a universal policy of accurate collection of information.

Failures

- Perhaps McGrigor's single greatest failure was his inability to persuade Wellington to provide an effective field medical unit to remove wounded soldiers from the battlefield. Furthermore, there was no provision for appropriate transport to transfer patients between regimental hospitals in the forward areas and general hospitals in the rear. An unsprung bullock cart was a very poor form of transport and not infrequently the sick and wounded were sent to the rear on mules and were tied on to prevent them from falling off. As a result many died during these journeys or soon after they had arrived at base in an exhausted and moribund state;
- Wellington would not entertain the use of transport for any purpose other than troop movements to engage the French in combat and McGrigor failed to influence this policy.

Reflecting on the inadequacy of the evacuation of British sick and wounded, William Fergusson, who was Inspector General of Hospitals for the Portuguese Army, and subsequently Principal Medical Officer of the British 2nd Division, was firmly of the view that the French did very much better:

> Our means of transporting sick and wounded have ever been deficient and cruel, as all can testify who attended the bullock cars of the Peninsula. We have indeed a few spring wagons, but not a tithe of what an army engaged on actual service would require; and as to a hospital corps, duly organized for the service of the hospitals in all its branches, we have yet to learn what it means. That of the French, which attended the grand armies in the last war, amounted to thousands in number, mounted and dismounted, with officers in graduated rank, and possessed every species of equipment, including horses, farriery, &c. which that branch of the service could require. A better organization, whether as it regards humanity, or the efficiency of our army, it is to be hoped will be made in future wars.[39]

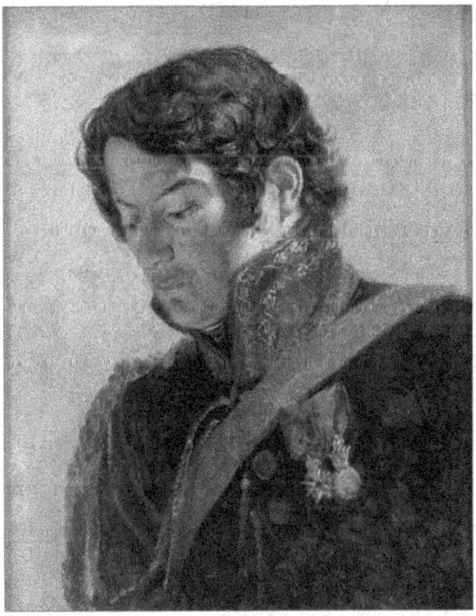

Figure 4.7. Portrait of Dominique Larrey (Courtesy of Bridgeman Art Library).

The French set the standard when Napoleon's Baron Dominique Larrey invented the flying ambulance for rapid evacuation and movement of sick and wounded.

Another important French military surgeon, Baron Pierre Francois Percy, also had firm ideas as to how the wounded should be evacuated from the battlefield. What Larrey and Percy meant by the word ambulance was a mobile military hospital with all the necessary equipment and personnel to perform the task of removing and treating battle casualties as quickly and efficiently as possible. It is only in Britain where the word ambulance has come to refer exclusively to the vehicle used to convey the sick or wounded to a hospital. In Larrey's time such a vehicle was an *ambulance wagon*.

During a previous campaign with Napoleon on the Rhine in 1792, Larrey documented his concerns with the evacuation of the wounded:

> I now first discovered the inconvenience to which we were subjected in moving our ambulances or military hospitals. The military regulations required that they should always be one league distant from the army. The wounded were left on the field, until after the engagement, and were then collected at a convenient spot, to which the ambulances repaired as speedily as possible; but the number of wagons interposed between them and the army, and many other difficulties so retarded their progress, that they never arrived in less than twenty four or thirty six hours, so that most of the wounded died for want of assistance. This suggested to me the idea of constructing an ambulance in such a manner that it might afford a ready conveyance for the wounded during the battle.[40]

Larrey developed his concept of a "flying ambulance" during Napoleon's campaign in Italy in 1797. The advantage of this system was that the ambulances could follow the movements of troops near the front area and were capable of separating into sub-divisions, heading off with a flying ambulance vehicle to deal with casualties from a smaller unit of soldiers, perhaps engaged in a diversion:

> With these ambulances, the most rapid movement of the advanced guard can be followed up, and when necessary, they can be separated into a great many divisions, every officer of the medical staff being mounted, and having at command a carriage, a mounted overseer, and everything necessary for affording the earliest assistance on the field of battle.[41]

All the personnel necessary for an ambulance formed a legion of about three hundred and forty men, comprising officers, sub-officers and privates. During the campaign, the flying ambulance treated all the wounded men and was divided into three equal divisions to deal with all the wounded efficiently. There were 113 men in each division, under the overall command of the chief surgeon.

Larrey summarised the composition of each of the three divisions of the flying ambulance as follows. Here is what he said:[42]

- One surgeon-major (First class), commanding with two senior surgeon's mates of second class;

- Twelve junior surgeon's mates of the second class, two serving as apothecaries;
- One lieutenant, steward of division of ambulance;
- One sub-lieutenant, inspector of police, acting as under-steward;
- One quartermaster general, of the first class, of ambulance;
- Two deputies of the third class of ambulance;
- One bearer of surgical instruments, with a trumpet;
- Twelve soldiers on horseback as overseers to care for wounded, among them a farrier, a saddler and a boot-maker;
- One commissioned sergeant major of the first class;
- Two commissioned officers of the second class to precede the ambulance;
- Three corporals, retained for the performance of various errands;
- One lad with a drum carrying surgical dressings;
- Twenty five foot soldiers as overseers to take care of wounded.

> There were twelve light and four heavy carriages to a division. This number of carriages required:

- One quarter master as general director;
- One assistant quartermaster;
- Two brigadiers, one of whom was a farrier;
- One trumpeter;
- Five soldiers as guides.

The total number of men per division of the ambulance was 113. If the reader adds the numbers, they do not come to 113, and Larrey did not specify what the additional men were used for.

The vehicles themselves used for evacuation were of two types:

(i) Smaller carriages were thirty-two inches wide and were drawn by two horses. Two patients could conveniently lie at full length in them. The frame resembled an elongated cube, curved on the top; it had two small windows on each side, a folding door opened before and behind.

(ii) The second, larger type was used for more rugged terrain, remembering that it was first used in the mountainous Italian Campaign:

> The second kind of light carriage, on springs, was a chariot with four wheels; the body of which was larger and longer than those with two wheels, but of similar form; it was also hung on four springs and furnished with an

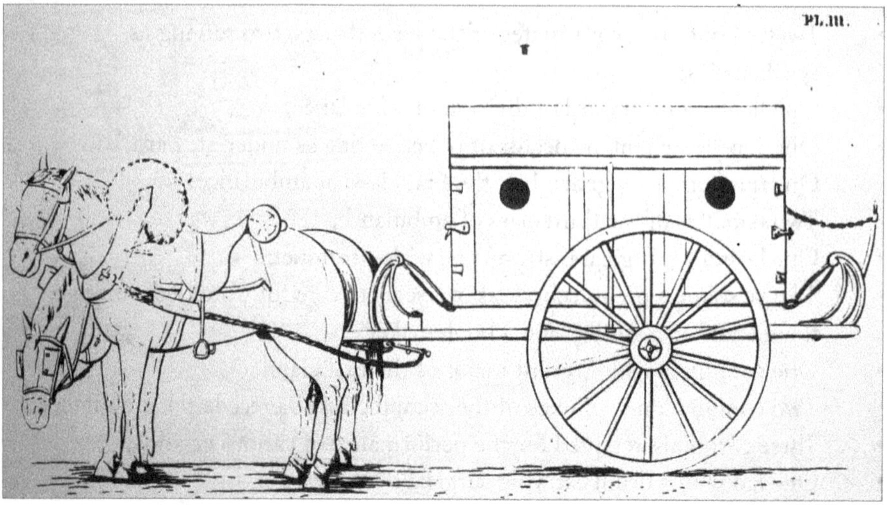

Figure 4.8. Larrey's two-wheeled ambulance vehicle, taken from a sketch in Larrey, D.J., *Memoirs of Military Surgery of Campaigns of the French Army* Vol. I, Translated by Hall R.W., Baltimore: J. Cushing, 1814.

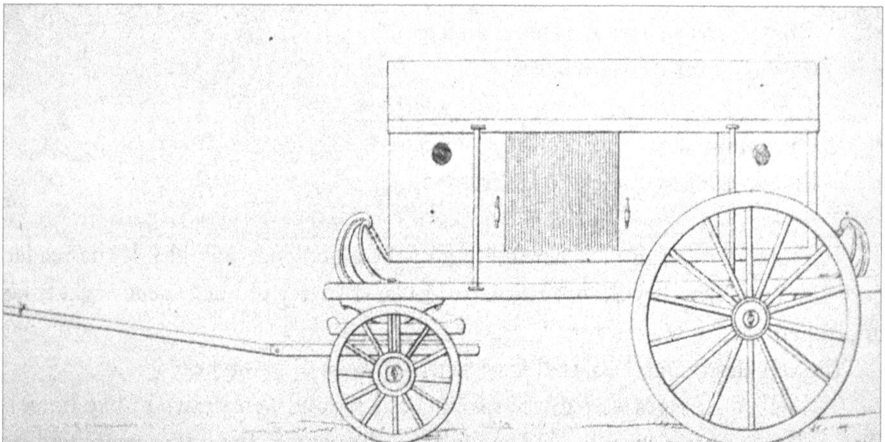

Figure 4.9. Larrey's four-wheeled ambulance vehicle, taken from a sketch in Larrey, D.J., *Memoirs of Military Surgery of Campaigns of the French Army* Vol. I, Translated by Hall R.W., Baltimore: J. Cushing, 1814.

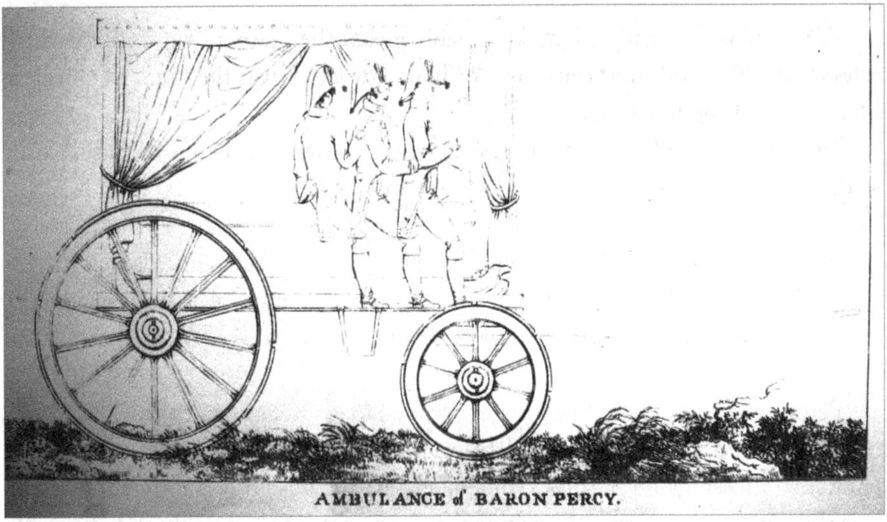

Figure 4.10. Ambulance of Baron Percy, taken from a sketch in Larrey, D.J., *Memoirs of Military Surgery of Campaigns of the French Army* Vol. I, Translated by Hall R.W., Baltimore: J. Cushing, 1814.

> immovable mattress, and the panels were stuffed a foot in height, like the bodies of the small carriages. The left side of the body opens almost its whole length, by means of two sliding doors, so as to permit the wounded to be laid in a horizontal position.[43]

The considerable planning and thought which went into Larrey's flying ambulance was in marked contrast to the unsprung bullock wagons grudgingly provided for the evacuation of Wellington's sick and wounded forces in the Peninsula. This must have made a significant difference to the morale of French troops, knowing that if sick or wounded, they would be rapidly evacuated to the rear in as comfortable a way as possible. Given the speed of evacuation, this may have made a difference to the outcome for the wounded.

Baron Percy was another of Napoleon's senior medical officers. He devised an alternative system, which Larrey refers to in his book.

> The project of the first surgeon of the army of the north, M. Percy, has but a single object; it is a kind of wurf, the staff officers attached to it being on horseback, in the same manner as the flying artillerists; it also carries the instruments, and preparations for dressing.[44]

When he wrote "wurf", Larrey probably meant the German word *wurtz* which refers to a "thick and short sausage". A "flying artillerist" was the French equivalent of a soldier of the horse artillery.

There was clearly a healthy rivalry between Larrey and Percy, because Larrey said:

> A view of the plate No VI, will give the reader a sufficient idea of this carriage to enable him to draw a comparison of these two plans and to judge of their respective advantages and disadvantages. [45]

Percy's vehicle was a light carriage intended to carry eight surgeons, attendants, hand litters and surgical dressings. The occupants of the vehicle sat on boxes which contained dressings for 1,200 wounded. Whilst the design was different, the aim was the same; to evacuate the wounded from the battlefield quickly and efficiently.

Whilst McGrigor was very much a medical administrator, Larrey and Percy were also prominent military surgeons of their day. George James Guthrie and John Hennen were the surgeons in the British army who were at the forefront of surgical practice and advances in war surgery.

It is of interest to note that both Larrey and Percy were made Honorary Members of the Aberdeen Medico-Chirurgical Society in 1817 at the instigation of McGrigor. [46]

SURGERY IN THE BRITISH ARMY IN THE PENINSULA

It is against the background of sickness and disease that battle casualties in the Peninsular War must be considered. It has already been shown that for every soldier who died of wounds, four died of disease. Deaths from wounds formed only the third largest of the ten commonest causes of death occurring in the British Army.

The surgical treatment of wounds received much attention by military surgeons and George James Guthrie and John Hennen made significant advances in the surgical management of wounds. They were also very much aware of what their French counterpart surgeons, Larrey and Percy, were doing with French casualties and the surgical advances they were making. Infection and sepsis were common problems encountered by surgeons during the Peninsular War. Indeed, inflammation of wounds was regarded as a normal part of wound healing.

Antisepsis was not used in surgery until 1865, when Joseph Lister tested the results of spraying surgical instruments, the surgical incision in the body's tissues and dressings, with a solution of carbolic acid solution. This was a tremendous advance which resulted in the destruction of harmful bacteria and Lister was able to demonstrate that carbolic acid solution swabbed on wounds reduced the incidence of hospital gangrene, a disease which was all too prevalent throughout the nineteenth century. Aseptic surgery, which involves the sterilization of instruments and dressings by steam, was developed subsequently and was almost a century away from surgical practice of the Peninsular War. Anti-sepsis in a military setting was used for the first time in the Franco-Prussian War (1870-1871).

Epidemics of hospital gangrene were all too common in crowded wards containing many wounded soldiers. There was a serious outbreak of hospital gangrene in February 1813 at Ciudad Rodrigo in Spain. Today, surgeons recognise gangrene as a potentially lethal infection which flourishes in deep seated locations such as the thigh or buttock, where after an injury or wound, the muscle has died. Under such circumstances, the organism Clostridium Perfringens (which used to be known as Clostridium Welchii) has an opportunity to proliferate, forming a toxin which causes further muscle damage and forms bubbles of gas within the dead muscle fibres (hence the name gas gangrene). Unless all dead muscle is radically removed, the infection spreads to the bloodstream with an invariably fatal outcome.

Hospital gangrene of the nineteenth century was a different disease entity from gas gangrene. It caused rapidly spreading and very extensive ulceration associated with tissue death, which attacked operation wounds a few days after surgery and could spread rapidly within a ward from one patient to another. John Bell (1763-1820) was a prominent Edinburgh-trained surgeon who described the typical course of the disease. A patient with a minor wound would at first make satisfactory progress and then, after a few days, everything would begin to go wrong. In his book, *The Principles of Surgery in Two Volumes* Bell provided an illustration of a patient with a gangrenous large ulcer, which he defined as hospital gangrene. There was a huge and deep ulcer which had its origin in small beginnings.[47]

Bell described what happened during the development of this progressive, ulcerating lesion as follows:

> The sore inflames, then come vomiting, diarrhoea and a distinct fever, and the disease seizes plainly in the wound part. In the first day, the wound swells, the skin retracts, wastes, has a dark erysipelatous redness verging to black, the cellular membrane is melted down into a foetid mucus, and the fascia is exposed but, in the second stage, the fascia and skin unable to bear

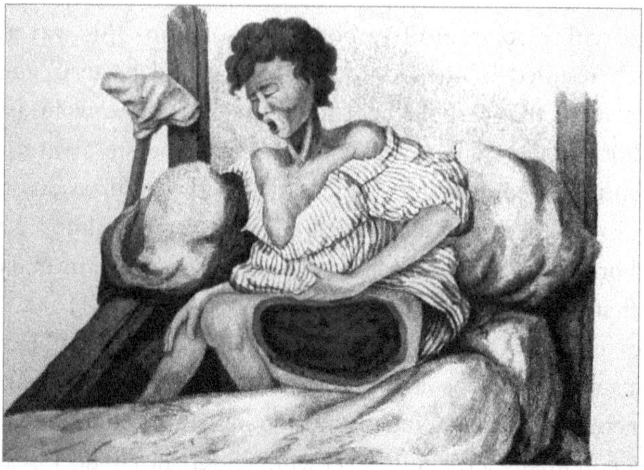

Figure 4.11. This shows the effect of hospital gangrene. A patient has a huge defect in his thigh caused by a very severe infection resulting in necrosis (death) of tissue which has sloughed off. Taken from a sketch in: Bell, J. *The Principles of Surgery in Two Volumes*. Edinburgh: for T Cadell & N. Davies; T.N. Longman & O. Rees & others; 1801, pp.107-109.

> the inflammation, and deprived of mutual support, become black, foetid, soft and fall into perfect gangrene.[48]

Sometimes the disease stopped there, and the patient's wound eventually healed up, but he continued:

> If the patient is to die, the gangrene proceeds; the skin first sloughs off; then the fascia which dive between the muscles to enclose, protect and nourish them are next affected; the muscles are divided from each other more and more. In many you could have laid your hand edgeways betwixt the several muscles of the thigh. Then the vomiting, diarrhoea, and nervous systems increase, the pain is dreadful; they are exhausted in the course of a week and die.[49]

What Bell described is a condition we would now recognise as necrotising fasciitis, rather than a deep-seated gas gangrene. Necrotising fasciitis is usually seen nowadays when it occurs as a complication of intravenous drug abuse using contaminated, dirty needles. There is extensive and rapidly spreading infection within the skin and subcutaneous planes, which quickly involves the deep fascia, and sub-fascial plane, before running unchecked through muscle planes, culminating in the death or necrosis of the body tissues it affects. Septicaemia, circulatory collapse and death may then occur. When it produces this type of clinical picture, the organism is referred to in lay terms as "a flesh-eating bug", a descriptive yet fitting term.

Bell recognised that hospital gangrene outbreaks occurred in surgical wards and that the best thing to do with any patient not affected when an outbreak occurred was to get that patient out as quickly as possible before he contracted the disease:

> Bear in mind that this is a hospital disease; that without the circle of infected walls men are safe; let him, therefore, hurry them out of this house of death; let him change the wards, let him take possession of some empty house, and so carry his patients into good air; let him lay them in a school-room, a church, on a dung-hill, or in a stable.[50]

James Syme (1799-1870) was Professor of Surgery at the University of Edinburgh and he commented about this disease that:

> This hospital gangrene, as it is named, no doubt depends on the unwholesome atmosphere exciting preternatural irritability, and the treatment, therefore, essentially requires removal from the sphere of this deleterious influence. Other means will hardly be required if this be afforded, while the most careful administration of dressings will be of little avail so long as the great desiratum is withheld.[51]

It is interesting to note that 200 years ago hospitals were regarded as dangerous places for a patient to be. In 2012, there are so-called "hospital superbugs." These are antibiotic-resistant bacteria which usually inhabit hospitals and tend to affect debilitated patients in places such as intensive therapy units. They may also cause antibiotic resistant wound infections in patients who have had joint replacements. Given the appropriate conditions, "hospital superbugs" can kill a patient today, just as surely as bacteria killed soldiers during the Peninsular War. While much may be done in modern times to reduce the likelihood of cross-infection, it cannot be completely eliminated and risks still exist for patients in hospitals.

PENINSULAR SURGEON GEORGE JAMES GUTHRIE

Born in 1785, George James Guthrie was descended from a Scottish family from Forfarshire. He was the only son of Andrew Guthrie, a well-known chiropodist

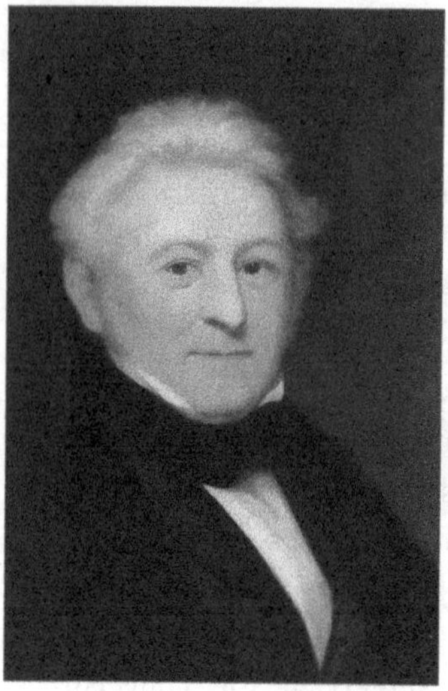

Figure 4.12. George James Guthrie (Courtesy of the Royal College of Surgeons of England).

practising in Lower James Street, Golden Square, London. He was articled to a Mr Phillips, a surgeon practicing in Pall Mall and then studied under a Dr Hooper, physician to the Marylebone Infirmary. In 1800, when he was just 15 years old, Guthrie was appointed as a hospital assistant to the York Military Hospital and became a member of the Royal College of Surgeons of England before his 16th birthday. He was appointed assistant regimental surgeon to the 29th Foot (later to become the Worcestershire Regiment) and spent time in North America. In 1808 the regiment moved to the Peninsula where he endured both wounds and disease. He was wounded in both legs by a musket ball, but continued to treat soldiers under his care. He caught a fever, which was either malaria or typhoid and nearly died.

He was invalided home in 1810, but soon recovered and returned to Portugal where he was attached to the 4th Division. He was the senior surgeon at the Battle of Albuera in May 1811, where the Fusilier Brigade lost 1,090 men out of 1,500 and the 57th Regiment (now the Middlesex Regiment) earned the nickname "Diehards".[52] Their commander, Colonel Inglis, had his horse shot from under him but although severely wounded himself and outnumbered by the French he called to his men "Die hard, 57th, die hard!" "Albuera" was the principal battle honour on the Middlesex Regiment's colours.

A description of his Peninsular experiences in which Guthrie often displayed the qualities of a soldier as well as of a surgeon was documented in the medical journal, *The Lancet*.[53]

A high proportion of war wounds which were treated in the early nineteenth century were musculo-skeletal and predominantly affected the limbs. There were no anaesthetics at that time, and consequently abdominal operations and operations within the chest cavity were never seriously considered. Patients either lived or died depending on whether vital structures within the chest and abdomen had been damaged.

Any surgical procedures had to be performed quickly and efficiently and wounds which most readily leant themselves to surgery with a prospect of survival were musculo-skeletal ones and Guthrie's experience and expertise enabled him to make many important contributions to military surgery. These are outlined below.

Early amputation was better than performing late surgery

The surgeon John Hunter (1728-1793) had taught that in severe wounds of the extremities, amputation should only be performed after suppuration (infection and formation of pus) had set in which was usually around six weeks after wounding had occurred. This was the established and accepted way of managing these casualties. Guthrie demonstrated conclusively that wounded soldiers stood a much greater chance of survival if amputation was undertaken at an early stage, often within hours of being wounded and not several weeks later as Hunter had recommended.

He set a pattern for future military surgeons to follow. During the Great War, one of the few recommended procedures performed at advanced dressing stations of field ambulances was amputation of the completely mangled and unsalvageable extremity using only local anaesthetic. The general condition of the patient immediately improved following removal of the extensively destroyed and devitalised limb.

Table 4.3 show the results for early and late amputations performed during the six months from 21 June to 24 December 1813. The second column shows the number of patients who died. The figures clearly demonstrate the advantage of performing early surgery.[54]

Table 4.3 Different outcomes between early and delayed amputations between 21 June and 24 December 1813.

	Delayed Amputations hospital stations between 21st June and 24th December 1813		**% Deaths**
Upper Extremity	296	116	39
Lower Extremity	255	149	58
Total number of operations	551	266	48

	Early Amputations in the Field between 21st June and 24th Dec 1813		**% Deaths**
Upper Extremity	163	5	3%
Lower Extremity	128	19	14.8%
Total number of operations	291	24	8.2%

From Guthrie, J.G., *A Treatise on Gunshot Wounds: On Inflammation, Erysipelas, and Mortification, On Injuries of Nerves.* London: Burgess and Hill, Third Edition, 1827, p.228.

One amputation which received particular attention was hip disarticulation. This involves removal of the lower limb through the hip joint. Previously considered impossible, Guthrie was of the opinion that this operation deserved the full attention of surgeons:

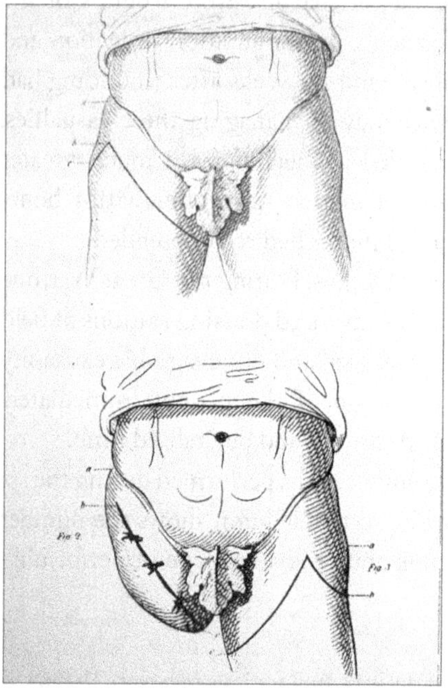

Figure 4.13. This shows the incision performed by Guthrie to perform the operation of hip disarticulation on François de Gay. Sketch taken from: Guthrie, J.G., *A Treatise on Gunshot Wounds: On Inflammation, Erysipelas, and Mortification, On Injuries of Nerves.* London: Burgess and Hill; Third Edition, 1827.

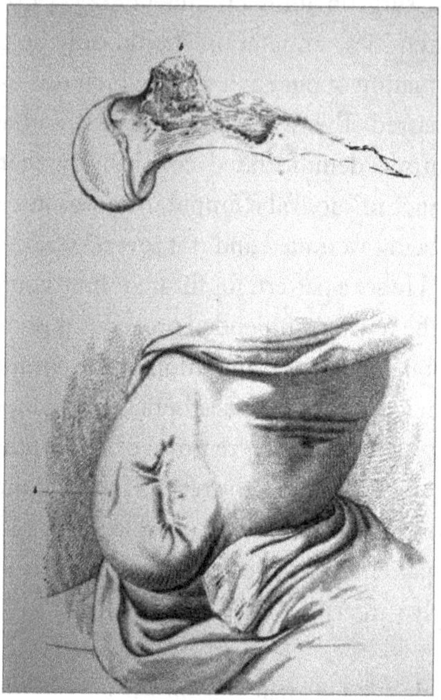

Figure 4.14. The hip wound of François de Gay, and the appearance of his upper femur where the bone had been fractured by a missile. Sketch taken from: Guthrie, J.G., *A Treatise on Gunshot Wounds: On Inflammation, Erysipelas, and Mortification, On Injuries of Nerves.* London: Burgess and Hill; Third Edition, 1827.

> The removal of nearly one fourth of the body must always be attended with the greatest danger, and must frequently be unsuccessful. It does not, however, follow that it should never be performed; on the contrary, when there is no chance of life, unless relief be obtained by removal of the injured part, the operation should be resorted to.[55]

Table 4.4 Summary of outcomes of seven cases of hip disarticulation performed on wounded soldiers by Baron Larrey.

Case Number	Mechanism of wounding	Complications	Outcome
Case 1			
Unidentified French Soldier	Shell splinter - severe upper thigh wound with fracture	Hurried journey from the front to base	Death within 24hrs
Case 2			
Officer of 18th Demi-Brigade	Shell fragment causing circumferential tissue loss and fracture at hip	Infection on stump	Death 8th day post op
Case 3			
Drummer of 2nd Demi-Brigade	Shell splinter carried away thigh. Fracture of femur extended to hip joint	Unknown. Patient lost to follow up during transfer	Died few days after surgery
Case 4			
Imperial Guard at Battle of Wagram	Severe thigh wound with fracture into hip joint Delayed decision to operate	Femoral artery tied. Limb removed in 15 seconds	Died after 3 hours
Case 5			
Imperial Guard at Battle of Wagram	Severe loss of soft tissue thigh Fracture into hip joint. Delayed decision to operate	Femoral artery tied and limb quickly removed	Died within 24 hrs.
Case 6			
Russian soldier at Witepsk	Shell splinter causing severe thigh wound. Suppuration already established	Dysentery on 11th post op day	Died 29th day post op
Case 7			
French dragoon Mosaizsk	Shell splinter	None known	Patient died on his way back to France; cause of death unknown

From Guthrie, J.G., *A Treatise on Gunshot Wounds: On Inflammation, Erysipelas, and Mortification, On Injuries of Nerves.* London: Burgess and Hill, Third edition, 1827, pp.318-322.

Larrey had performed the operation seven times in severely wounded soldiers and none of his patients survived. They are summarised in Table 4.4.[56]

After the Battle of Waterloo, Guthrie performed the operation successfully on a French soldier, François de Gay, who had lain on the battlefield for several days without food or water. He was wounded on 18 June 1815 and admitted to hospital on 5 July 1815! Figures 4.13 and 4.14 show the incision Guthrie used for the amputation, and demonstrates a fracture through the upper femur.

A musket ball entered behind his hip and fractured the neck of his femur, making its exit anteriorly about four inches below the groin. He was admitted to the Elizabeth Hospital in Brussels on 5 July 1815, by which time he had an extensive pressure sore on his sacrum. Surgery was performed on 7 July 1815, nineteen days post-wounding. He had a long and stormy post-operative course but he survived. He was transferred to the York Hospital in London before being moved to Les Invalides in Paris, where he was fitted with an artificial limb:

> He is capable of walking as much as three miles at a time, the wooden leg which he has attached to his body being thrown forward by an exertion of the muscles of the trunk. He is in very good health.[57]

Without doubt, if he had not had surgery this soldier would have died. The problem which led to the very high mortality of this procedure was that soldiers with extremely severe wounds, and who had lost a great deal of blood then had to undergo a major operation. The operation itself was inevitably associated with a great deal of further blood loss. They had to endure the procedure without anaesthesia and without intravenous fluid and blood replacement, all of which would be available with modern surgery and would enable the procedure to be carried out more successfully.

Hip disarticulation is an operation which is still performed today. On very rare occasions it may be used in cases of major trauma. More commonly it is performed in patients who have advanced cancers located around the hip area and in whom it is not possible to remove the tumour and save the limb from being amputated. It is a procedure which would probably take an experienced surgeon somewhere between an hour and a half to two hours to perform and it would be done under general, or spinal, anaesthetic, with full support including specialised monitoring equipment, skilled anaesthetic administration and appropriate intravenous fluid replacement including blood if necessary.

When Guthrie performed this operation, it was done without anaesthesia. All he had was a very sharp amputation knife and a ligature to tie off the femoral artery

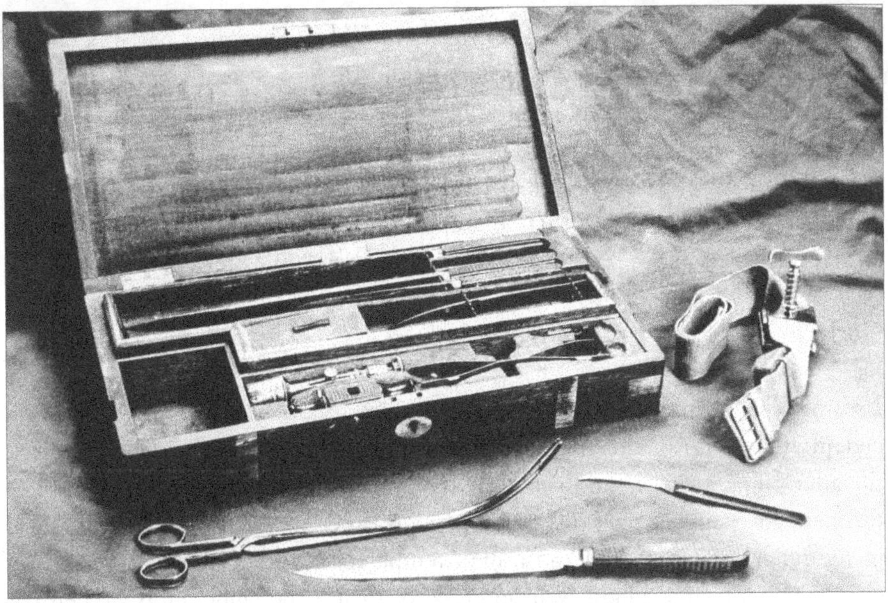

Figure 4.15. A typical set of surgical instruments. In the foreground is a typical amputation knife. There is also a tourniquet. The screw can be tightened against the main artery of the arm or leg after the strap of the tourniquet has been applied to the limb. (Courtesy of Aberdeen Medico-Chirurgical Society).

and vein to stop the patient from bleeding to death. Instead of taking one or two hours, he took several minutes to perform the amputation. Precision of movement and great speed and accuracy were essential. This was pioneering surgery indeed! The amputation knife used by Guthrie would be similar to the one shown in the foreground of the set of surgical instruments in Figure 4.15.

Even when general anaesthesia became available, surgeons accustomed to operating at great speed often found it impossible to slow down. On 21 December 1846, the first British operation under general anaesthesia was performed by Robert Liston at University College Hospital in London. Liston used ether during an operation to amputate the leg of a butler, Frederick Churchill. The amputation allegedly took 28 seconds. Liston's admirers claimed that:

> The gleam of his knife was followed so instantaneously by the sounds of sawing as to make the two actions appear almost simultaneous.[58]

Liston was a surgeon who prided himself in the great speed of his surgery. Accuracy came second. In his most famous case, it is alleged that he performed an amputation of a leg in under 2½ minutes. The patient died post-operatively of hospital gangrene, as patients frequently did in the first half of the nineteenth century. In his haste, he amputated some of the fingers of his young assistant, who also died from hospital gangrene some days later. It is said that he slashed through the coat tails of a distinguished surgical spectator, who was so terrified that the knife had pierced his "vitals" that he dropped dead from a heart attack. This is the only recorded operative procedure in the world with 300% mortality!

Guthrie's treatment of erysipelas

Erysipelas is a streptococcal infection of skin, resulting in discolouration and oedema (swelling) of the skin and subcutaneous tissues. Guthrie observed that the affected part swells rapidly and the tissues may be under great tension. When this happens, pain becomes severe and patients experience systemic manifestations including rigors (shivering) and a high temperature. If the condition progresses unchecked, infection might well progress to involve the whole limb. Sometimes there might be a localised collection of pus or serous fluid within the affected limb, while in other cases suppuration might not be circumscribed. The membrane investing the muscles (called deep fascia) of the limb sloughs and the undermined skin loses its blood supply (which comes via blood vessels traversing the muscle) and dies off, often with fatal consequences.

Guthrie devised an operation to prevent death of tissues caused by excessive pressure which involved making a long relieving incision to decompress the muscle deep to the fascia, in order to relieve the dangerous build-up of pressure:

> On making an incision at an early period, the leaden coloured and slightly gelatinous appearance of the cellular membrane will be readily perceived, and the state of tension of the skin will be immediately estimated by the retraction of the edges of the wound, one of four inches in length separating two in width.[59]

Presumably when Guthrie talked about the "cellular membrane" he was referring to the investing deep fascia, a thin but very strong membrane which invests the muscle groups as already explained. This deep fascia would have to be incised to decompress the muscle and relieve pain.

Commenting on delay in treatment he went on to say:

> If the operation has been delayed, the cellular membrane will have been destroyed, the skin will be undermined, a part of it must be lost, in spite of the operation, which will only be in time to allay the constitutional symptoms, and thereby perhaps save the patient.[60]

Control of arterial haemorrhage

Prior to the Peninsular Campaign, it had been thought that it would be quite impossible to "command the flow of blood through the great arteries". Guthrie's experience completely discredited this notion. It was perfectly possible to control the blood flowing through an artery by putting direct local pressure on the artery when it could be felt through the skin, or identified at operation. In August 1808, while amputating a limb, a tourniquet buckle broke. Guthrie immediately compressed the bleeding artery and realised that he could control bleeding by directly compressing the femoral artery at the groin where it is easily palpable. He rarely used the tourniquet again in his surgical practice.[61]

Guthrie illustrated his point with the following statement:

> On the return of the medical officers of the army to London in 1814, it was not a little amusing to hear the teachers of surgery gravely informing their students, that amputation at the shoulder joint was a most formidable operation, on account of the impossibility of effectually preventing the flow of blood through the arteries; and when they did notice amputation at the hip joint, it was only to declare it a murderous operation.[62]

Because it was so easy to control arteries by direct pressure, Guthrie became concerned that amputations would be performed unnecessarily, when a technically more challenging, limb preserving procedure involving more blood loss would be avoided because it was more difficult to do.[63]

Limb preserving surgery versus amputation

Guthrie preserved limbs where at all possible, even when very major wounds had been sustained. As his experience grew, he performed fewer upper limb amputations, opting for a limb sparing excision of head of humerus for comminuted fractures involving the shoulder joint, and excision of the elbow joint for similar wounds involving the elbow.

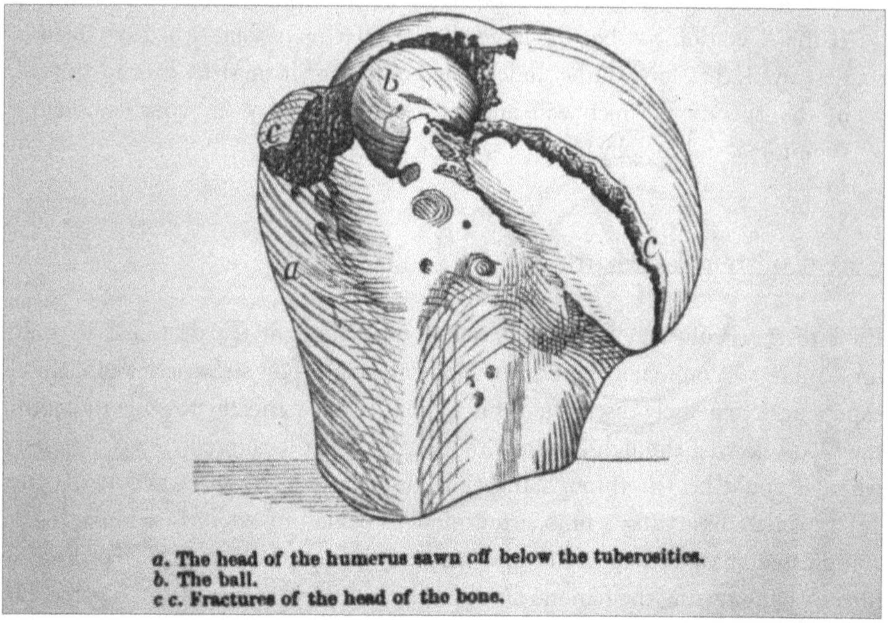

Figure 4.16. This diagram shows the head of a humerus, which has been damaged by a musket ball. The bone has been excised, leaving an unstable arm, but better than having an amputation. Guthrie et al employed this limb sparing procedure with increasing frequency. Sketch taken from: Guthrie J.G., *Commentaries on the Surgery of the war in Portugal, Spain and the Netherlands.* Philadelphia: J.B. Lippincott & Co; 1862.

Such operations would have left the patient with a "flail" arm, which lacked stability, but the arm still retained a functioning hand which was very much better than an amputation.[64]

The Battle of Toulouse in 1814 was the last battle to be fought in the Peninsular War and took place after French forces had been driven out of Spain and into France. During this battle, out of 1,242 capital (major) operations, only 48 amputations were performed which was 4% of the total cases. Of 304 wounds of the upper extremities, there were 7 amputations, representing 2-3% of the total operations performed.

Larrey performed excision of the head of the humerus on 10 occasions, and Percy on nine occasions.[65]

Larrey said that:

> I have had the good fortune, in ten cases, to prevent the unfortunate result (amputation) by extracting either the head of the humerus or its fragments without delay.

> This operation should be performed as soon as possible, as it prevents irritation, inflammation, abscesses, sinuses, and excessive caries of the humerus that would require amputation of the arm.[66]

In his writing, it is quite clear that Guthrie held both Larrey and Percy in the highest esteem. There was a professional respect between these surgeons that transcended the inconvenience of being enemies with opposing armies for much of the time.

Control of arterial haemorrhage by ligating both ends of an artery

Guthrie documented that it was important to tie off both ends of a divided artery with ligatures in order to control bleeding from it. Just tying off the vessel proximal to where the damage had occurred was insufficient to stop the bleeding completely. Previous practice was based on the teachings of John Hunter. Guthrie demonstrated that bleeding would continue from the other end of the artery, because there are usually many inter-connecting arteries from different source vessels, particularly around joints, which create a network of vessels called an anastomosis. If only one end of the artery is tied, the anastomotic vessels communicating with the artery below the tie will allow it to continue to bleed from the untied lower end of the vessel. This all seems obvious to surgeons today, but it was ground-breaking work at that time:

> My paper in the *New Medical and Physical Journal*, demonstrated the necessity for performing the operation at the wounded part of the vessel, and not at a distance. It showed, what is not yet well understood by many, that in no case (and this is without exception) should one ligature above the wound be depended upon, but that another should be applied below.[67]

Splinting of fractures of the femur (thigh bone)

In 1813 Guthrie used a long splint for fractures of the thighbone, in an attempt to prevent some of the deformity which inevitably resulted from this wound. These long splints crossed two joints, i.e. the one above and the one below the fracture, which helped to immobilize the fracture a little better, although it was not a particularly satisfactory solution, because the muscles of the thigh are so strong, that deformity of the limb due to muscle spasm almost inevitably occurred, with over-riding of bone ends. The Thomas Splint, introduced during the Great

War for treating fractures of the femur was much better, since its design allowed longitudinal traction to be applied to the limb which overcame muscle spasm, and reduced shortening.

At the Battle of Toulouse, Guthrie documented 43 fractures of the femur:

- 20 died, 7 having suffered amputation;
- a further 5 were amputated;
- 18 were cured and under treatment. Of the 18 cured and under treatment, 5 only can be considered well or as using their limbs. Two more consider their limbs more valuable and serviceable, than a wooden leg; and the remaining 11 wish they had been amputated at first, as they are not likely to do well; and if they recover, the limbs will be distorted and unserviceable.[68]

John Hennen commented on Guthrie's experience with fractures of the femur[69] and his general observations on fractures of the femur will be dealt with in discussing his career in the next section.

It is of interest to note that fractures of the femur remained very troublesome wounds in the first part of the twentieth century, where they continued to have a high mortality in the first two years of the Great War.[70]

Tables 4.5 (a) and 4.5 (b) give an outline of the range of cases Guthrie saw and treated, with a summary of the outcomes for each type of wound. They are from his experience at Toulouse in 1814. There are separate tables for officers and enlisted men.

One of the most notable features is the absence of any cases of hospital gangrene in any of the wounded following the Battle of Toulouse. This was probably due to improved facilities provided for surgeons by James McGrigor. Overcrowding was one of the main predisposing factors to outbreaks of hospital gangrene. The overall percentage death of wounded officers was 3% compared with 12% for enlisted men. Guthrie was unable to explain the different survival percentages. He was adamant that officers did not get better treatment than the men.

By way of contrast, between 21 June and 24 December 1813, in the general hospitals of Vitoria, Santander, Bilbao, Passages and Vera, there were 584 capital operations of whom 287 died, an overall mortality of 49%. Overcrowding was probably the cause for this extremely high death rate.

Over the same period, in divisional hospitals, 317 capital operations were performed with 27 deaths, which was a mortality of 8.5%.[71] One possible explanation for the significant difference between the respective percentage figures

Table 4.5(a) Results of surgical cases treated and capital (major) operations performed, amongst officers at Toulouse from 10th April to 28th June 1814.

Location of wounds	Total Treated	Discharged	Transferred to Bordeaux	Died	Remaining	% Deaths
Head	6	4	1		1	
Thorax	10	2	2		6	
Abdomen	1				1	
Upper limb	33	9	15		9	
Lower limb	49	12	21	1	15	2
Compound Fractures	7		1	2	4	29
Minor wound	11	7	2		2	
Gangrene	0	0	0	0	0	
Totals	117	34	42	3	38	3

From Guthrie, J.G., *A Treatise on Gunshot Wounds: On Inflammation, Erysipelas, and Mortification, On Injuries of Nerves*. London: Burgess and Hill; Third edition, 1827, p.155.

Table 4.5(b) Results of Surgical cases treated and capital operations performed in enlisted men at Toulouse between April and June 1814.

Location of Wound	Total treated	Died	Discharged to duty	Transferred Bordeaux	% Deaths
Head	95	17	25	53	18
Thorax	96	35	14	47	36
Abdomen	104	24	21	59	23
Upper limb	304	3	96	205	1
Lower limb	498	21	150	327	4
Compound fractures	78	29		49	37
Gangrene	0	0	0	0	
Spinal injury	3	3			100
Joints	16	4		12	25
Amputations (7 arm;41 leg)	48	10		38	21
Total	1242	146	306	790	12

From Guthrie, J.G., *A Treatise on Gunshot Wounds: On Inflammation, Erysipelas, and Mortification, On Injuries of Nerves*. London: Burgess and Hill, Third edition, 1827, p.155.

is that by the time the wounded reached general hospitals for surgery, it was too late for many of them. Alternatively, perhaps only the most seriously wounded were sent to general hospitals.

During this period, there were 1,614 cases of hospital gangrene, of which at least 502 died, there being 85 cases still under care at the time the analysis was published. Some of them may have died subsequently. A total of 282 underwent surgery and Table 4.6 gives breakdown of these figures.[72]

Table 4.6 Return of the number of cases of hospital gangrene which appeared at the hospital stations in the Peninsula between 21 June and 24 December 1813.

Stations	Number of cases	Discharged cured	Died	Under observation	Number operated on
Santander	160	72	35	53	25
Bilbao	972	557	387	28	183
Vitoria	441	349	88	4	74
Passages	41	2	2		37
Vera					
TOTAL	1614	980	512	85	282

From Guthrie, J.G., *Commentaries on the Surgery of the war in Portugal, Spain and the Netherlands.* Philadelphia: J.B. Lippincott & Co, 1862.

Surgical anecdotes

There are one or two interesting anecdotal comments in Guthrie's writing. The first relates to penetrating wounds of the chest, on which subject Guthrie wrote:

> The advantages derived from the closure of punctured wounds of the chest in former times led to the practice of sucking them by the mouths of irregular practitioners, generally the drum major of the regiment, and the consequences, although in some cases miraculous, were in others quite unfortunate. Punctured wounds of small size may be sucked chirurgically, if anyone be willing to do it, after which a bit of dry lint should be placed on the wound. [73]

This is not something that would be done today.

Guthrie made a very interesting observation on bayonet wounds. He said:

> A great delusion is cherished in Great Britain on the subject of the bayonet - a sort of monomania very gratifying to the national variety, but not quite in accordance with matter of fact. Opposing regiments, when formed in line, and charging with fixed bayonets, never meet in a struggle, hand to hand, foot to foot, and this for the very best possible reason, that one side turns round and runs away as soon as the other comes close enough to do mischief.[74]

He went on to say that perhaps the victims have been killed but their bodies were never found. In more recent times, during the Great War, bayonet wounds were also conspicuous by their absence, being responsible for only 0.32% of 212,659 cases admitted to the medical services.[75]

In 1814, after the Peninsular War drew to a close, Guthrie retired on half-pay and returned to London. Wounded soldiers from the Peninsula were sent to the York Hospital which was situated where one end of Eaton Square now stands. Guthrie gave lectures and took charge of two wards in which soldiers whose wounds were interesting could be used for teaching purposes.

After Napoleon's defeat at Waterloo in 1815, Guthrie was appointed as a Surgeon to the Westminster Hospital and was elected to the Council of the College of Surgeons of England in 1824. He was appointed to the Chair of Anatomy the following year and became President of the Royal College of Surgeons of England on three occasions, in 1833, 1841 and 1854.

He was appalled that there was no Professor and School of Military Surgery in London, especially since there was just such a position in Edinburgh, where Professor John Thomson held the post from 1806 to 1822.

Guthrie formed an association with Professor Thomson and delivered lectures to packed military audiences both in Edinburgh and London. Guthrie's book, *A Treatise on Gunshot wounds: on Inflammation, Erysipelas, and Mortification, on Injuries of Nerves* was first published in 1815. By the time the 6th edition of the book was published in 1862, it had been transformed into a series of comprehensive lectures under the title, *Commentaries on the Surgery of the War in Portugal, Spain, France and the Netherlands from the Battle of Rolica in 1808 to that of Waterloo in 1815, with additions relating to those in the Crimea in 1854-1855.*

Guthrie was elected to be a member of the Royal Society in 1827 and turned down a knighthood saying that he could not afford it. He died aged 71 on 1 May 1856.

If McGrigor was the father of Army Medical Services, then Guthrie was surely the father of British Military Surgery.

PENINSULAR SURGEON JOHN HENNEN

John Hennen was descended from a family which originated from County Mayo and was born in Castlebar in 1779. He attended school at Limerick and was apprenticed to Mr J Hennen, his father, who was also a surgeon. In 1797, he went to Edinburgh to continue his studies under Munro Secundus and he obtained the diploma of the Royal College of Surgeons of Edinburgh in 1798. In 1799, he joined the army of Sir Ralph Abercromby, with the rank of hospital mate. He was promoted to the position of assistant surgeon to the 40th Regiment of Foot and he went to Egypt with them in 1800. He was subsequently stationed at Malta and Gibraltar.

On his return to the United Kingdom, he spent time in Ireland with 7th Garrison Battalion. In the spring of 1806, he was appointed surgeon to 2nd Battalion of 30th Regiment of Foot and went to Portugal under Sir Arthur Wellesley in 1807, where he dealt with the sick on a regular basis and with the wounded from many of the Peninsular Campaign battles.[76] Hennen's uncommon zeal, activity and professional attainments soon attracted the notice of James McGrigor.

Hennen performed his medical duties with great diligence and he documented every case of interest which passed through his hands. This provided the clinical material for his book *Principles of Military Surgery*, which gives the modern reader great insight into the practice of military surgery during the Peninsular War. All of the descriptions which follow are based on Hennen's clinical experience, as are the particular cases described below and are taken from the third edition of his book *Principles of Military Surgery*, which was published after his death in 1829. [77]

Indications for performing an amputation

It has already been noted that amputation was a frequently performed major, or "capital" procedure. Guthrie was concerned that it was performed too frequently. There was a popular belief, prevalent at the time, that amputation was the surgical solution employed for most wounds of the extremities. John Hennen laid down clear guidelines and specific indications for amputation, which he summarised as follows:

1. In situations where the limb has already been carried off by a ball, then tidying up of the amputation should be performed.

It frequently happens that an arm or leg, or perhaps both, are carried completely off by round shot, leaving an irregular surface of jagged and lacerated soft parts, and a projecting bone shivered to pieces. The obvious plan to be followed in this case is to reduce this horrid-looking wound to the simple state of a limb which has been separated by art.[78]

2. Where there has been extensive joint involvement, then amputation is the treatment of choice.

Extensive Injuries of the Joints form an urgent class of cases for immediate amputation. I am well aware that some very favourable joint cases have ended successfully without removing the limb; but 1 will venture to assert, that the pain and inconvenience of the cure, the subsequent inability of the member, and its proneness to disease, have infinitely counterbalanced the benefit derived from saving it.[79]

3. Amputation should be performed when there has been an extensive compound fracture close to a joint.

Under the same law are included, by the best and most experienced army surgeons, all compound fractures close to the joints, especially if conjoined with lacerated vessels or nerves or much comminution of the bone, particularly if the femur is the injured bone.[80]

4. Amputation is indicated when there has been extensive vessel or nerve damage.

Extensive loss of substance, or disorganization of the soft parts, by round-shot, leaving no hope of the circulation and other functions being carried on, in consequence of torn arteries, nerves, &c[81]

5. Amputation should be performed when there is complete disorganisation of structures, even with the skin still intact.

Cases where the bones have been Fractured or Dislocated, without rupture of the skin or great loss of parts, but with great injury or disorganization of the ligaments, &c., and injuries of the vessels, followed by extensive internal effusions of blood among the soft parts. [82]

In other instances, Hennen stated that the wound should be explored and all splinters of shell and bone fragments removed, as well as bits of clothing and dirt etc. His scientific approach discredited the notion that amputation was relied upon all too frequently:

> It is a very prevalent idea among the uninformed private soldiers, and some of the junior officers, that the surgeons "lop off," as their phrase is, limbs by cart-loads, to save trouble; and sorry am I to say, that some private practitioners, whether from ignorance or design, have assisted in propagating the scandal. I shall not descend to a formal refutation of this opinion; as well might the army surgeons be charged with the deaths that occur on the field. Where the greatest number of serious injuries occur, there will the most lives and the most limbs be lost, and one day's action may occasion a greater destruction of both, than the best employed civil practitioner could witness in a lifetime. To form comparisons, therefore, between the amputations called for in civil and in military life, is not only absurd, but places the person who makes them, however high in rank, upon a level in point of intellect with the lowest vulgar.[83]

It has already been noted in an appraisal of Guthrie's work, that the developing principles of surgery and their applications were far ahead of any general supportive measures available at the time, which were not only illogical and without any scientific basis, but were also potentially very harmful:

> We bleed the patient in proportion to the violence of the injury, administer a purge, and lay him on a litter, or in the wagon, that is to carry him to his ultimate destination.[84]

Bleeding a patient who had already lost a great deal of blood from a major wound would precipitate shock secondary to blood loss and administering a purgative to make the poor soldier's bowels move would achieve nothing other than add to his misery. The serious problems associated with patient transport have already been considered at length.

Hennen's book is very different from a surgical textbook today, since it is a collection of case histories, and anecdotal in its presentation. Here are some examples to give the reader some insight into what sort of work Peninsular War surgeons were doing.

Hennen's treatment of wounds caused by sabres and swords

These were dealt with by removing filth of the battlefield as much as possible, before opposing the skin margins:

> In open sabre cuts, thrusts from pikes, bayonets, or small swords, in muscular parts, we may commence our plan of cure upon the field. After cleaning away the blood and filth, and removing any extraneous matter within our reach, we lay the lips of the wound neatly together with straps, or, if necessary and practicable, with ligatures, and support the part with a bandage; or, if it is a deep thrust, we lay a compress along its course, and bind it up moderately tight. If the joints or cavities are injured, we employ the lancet unreservedly, and administer a brisk purgative: if the intestines are cut, and hang from the wound we secure them to its lips by a few close stitches: if they are sound, we replace them, and close the orifice with ligatures and straps.[85]

Removal of foreign bodies

Hennen realised that when a soldier sustained a penetrating wound from a musket ball, then dirt and debris from the battlefield was forced into the depths of a wound as well as the ball. Furthermore, the ball caused destruction of the wounded soldier's own tissue as it passed through it, thereby aggravating the problem. This is a lesson that surgeons of every new generation have to "re-learn" when they deal with battle casualties for the first time:

> These bodies naturally divide themselves, first, into the inflicting body itself, or the articles attached to it; secondly, substances forced in with the inflicting body; thirdly, component parts of the limb or organ wounded, but which have been rendered extraneous by their total or partial death. All these may be found either in or near the wounds themselves; or by their gravitation, by muscular action, or by other causes, may have been carried from their original situation, and deposited in or near other distant organs.[86]

Sometimes, the foreign body might be very large and Hennen illustrated his point with the following case:

> A shot from a heavy gun came rolling along the ground, like a spent ball, towards the trenches. It rolled over that part of the banquet under which Lieutenant F happened to be lying down, and buried itself under the skin and muscles of his hip. He was immediately put into a dooly and carried to Dr Anderson's tent. Upon laying down the dooly, the bearers complained of the difficulty they had found in carrying it from the trenches, owing to its having been unusually heavy on one side. Dr Anderson, upon running his fingers into the wound, was surprised to find a mass of iron of such unusual size, that he concluded it must be part of a large shell which was lodged there. Lieutenant F being then moribund the shot was not cut out till after he died, when it proved to be what Dr Anderson called to me unequivocally a thirty-two pound shot. One circumstance only throws any doubt upon its having been actually a shot of this calibre, and it is this. It was afterwards said that this shot had been fired from a gun very conspicuous, during the siege, both from its being mounted upon a high cavalier, and also from the mischief it did, and it was also said, that after the place was taken, this gun was found to be only a French 24-pounder, which gives a calibre of nearly twenty-eight pounds English.[87]

Hennen removed various foreign bodies from soldiers, including coins, other soldiers' teeth and bits of bone of varying sizes:

> A soldier of the 52nd Regiment was wounded at Badajoz by a ball, which carried off his arm. He lay for some time in the breach among the heaps of his wounded comrades, the enemy keeping up an incessant fire upon them. When brought into the hospital at Elvas, several fragments of the bones of a cranium were taken from a lacerated wound on his thigh.[88]

Hennen stated that the surgeon's exploring finger was the best instrument for probing a wound, rather than any particular surgical instrument, a principle that most surgeons can relate to and agree with. A good operating finger is an essential prerequisite to a good operating technique! There have been occasional surgical fads where a "no touch technique" has been employed, when only instruments are allowed to make contact with the wound. It is absolutely essential for a good surgeon to be able to handle tissues firmly, yet gently, moving confidently and safely and not poke at the wound with forceps or other metallic objects:

> The experience of all ages has confirmed the dictates of common sense in giving the preference to the finger over all other instruments, for probing a wound.[89]

However, it was not the surgical practice of the day to enlarge wounds, and therefore on many occasions there must have been residual dead tissue and foreign material left behind which must have led to suppuration. Modern surgical practice dictates that entry and exit wounds should be greatly enlarged, to allow direct inspection and excision of all dead and devitalised tissue. This practice has its origins in the surgery of the Great War and reduces the risk of serious infection developing from any fragments of retained dead or foreign material. The absence of anaesthesia was a limiting factor in the days of Hennen and Guthrie which must have restricted what they could do and achieve.

Compound fractures of the femur

Throughout the nineteenth century, the compound fracture of the thigh bone or femur was one of the most difficult wounds to treat. Hennen wrote:

> But the most serious accidents of all are Compound Fractures, particularly of the Femur; that bone, whose fracture, as observed by Pott, "so often lames the patient, and disgraces the surgeon." Everything connected with these injuries is worthy of the most particular attention.[90]

Fractures of the femur carried a very high mortality. Splints were only used occasionally, although Guthrie made an effort to improve the treatment of compound fractures of the femur, as discussed earlier in this chapter, by employing a long splint. Patients usually just lay unsupported in bed:

> That lying on the back, with the limb extended, is by far the most tolerable to the patient, and admits of much easier access and dressing; and, what is still more important, is, in its ultimate success, equal, if not superior, to either the bent position of Pott, the patient on his side; or the semi flexion of the knee, the patient on his back, and the limb in a fracture box.[91]

It is of interest to note that during the Great War, compound gunshot fractures of the femur carried high percentage mortality, some estimates putting this at around 80% in 1914 and 1915.[92]

In 1829, Hennen wrote:

> The estimate of the mortality occasioned by compound fractures of the thigh from gunshot is most melancholy. In the French army, Baron Percy has calculated that scarcely two in ten recover. In the English army in the Peninsula, Mr. Guthrie found, that, on a review of his cases, not more than one-sixth recovered, so as to have useful limbs; two thirds of the whole died, whether amputation was performed or not; and the limbs of the remaining sixth were not only useless, but a constant source of uneasiness to them for the remainder of their lives.
>
> Not a single case has done well where amputation was deferred, and even where it has been performed, two out of three have died. [93]

The first stage of treatment, according to Hennen should be as follows:

> The first stage, therefore, of compound fracture, is one demanding the most rigid antiphlogistic treatment, the most perfect ease and quiet of the patient, and, except in regulating the fever, requiring but little aid from mere surgery, beyond the removal of detached splinters and extraneous bodies.[94]

Experience gained during the Great War dictated that early wound excision, removing all dead and devitalised tissue, was an essential step in the management of compound fractures of the femur. Since surgeons in Hennen's day did not have the experience or the ability to do this, given that there were no anaesthetics, then amputation would have provided the best chance of survival. He went on to discuss management of those in whom amputation was not performed:

> Much, however, may be done by proper management, particularly of the beds. As the irregularities of an ordinary paillasse would obviously injure our patients, one great source of comfort and ease to them will be, preparing a set of well stuffed cases of combed straw, wool, chaff, or any other material that may be procured, and placing them on the firmest wooden bedsteads we can get, or on boards and tressels. [95]

Hennen then placed the patient on his back and said:

> I then proceed more accurately to adjust the fractured bone; and to this end, place the patient on his back, a change of posture which invariably gives relief.[96]

To gain some control over the position of the bones, Hennen stated:

> I stretch out and retain the limb by means of tape fixed to the bottom, or what I have found answer still better, by a common tourniquet, the centre of its strap firmly fixed round the knee or ankle, and buckled over the bed post, so that, by turning the screw, the extension may be moderately made and increased as circumstances demand. This, which was suggested to me by Professor Thomson, at Brussels, I have found of very great assistance in some obstinate cases.[97]

Hennen effectively made the patient more comfortable using this technique by applying longitudinal traction to the limb and overcoming muscle spasm.

The greatest problem in treating compound fractures of the femur was to be able to dress the wound, while at the same time keep some control over the position of the fracture.

> The great error of all the machines for fractures is their complication, and their not admitting of the limb being freely dressed without disturbance, added to which, their price forms a very great barrier to their general introduction.[98]

In summary, it was very difficult to immobilise the fractured femur, while at the same time allowing access to dressings. There was no splint available to adequately immobilise a fractured femur at this point in time and it would not be until the Thomas Splint was used during the Great War that results of treatment of this difficult wound would improve.

Abdominal wounds

Hennen summed matters up by the opening statement in the chapter in his book:

> These injuries are extremely severe in their nature, and very dubious in their results. In a penetrating wound of the abdomen, whether by gunshot or by a cutting instrument, if no protrusion of intestine takes place, and this, it

> must be observed, in musket or pistol wounds rarely occurs, the lancet, with its powerful concomitants, abstinence and rest, particularly in the supine posture, are our chief dependence.
>
> Great pain and tension, which usually accompany these wounds, must be relieved by leeches to the abdomen.[99]

Application of leeches to a patient with a penetrating abdominal wound would achieve nothing. Patients occasionally survived, with fistulous tracts discharging bowel contents to the exterior by a naturally formed enterostomy or colostomy (where the bowel contents drain directly onto the skin), but surgeons were merely interested bystanders and observers of what had happened without any ability to intervene in any way.

Blunt injuries to the abdomen associated with intestinal rupture were also seen. They were often not diagnosed till post mortem examination. Hennen described a young soldier who was kicked by his horse, and he complained of severe pain in the epigastric region. His condition progressively deteriorated, during which time he was given purgatives to try and make his bowels move, and he was bled as was the usual treatment. His abdomen became progressively distended, and he died two days after injury. Post mortem examination revealed a rupture of the intestines, with much free fluid and pus within the abdominal cavity. The need for extremely rapid surgery (since there was no anaesthesia) meant that abdominal surgery was not considered as a feasible proposition and was therefore given no consideration during this phase of surgical development in the early 19th century.

Chest wounds

By the same token, wounds of the chest were either "survivable" or fatal depending on structures damaged within the thoracic wall. Surgeons were largely unable to deal with these wounds.

Wounds of the skull and brain

The general opinion of wounds of the skull and brain may be summed up in the words of George James Guthrie, the British surgeon-in-chief in the Peninsular War and at the Battle of Waterloo:

> Injuries of the head affecting the brain are difficult of distinction, treacherous in their course and, for the most part, fatal in their results.[100]

Hennen referred to the usual treatments of leeches and bleeding and purgatives, so once again, surgeons were observers, without the knowledge or expertise to intervene in a meaningful way:

> I certainly think we but too often omit making ourselves perfectly acquainted with their state, by being content with a superficial incision, and clipping the hair surrounding an injury, instead of a free opening, and shaving to a sufficient extent, as practised by our forefathers.[101]

This seems quite a sensible move, but it was to make the application of leeches easier, rather than to permit any logical management of the wound of the skull and brain.

Bayonet thrusts through the mouth or orbit of the eye were generally fatal. Of sabre wounds of the skull he wrote:

> Where a large portion of bone is removed from the cranium by a wound, nature supplies its place by a tough ligamentous membrane.[102]

Perhaps patients survived in spite of the attentions of the surgeon rather than because of it!

Of gunshot wounds of the skull and brain he wrote:

> Fractures from gunshot are almost universally of the compound kind, and are rarely unaccompanied with great depression of the skull. The difficulties of elevating or extracting the depressed portions of bone beat in upon the brain by gunshot, or the extraneous matter carried into its substance, are often very embarrassing.[103]

There was no logical protocol, and penetrating wounds were often treated by methods we would consider quite absurd today. Hennen wrote:

> It can never be too often repeated to the young surgeon, that by the lancet, purgatives, cold applications to the part, and rigid abstinence, he may prevent infinitely more fatal events, than he ever can by the most dexterous application of the trephine or the saw.[104]

Yet there were occasional logical applications of surgical principles emerging. Larrey removed a ball from within a soldier's skull:

> M. Larrey asserts that it can be done with safety and with effect. He informs us, that he traced a ball which entered the frontal sinus of a soldier during the insurrection at Cairo, by means of an elastic bougie, from the orifice to the occipital suture, in the direct course of the longitudinal sinus; and by a corresponding measurement externally, he was enabled successfully to apply a trepan over it and extract it.[105]

There is no doubt that Larrey was a surgeon of quite exceptional ability, and much quoted by both Hennen and Guthrie in their writings.

Depressed fragments of bone were removed, but often in a fairly haphazard kind of a way, and death from brain abscess was a frequent outcome. The systematic treatment of head injuries would have to wait for future conflicts.

In the peace of 1814, Hennen returned to Scotland and established himself as a general practitioner in Dumfries, the birth place of his wife. It was not long, however, before he had a further opportunity to exhibit his surgical skills at Waterloo in 1815.

After Waterloo, he became deputy inspector of hospitals in Portsmouth, during which time he completed his book, *Principles of Military Surgery*. In 1820, he moved to Edinburgh, took his MD degree and became editor of the Edinburgh Medical and Surgical Journal and lectured on military surgery. In 1825, he was appointed Principal Medical Officer in Malta and the Ionian Islands, moving to Gibraltar in 1826. While there, there was an outbreak of yellow fever, which Hennen contracted and he died on 3 November 1828 at the age of 48 years.

CONCLUSIONS

James McGrigor made a huge difference to the health and well being of soldiers during the Peninsular War. He recognised that prompt management of war wounds was essential and he developed the regimental hospital system to provide this early treatment and to avoid long and debilitating journeys of the sick and wounded to distant base hospitals. He segregated the wounded from the sick and avoided overcrowding at all costs since he realised that outbreaks of diseases such as typhus fever were much more likely to occur when men were crowded together in squalid conditions.

He installed beds in hospitals and put a stop to wounded and sick soldiers lying in straw. He established convalescent hospitals to reduce the probability of early relapse and death from disease. He especially used his brilliant organisational skills over the winter months of 1812/13 when Wellington's army was demoralised and suffering a great deal from sickness and disease after the long retreat from Spain into Portugal. As a result of his efforts, Wellington's army was fit to continue the campaign by the spring of 1813. Wellington had complete faith in McGrigor's ability. McGrigor became Director General of Army Medical Services in 1815 and would justifiably be called the father of Army Medical Services.

George James Guthrie was a brilliant surgeon and his work during the Peninsular War on early amputation, the surgical management of erysipelas, the control of arterial haemorrhage and on limb sparing surgery of the upper extremity established him as one of the outstanding surgeons of his era. Wounds of the abdomen were outwith the expertise of Peninsular War surgeons and the treatment of such wounds would not make significant progress until the early twentieth century. Similarly soldiers who had sustained significant chest wounds and head wounds were not dealt with surgically.

Both McGrigor and Guthrie lived long and productive lives. John Hennen, alas, was not so lucky. He died, a victim of yellow fever in Gibraltar, while looking after others suffering from an outbreak of that same disease. It was a hard life in the army and medical officers were no more immune to diseases than those they were looking after. It was a young man's game, as Guthrie pointed out:

> Doctors of fifty years of age cannot do it; they are physically unequal to the labour. A staff surgeon half a century old on a field of battle is almost an absurdity in the art, if not in the science of surgery: he ought to be promoted to the rank of inspector.[106]

ENDNOTES

1. Harvey, R., *The War of Wars.* London: Constable, p.582.
2. Horne, A., *How far from Austerlitz?* London: Macmillan, 1996, pp.237-239.
3. *Ibid*, p.242.
4. *Ibid*, pp.254-255.
5. *Ibid*, p.293.
6. Milne, G.P., *Aberdeen Medico-Chirurgical Society A Bicentennial History 1789-1989.* Aberdeen: Aberdeen University Press, 1989, p.23.
7. *Ibid.*

8. Hodge, W.B., "On the Mortality arising from Military Operations". *Journal of the Statistical Society of London.* 1856:19; pp.219-271.
9. *Ibid*
10. *Ibid*, p.247.
11. Cantlie, N., *A History of the Army Medical Department.* Edinburgh: Churchill Livingston, 1974, Volume 1, p.334.
12. *Ibid*, p.335.
13. Hodge, *op. cit.*, p.248.
14. *Ibid*, p.267.
15. McGrigor, J. "Sketch of the Medical History of the British Armies in the Peninsula of Spain and Portugal during the late campaigns". *Medical and Chirurgical Transactions.* 1815; 6: pp.381-489.
16. McGrigor, J., *op. cit.*, pp.482-486.
17. McGrigor, M., *The Scalpel and the Sword. The Autobiography of the Father of Army Medicine* .Dalkeith: Scottish Cultural Press, 2000, p.167.
18. Cantlie, *op. cit.*, p.340.
19. *Ibid*, p.341.
20. McGrigor M., *op. cit.*, p.169.
21. *Ibid.*
22. McGrigor, M., *op. cit.*, p.170
23. Cantlie, *op. cit.*, p 346.
24. *Ibid*, p.343.
25. McGrigor, M., *op. cit.*, p.191.
26. *Ibid*, p.192.
27. *Ibid*, p.193.
28. Cantlie, *op. cit.*, p.347.
29. *Ibid*, p.348.
30. McGrigor, M., *op. cit.*, p.202.
31. *Ibid*, p.206.
32. Cantlie, *op. cit.*, pp.352-3.
33. McGrigor, J., *op. cit.*, pp.482-486.
34. McGrigor, M., *op. cit.*, p.218.
35. Cantlie, *op. cit.*, p.352.
36. *Ibid*, p.353.
37. McGrigor M., *op. cit.*, p.221.
38. Cantlie, *op. cit.*, p 357.
39. Fergusson, W., *Notes and recollections of a professional life.* London: Longman, Brown and Green, 1846, p.62.

40. Larrey, D.J., *Memoirs of Military Surgery of Campaigns of the French Army* Vol. I Translated by Hall R.W., Baltimore: J. Cushing, 1814, pp.23-24.
41. *Ibid*, pp.78-83.
42. *Ibid.*
43. *Ibid*, p.82.
44. *Ibid*, p.83.
45. *Ibid*, p.83.
46. Riddel, J.S., *The Records of the Aberdeen Medico-Chirurgical Society from 1789 to 1922.* Aberdeen: W & W Lindsay, 1922, p.78.
47. Bell, J., *The Principles of Surgery in Two Volumes.* Edinburgh: for T. Cadell & N. Davies; T.N. Longman & O. Rees & others, 1801, pp.107-109.
48. *Ibid*
49. *Ibid.*
50. *Ibid*, p.117.
51. Syme, J., *The Principles of Surgery.* Edinburgh: MacLauchlan and Stewart, 1832, p.69.
52. Watts, J.C., "George James Guthrie Peninsular Surgeon". *Proceedings of the Royal Society of Medicine* 1961 September; 54(9) pp.764-768.
53. "Biographical Sketch of G J Guthrie". *Lancet* 1850, i. pp.726-36.
54. Guthrie, J.G., *A Treatise on Gunshot Wounds: On Inflammation, Erysipelas, and Mortification, On Injuries of Nerves.* Third edition: London: Burgess and Hill, 1827, p.228.
55. *Ibid*, p.312.
56. *Ibid*, pp.106-110.
57. *Ibid*, pp.342-350.
58. Gordon, R., *Great Medical Blunders.* Cornwall: Stratus Books Ltd, 1983.
59. Guthrie, *op. cit.*, p108.
60. *Ibid.*
61. *Ibid*, p.viii.
62. *Ibid*, p.viii.
63. *Ibid*, p.ix.
64. Cantlie *op. cit.*, p.374.
65. Guthrie, *op. cit.*, pp.476-477.
66. *Ibid.*
67. *Ibid*, p.ix.
68. *Ibid*, p.154.
69. Hennen, J., *Principles of Military Surgery* 3rd Edition. London: John Wilson, 1829, pp.109-110.

70. Scotland, T.R., S.D. Heys, *War Surgery 1914-1918*. Solihull: Helion and Company, 2012.
71. Cantlie, *op. cit.*, p.375.
72. Guthrie, J.G., *Commentaries on the Surgery of the war in Portugal, Spain and the Netherlands* Sixth Edition: Philadelphia: J.B. Lippincott & Co, 1862.
73. *Ibid*, pp.414-5.
74. *Ibid*, pp.38-39.
75. Mitchell T.J., G.M. Smith, *History of the Great War Medical Services Casualties and Medical Statistics*. London: His Majesty's Stationery Office, 1931, p.40.
76. Edwards, D.O., *Biographical Sketch of the Late John Hennen in the Lancet MDCCCXXVIII-IX*. In Two Volumes, Volume II. Edited by Wakely, T., London: Mills, Jowett and Mills; Printed for editor by Mills, Jowett and Mills; pp.44-46.
77. Hennen, J., *Principles of Military Surgery* 3rd Edition. London: John Wilson, 1829.
78. *Ibid*, pp.38-42.
79. *Ibid*.
80. *Ibid*.
81. *Ibid*.
82. *Ibid*.
83. *Ibid*, p.47.
84. *Ibid*.
85. *Ibid*, p.48.
86. *Ibid*, p.77.
87. *Ibid*, pp.79-80.
88. *Ibid*, p.86.
89. *Ibid*, p.88.
90. *Ibid*, p.109.
91. *Ibid*, p.111.
92. Gray, H.M.W., *The Early Treatment of War Wounds*. London: Henry Frowde and Hodder & Stoughton, 1919.
93. Hennen, *op. cit.*, p.109.
94. *Ibid*, p.115.
95. *Ibid*.
96. *Ibid*, p.116.
97. *Ibid*.
98. *Ibid*, p.117.

99. *Ibid*, p.405.
100. Crockard, H.A., "Bullet injuries of the brain". *Annals of the Royal College of Surgeons of England.* 1974 Sept; 55(3): pp.111-123.
101. Hennen, *op. cit.*, p.282.
102. *Ibid*, p.286.
103. *Ibid*, p.288.
104. *Ibid*, pp.287-8.
105. *Ibid*, p.291.
106. Guthrie, J.G., *Commentaries on the Surgery of the war in Portugal, Spain and the Netherlands.* Sixth Edition: Philadelphia: J.B. Lippincott & Co, 1862.

5

The Battle of Waterloo

18 June 1815

When the Peninsular War came to an end in 1814 and Napoleon was sent into exile on the island of Elba, James McGrigor returned to Great Britain. He was received by the Duke of York and was warmly greeted by the three members of the Medical Board, the Director General Dr John Weir, Sir Charles Kerr and Sir William Franklin. The Duke of Wellington insisted that McGrigor should wait on him every day to clear up various matters relating to the medical aspects of the Peninsular campaign. As a result of Wellington's influence, the Duke of York bestowed a knighthood on McGrigor, who then set off to visit his family in Aberdeen and Speyside and at the same time he began to seek employment.

McGrigor didn't have to wait long because Dr John Weir was taken ill and was forced to retire from the Medical Board. McGrigor, at the age of 44, was appointed Director General as his successor on 13 June 1815. His first job was to make the necessary preparations for the Battle of Waterloo fought less than a week later on Sunday 18 June.

McGrigor selected Inspector of Hospitals James Grant as the Principal Medical Officer for the Waterloo campaign and allocated 52 medical officers as administrative heads of the field formations and general hospitals. Six general hospitals were made ready to treat the wounded in Brussels and other general hospitals were opened at Ostend, Antwerp, Bruges and Ghent. A complete garrison company of four officers and 107 non-commissioned officers (NCOs) and men who were veterans were sent over to act as hospital attendants. Waterloo was the bloodiest battle of the Napoleonic Wars and medical resources were stretched to the limit.

Napoleon and his army crossed the River Sambre at Charleroi on 15 June 1815 and marched north towards Brussels. Napoleon's total force of 128,000 men was opposed by two armies; a Prussian army of 123,000 was commanded by Gebhard von Blucher and an Anglo-Allied coalition army of around 107,000 men was commanded by the Duke of Wellington. Wellington's coalition army consisted of troops from Britain, Netherlands, Hanover, Nassau and Brunswick. Many of his experienced troops from the Peninsular War were by then serving in America and Canada.

Napoleon aimed to strike at the junction of the Allied and Prussian armies, driving them apart and then destroying each in turn. On 16 June 1815, he engaged the Prussians at Ligny, while the British held their ground at Quatres Bras, before withdrawing in a northerly direction towards Brussels to the top of a gentle ridge just south of the village of Mont St Jean adjacent to the larger village of Waterloo.

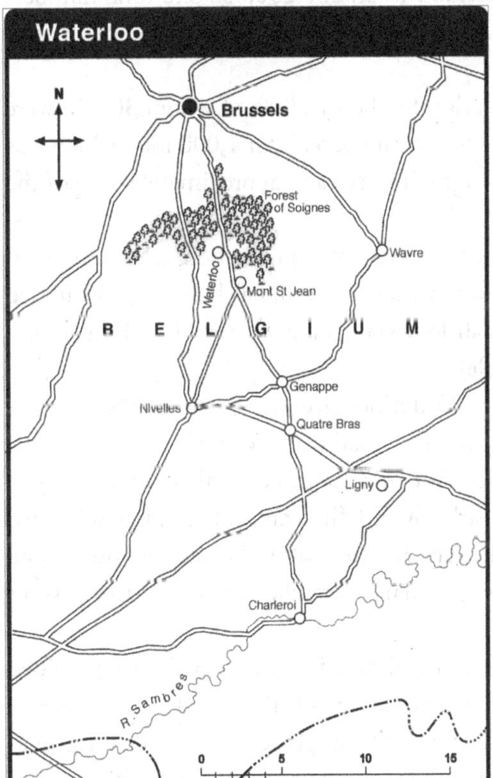

Figure 5.1. Map showing the area around Waterloo as it was on 18 June 1815.

Napoleon failed to destroy the Prussians at Ligny, who were able to withdraw to Wavre only 15 miles east of Waterloo. The Battle of Waterloo was fought on Sunday 18 June 1815 between Wellington's allied forces and the French. According to Wellington it was "a damned close run affair" and the outcome of the battle depended on the arrival of the Prussian army late in the afternoon on that very day.

It is difficult to obtain the precise number of troops under Wellington's command, since different reference sources give different information. The British contingent at Waterloo and Quatres Bras, was estimated to be around 49,900,[1] while the rest of his army comprised German Legion, Belgian, Hanoverian, Brunswick and Nassau troops and made up a total force of between 67,000 to 92,000[2,3] men. It is generally agreed, however, that he had 192 artillery pieces at his disposition.

According to Hodge, British casualties including those at Quatres Bras amounted to 10,266, of whom 2,126 were killed and 8,140 wounded. It is estimated that 1,119 of the wounded died, giving a total of 3,245 dead. The British casualty rate per 1,000 soldiers engaged amounted to 206 per 1,000 men. Losses at Waterloo may be found in Table 4.1 which compares losses at Waterloo with three battles from the Peninsular War and with the Battle of New Orleans. This comparison with other battles highlights the high number of casualties sustained at Waterloo.

The combined total of numbers of Allied and Prussian soldiers who fought at Quatres Bras, Ligny, Wavre and Waterloo was around 230,600 and total numbers killed and wounded were 36,590, giving an overall casualty figure rate of 159 per 1,000 engaged.[4]

French forces on the field of Waterloo totalled 72,000, of whom 30,000 were killed and wounded, giving a casualty figure rate of 417 per 1,000 men which was more than double the figure for Wellington's forces and approximately 42% of the total force.[5]

The only other battle where French losses were proportionately as high as Waterloo was at Trafalgar in 1805, when there were 8,000 killed and wounded out of a force of 20,000 (40%). British losses at Trafalgar were 1,700 killed and wounded out of a total of 12,000 (11%).

The medical task was formidable at Waterloo, given the huge number of dead and wounded. A total of 15,000 hospital beds had been provided. Every suitable building available out of cannon range was commandeered for this purpose. Many dressing stations were located in nearby Mont St Jean and walking wounded made their way back there during the day of battle, often helped by unwounded comrades. There was a clear need for designated stretcher bearers, but provisions for these had not been made.

Regiments had an establishment of medical officers and each was provided with a sprung wagon to evacuate the wounded. Each brigade had a staff surgeon, as Senior Medical Officer and each division a Deputy Inspector or staff surgeon as Principal Medical Officer. Many of them had served previously in the Peninsula.[6]

An assistant surgeon went with every unit into the battle zone and he was equipped with a tourniquet to staunch blood flow from major bleeding vessels. He was very much in the thick of the fighting and he attended to the wounded within the infantry squares which were formed during French cavalry attacks. Surprisingly, only one medical officer was wounded during the battle.

Figure 5.2 shows the track which led to Wellington's right wing at Hougoumont Chateau. French cavalry attacked from a valley to the left during the afternoon of

18 June 1815. In response, the British infantry formed squares in the field to the right of the narrow road to defend themselves against incoming cavalry. British artillery batteries were lined up on the right margin of the road, firing grapeshot and canister into the on-coming horsemen. When the French cavalry came near, artillerymen ran to shelter within the squares until the cavalry withdrew to re-group, at which point they returned to their guns.

The French cavalry could have spiked the British guns by hammering a sharpened stake into the hole used to ignite the powder, which in turn propelled the shot from the cannon. Had they done so they would have made the guns unusable and they would not have sustained such heavy casualties. As it was, when they withdrew to regroup before attacking again they faced British artillery every time they charged.

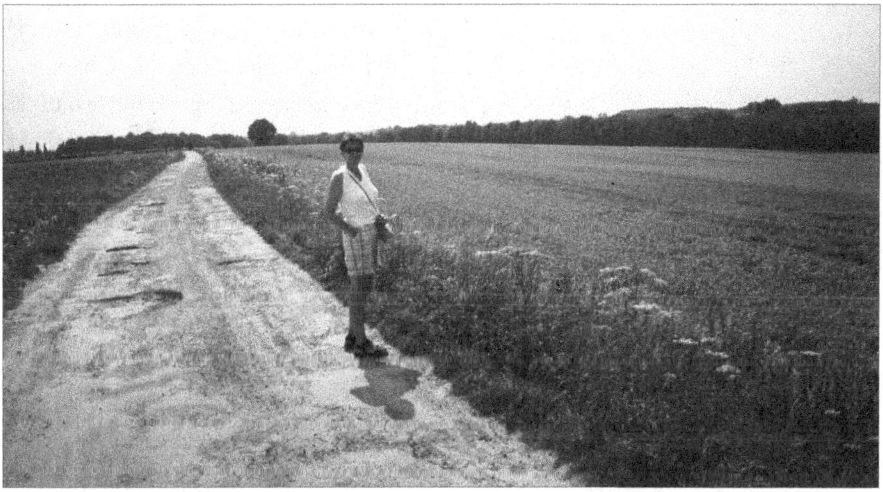

Figure 5.2. The lane leading from Wellington's centre towards Hougoumont on his right wing. The French cavalry attacked from the left in the afternoon of Sunday 18 June 1815 and British infantry formed squares in the open ground to the right. (Authors' photograph).

Hougoumont is a quarter of a mile further along the track, and marked Wellington's right wing, It was fiercely fought over for the whole day and was stoutly defended by Scots Guards and Coldstream Guards under the command of Colonel Macdonnel. At one critical moment, French infantry force open the north gate into the courtyard and burst through (Figure 5.3). Fortunately, the defenders managed to force the gate shut behind the assaulting troops and killed them all except one, a young drummer boy, whom they spared.

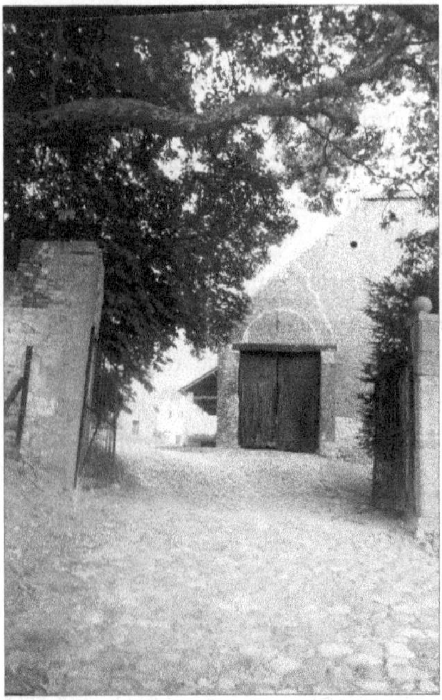

Figure 5.3. The gate at Hougoumont- the French managed to briefly enter the grounds through this gate before it was shut behind the troops who had fought their way through. They were all killed apart from a drummer boy. (Authors' photograph).

The Chateau at Hougoumont was set ablaze, and was burned to the ground. The adjacent chapel was not destroyed and many wounded were put in here until the battle was over.

Many of those killed at Waterloo were buried in mass graves, one of which is a few yards outside the back gate of Hougoumont in the foreground of Figure 5.5.

French wounded often lay on the battlefield for many days afterwards and kept themselves alive by eating the flesh from dead horses. While Larrey's ambulance system (detailed in Chapter 4) was very effective in removing wounded from the battlefield it was only operational when a battle had been won.

One of these French soldiers was François de Gay, (already referred to in Chapter 4), a private in the 45th Regiment of Foot. He had been wounded by a musket ball which had struck him from behind, had fractured the neck of his femur, close to the hip joint and exited anteriorly, four inches below the groin. He lay on the battlefield for several days and had developed a large sacral pressure sore. He was evacuated by the British and given medical care. He was taken to the Elizabeth Hospital in Brussels, where hip disarticulation was performed at 2pm on 7 July 1815, 19 days after he sustained the wound. His surgeon was George James Guthrie, who had returned to military duty and made his base in Brussels. John Hennen, the other great military surgeon of the era, assisted Guthrie in performing this procedure.

After a stormy post operative course the patient finally recovered and was sent from Brussels to York Hospital in London, where after a prolonged convalescence he was transferred to Les Invalides Hospital in Paris.

As a general rule, patients in need of an amputation and who had surgery early tended to do better that those operated on several days, or even weeks, later. The

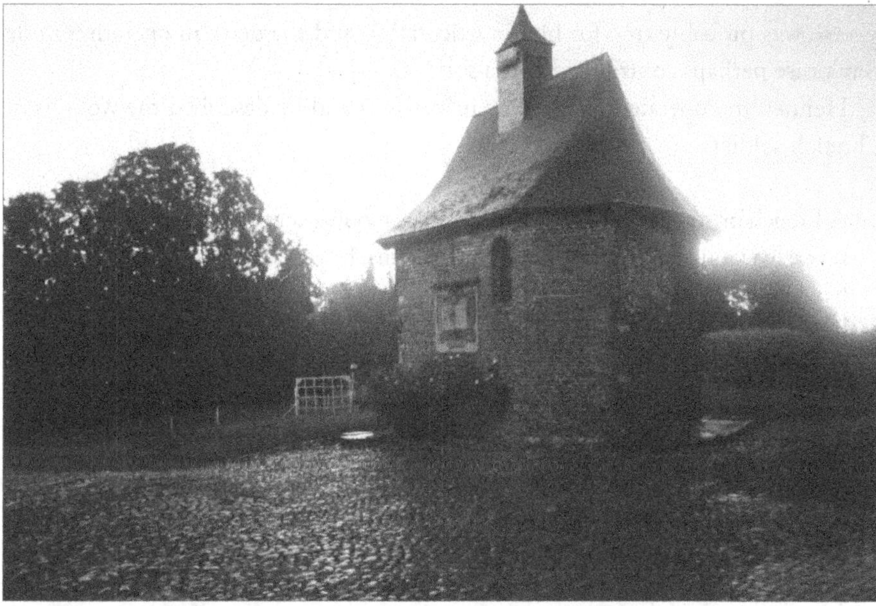

Figure 5.4. The chapel within the grounds of Hougoumont Chateau. It was used to house the wounded in relative safety until the battle was over. (Authors' photograph).

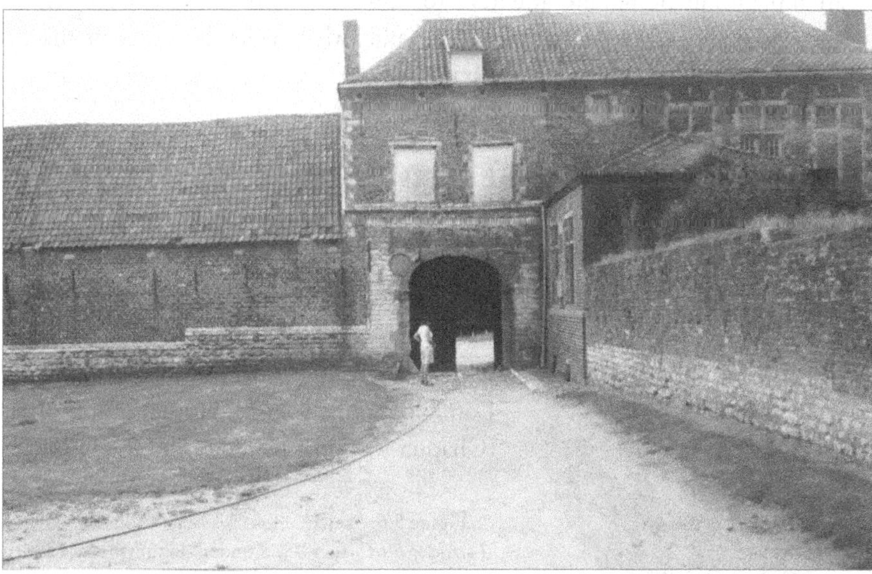

Figure 5.5. The area outside the back gate at Hougoumont. One of the mass graves is located here. (Authors' photograph).

reverse was probably true for hip disarticulation and the delay in operating in de Gay's case perhaps contributed to his survival.

Hennen too operated on patients in Brussels and he described the wounds of a French soldier:

> A French prisoner was brought into Brussels soon after the battle of Waterloo, severely wounded in action with the Prussians; he received after he fell several bayonet and sabre thrusts, and one lance wound through the chest; but the most serious injury was a compound fracture of the right thigh from gun-shot. Three musket balls had struck nearly at the same time on the outer side of the limb, splintering the os femoris from the middle of the upper third of the bone to within two inches of the condyles. The discharge, as might be expected, was enormous; but his appetite fortunately remaining good, he was enabled to support a waste of fluids scarcely to be credited. Whilst under cure, many extensive incisions were made to extract bones and balls; but with most extraordinary want of success. After the failure of these incisions, one of the balls spontaneously presented at the orifice, and another came away in a cataplasm. Although a recurrence to more ample incisions was pronounced the only chance for the poor fellow's recovery, no further operation was attempted; but by minute attention to dressings, supporting his strength, and, above all, moving him to another hospital which enjoyed a purer air, the fracture consolidated, a very few minute splinters were easily removed by the dressing forceps, and the man recovered.[7]

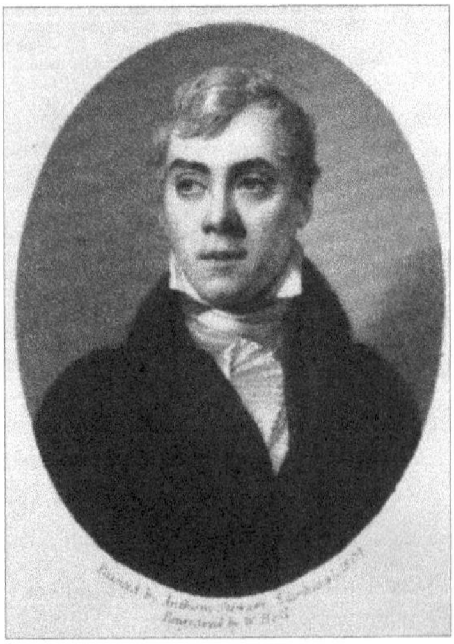

Figure 5.6. Sketch of Charles Bell. (From Bell, C., *Letters of Sir Charles Bell.* London: John Murray, 1870).

Some civilian surgeons travelled to Brussels from Britain, clearly seeking a spot of excitement, believing that this was too good an opportunity to miss. When news of the Battle of Waterloo reached London, surgeon Charles Bell, a Scot who was working in London and the younger brother of John Bell (Chapter 4), exclaimed to his brother-in-law:

Johnnie! How can we let this pass? Here is such an occasion of seeing gunshot wounds come to our very door! Let us go! [8]

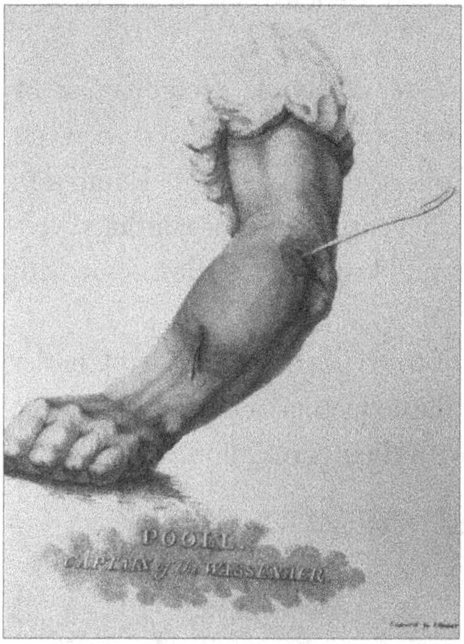

Figure 5.7. A contemporary sketch of a forearm missile wound. The probe demonstrates the entry and exit wounds. The forearm is swollen, red and clearly infected. Most wounds became infected, since treatment involved limited surgical exposure, and while attempts were made to remove foreign material, the extent of the surgery was much less than would be regarded as acceptable by modern standards. This sketch is an illustration for the book written by John Bell, the brother of Charles. (From Bell, J., *The Principles of Surgery in Two Volumes*. Edinburgh: for T. Cadell & N. Davies, T.N. Longman & O. Rees & others, 1801).

On 26 June 1815, he and John Shaw started for Brussels, and on arriving there he started to see and treat the wounded:

> The force with which the cuirassiers came on is wonderful. Here is an officer wounded; a sword pierced the back and upper part of the thigh, went through the woodwork and leather of the saddle, and entered the horse's body, pinning the man to the horse.[9]

He worked for many hours a day, treating the wounded and it became abundantly clear that the numbers had completely overwhelmed the medical services:

> It was thought that we were prepared for a great battle, yet here we are, eleven days after it, only making arrangements for the reception of the wounded. The expression is continually heard, "we were not prepared for this".[10]

He was so concerned about the plight of French soldiers, that on the morning of 3 July 1815 he wrote:

> I could not sleep for thinking of the state of the wounded French. I rose at four o'clock, and wrote to the surgeon-in-chief, and have taken on me to perform all the capital operations on the wounded French-no small effort.[11]

Bell inserted his surgical notes into a separate notebook, accompanied by sketches of the wounded. These sketches were afterwards reproduced in water colour. Some were deposited with the Royal College of Surgeons in Edinburgh and others with University College in London. Seventeen of the paintings were presented subsequently by Bell's widow to the Royal Hospital in Netley, along with his notebook.

Figures 5.8 to 5.11 inclusive show examples of the types of wound that Charles Bell saw after the Battle of Waterloo. They are in the collection of the Royal College of Surgeons of Edinburgh and are reproduced with their permission.

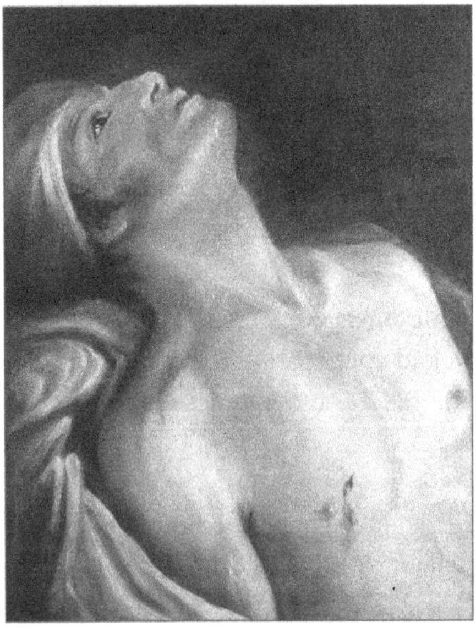

Figure 5.8. Watercolour by Charles Bell of a chest wound. This is a stab wound which has penetrated the chest wall. Patients with such wounds lived or died depending on whether any vital structure within the chest cavity had been significantly damaged. Surgeons were usually unable to intervene operatively. (Courtesy of the Royal College of Surgeons of Edinburgh).

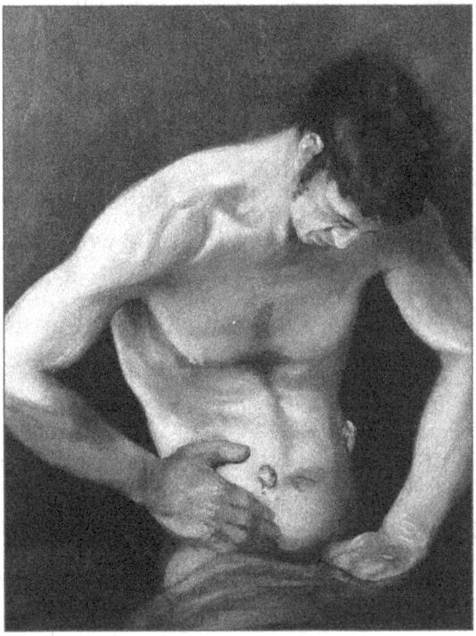

Figure 5.9. Watercolour by Charles Bell of an abdominal wound. This painting shows a soldier with two wounds in the abdominal wall through which bowel is protruding. Even if the intestine was not directly damaged and perforated by a missile or stab wound, the fact that the abdominal cavity had been breached would predispose the victim to peritonitis and death. Surgeons neither had the opportunity nor the surgical expertise to deal with such wounds. (Courtesy of the Royal College of Surgeons of Edinburgh).

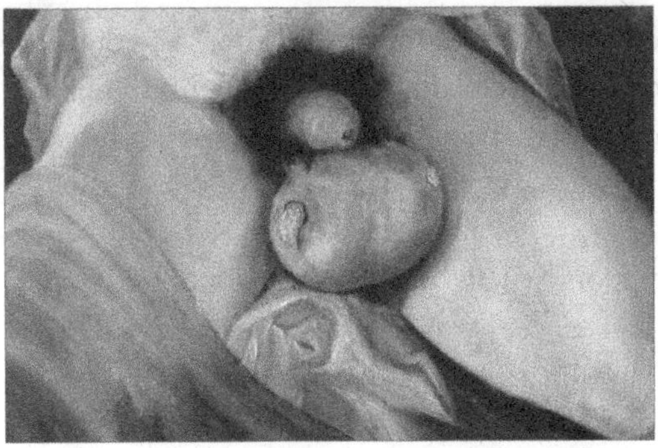

Figure 5.10. Watercolour by Charles Bell of a wound in the scrotum. The scrotum has two wounds and is grossly swollen. Pus can be seen discharging from the larger of the wounds, and the scrotum appears to contain much pus. Commonly this would lead to gangrene of the scrotum and death. (Courtesy of the Royal College of Surgeons of Edinburgh).

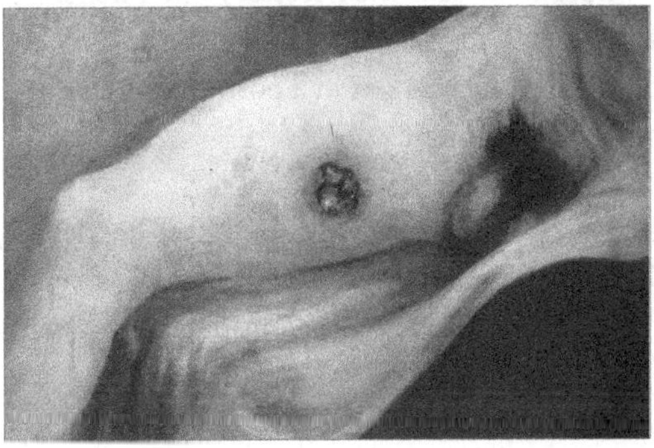

Figure 5.11. Watercolour by Charles Bell of a wound in the thigh. The wound looks infected and would often be followed by gangrene and death. (Courtesy of the Royal College of Surgeons of Edinburgh).

James Guthrie and Charles Bell did not see eye to eye, and there is evidence for this in Guthrie's book *A Treatise on Gunshot Wounds: On Inflammation, Erysipelas, and Mortification, On Injuries of Nerves*. Guthrie believed that excision of the head of the humerus (the bone in the upper part of the arm) was a good limb-saving procedure in situations where damage to the limb was confined to the upper humerus. He had considerable experience in performing this operation. Charles Bell saw fit to make some critical remarks about how the procedure had been performed in a patient under Guthrie's care at York Hospital in London. Guthrie wrote:

> If Mr Charles Bell had been thoroughly acquainted with the subject upon which he was writing, he would not have hazarded the criticism he has done. Mr Charles Bell has charged the medical officers of York Hospital with having confused notions on the subject of this operation, and with negligence of the anatomy of the parts. I now appeal to the profession to decide with whom the confusion of ideas, and the negligence, really exists.[12]

Guthrie was clearly annoyed that Bell had appeared in Brussels after Waterloo and had started to express his own opinions on matters that, perhaps with his somewhat limited knowledge and experience, might have been better kept to himself, because Guthrie went on to write:

> Instead of 30 cases needing operation he had seen 300, thrown upon him without the means of obtaining assistance, I would ask him what he would think of any man, who, at the end of a few days, should state what he saw in this peculiar situation to be Mr Bell's practice in more favourable circumstances. He could not even have done half the necessary operations. It was under such circumstances that Mr Bell saw the wounded a few days after the Battle of Waterloo, and therefore he was not in a position to draw one general inference as to the mode of treatment.[13]

Napoleon Bonaparte had dominated Europe for many years, but after his defeat at Waterloo he was sent to spend the rest of his life in exile in St Helena, a small island in the South Atlantic. He died on 5 May 1821, with considerable mystery surrounding the cause of his death.

One of the possessions of the Aberdeen Medico-Chirurgical Society is a copy of the death mask of Napoleon. It was found by an anatomist called Dr Reid, who subsequently went on to become Professor of Anatomy at the University of Aberdeen. The mask was found under a seat by Dr Reid while he was a lecturer in Anatomy in London.

The Aberdeen Medico-Chirurgical society also has a copy of Napoleon's post mortem report. It bears the signatures of five British medical officers who were in St Helena at the time and witnessed the post mortem examination performed by Corsican doctor Francesco Antommarchi. One of these was Charles Mitchell MD, an Aberdeen graduate. [14] Here are the findings of the post mortem, which concluded that Napoleon had died from cancer of the stomach.

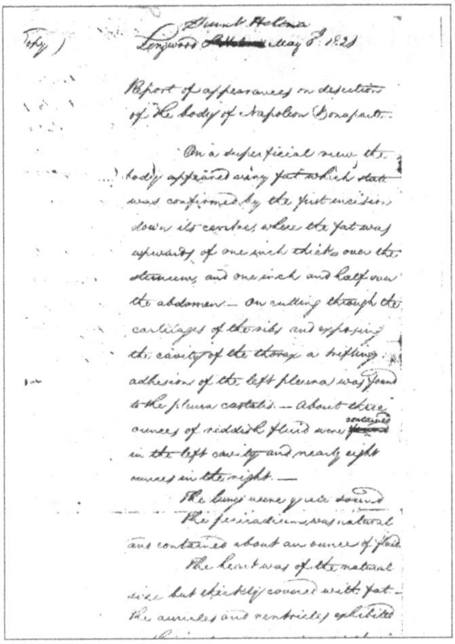

St Helena
Longwood May 8th 1821

Report of appearances on dissection of the body of Napoleon Bonaparte.

On a superficial view the body appeared very fat which state was confirmed by the first incision down its centre, where the fat was upwards of one inch thick over the sternum, and one inch and half over the abdomen — On cutting through the cartilages of the ribs and exposing the cavity of the thorax a trifling adhesion of the left pleura was found to the pleura costalis. — about three ounces of reddish fluid were contained in the left cavity and nearly eight ounces in the right. —

The lungs were quite sound.

The pericardium was natural and contained about an ounce of fluid.

The heart was of the natural size but thickly covered with fat. The auricles and ventricles exhibited

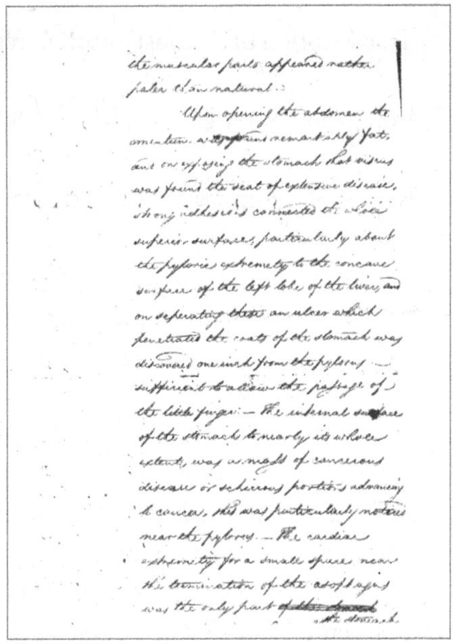

the muscular parts appeared rather paler than natural.

Upon opening the abdomen the omentum was found remarkably fat, and on exposing the stomach that viscus was found the seat of extensive disease, strong adhesions connected the whole superior surface, particularly about the pyloric extremity to the concave surface of the left lobe of the liver, and on separating these an ulcer which penetrated the coats of the stomach was discovered one inch from the pylorus — sufficient to allow the passage of the little finger. — The internal surface of the stomach to nearly its whole extent, was a mass of cancerous disease or schirrous portions advancing to cancer, this was particularly noticed near the pylorus. — The cardiac extremity for a small space near the termination of the oesophagus was the only part of the stomach

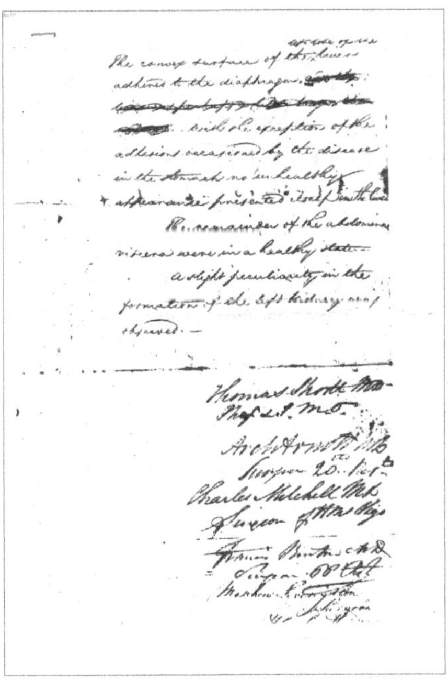

The convex surface of the liver adhered to the diaphragm. with the exception of the adhesions occasioned by the disease in the stomach no unhealthy appearance presented itself in the liver.

The remainder of the abdominal viscera were in a healthy state.

A slight peculiarity in the formation of the left kidney was observed. —

Thomas Shortt MD Phys & C. M. O.
Archd Arnott MD Surgeon 20th Regt
Charles Mitchell MD Surgeon of HMS Vigo
Francis Burton MD Surgeon 66th Regt
Matthew Livingstone Surgeon H. C. S.

Figure 5.12 (a), (b) and (c). Napoleon Bonaparte's post mortem. One of the signatories, Charles Mitchell, was an Aberdeen graduate, which is why the post mortem report came to be in the pathology department in University of Aberdeen. (Courtesy of the Aberdeen Medico Chirurgical Society).

Transcription of the post-mortem report on Napoleon with the five signatories:

Longwood Saint Helena, May 8 1821:

Report of the appearances on dissection of the body of Napoleon Bonaparte

On a superficial view the body appeared very fat which state was confirmed by the first incision down the centre where the fat was upwards of an inch thick over the sternum, and one inch and a half over the abdomen- On cutting through the cartilages of the ribs and exposing the cavity of the thorax, a trifling adhesion of the left pleura was found to the pleura costalis - about three ounces of reddish fluid were contained in the left cavity and nearly eight ounces in the right.- The lungs were quite sound. The pericardium was natural and contained about an ounce of fluid. The heart was of the natural size but thickly covered with fat. The auricles and ventricles exhibited nothing extraordinary except that the muscular parts appeared rather paler than natural. Upon opening the abdomen the omentum was found remarkably fat. And on exposing the stomach that viscus was found the seat of extensive disease, strong adhesions connected the whole superior surface particularly about the pyloric extremity to the concave surface of the left lobe of the liver, and on separating these an ulcer which penetrated the coats of the stomach was discovered one inch from the pylorus - sufficient to allow the passage of the little finger-the internal surface of the stomach to almost its whole extent, was a mass of cancerous disease and scirrhous portions advancing to cancer, this was particularly noticed near the pylorus -The cardiac extremity for a small space near the termination of the oesophagus was the only part appearing in a healthy state, the stomach was found nearly filled with a large quantity of fluid resembling coffee grounds. The convex surface of the left lobe of the liver adhered to the diaphragm. With the exception of the adhesions occasioned by the disease in the stomach no unhealthy appearance presented itself in the liver. The remainder of the abdominal viscera were in a healthy state. A slight peculiarity in the formation of the left kidney was observed.

Thomas Shortt MD
Arch Arnott MD
Charles Mitchell MD
Thomas Burton MD
Matthew Livingston Surgeon.

SIR JAMES MCGRIGOR'S LEGACY

After Waterloo there were no major wars to contend with and this gave McGrigor the opportunity to develop and implement his ideas. He was to be Director General of Army Medical Services for the next thirty-six years. He made significant improvements, and his various contributions are summarised below.

Education

- Medical candidates for a 1st Commission now had to produce certificates of regular study at an established school and had to demonstrate satisfactory performance in stipulated subjects, including anatomy, surgery, practice of medicine and chemistry for one year of study; they had to provide evidence of study in materia medica and botany for six months; they also had to have had experience in the practice of medicine and surgery for one year in a hospital with a full apprenticeship, or for three years without an apprenticeship. A period of five years would then be spent in junior ranks before becoming eligible for promotion to the rank of regimental surgeon;
- No candidate for assistant surgeon or hospital assistant was eligible to apply unless he had passed the examinations of the Royal Colleges of Surgeons in England, Edinburgh, or Dublin. Certificates of attendance at courses were no longer acceptable;
- Promotion would be judged on ability and not on the basis of status or patronage. A higher standard was required than for Royal Navy or Honourable East India Company, because these organisations still accepted certificates of attendance as adequate proof of competence;
- Those medical officers already in the service would be expected to add to their knowledge by attending courses and would have to be prepared for further examination in surgery before seeking promotion.

Improved status for medical officers

- The status of medical officers compared with combatant officers was an on-going bone of contention. In 1815, doctors were considered neither officers nor "gentlemen" and they had no power to make representation to higher authority. No medical officer could preside at any Court of Enquiry, for he was regarded as junior to the most junior ensign. Doctors were often barred from attending officers' social functions. McGrigor tried hard to obtain appropriate recognition for medical officers, but it would be many years after his death before that came about.

Improved Hospital Administration and Education facilities

- York Hospital in London was closed. Its location in the centre of London was inconvenient for the transport of cases. A site immediately accessible to shipping was required;
- A new hospital was opened at Fort Pitt in Chatham, with nine wards capable of accommodating 200 patients. The reason for this change was solely a question of convenience of site, since Chatham is at the mouth of the River Medway;
- New medical officers were put through an induction course where they had a probationary period during which they received instruction in medical administration, in the general duties of an officer and in military medicine and surgery;
- McGrigor opened a museum in Fort Pitt, which was visited by distinguished scientists and surgeons. It had an anatomical and pathological section, as well as an anthropological and botanical collection;
- One of his ambitions was to establish an Army Medical School. However, because of the financial expenditure during the Peninsular War, it would be 50 years before that actually happened.

Medical Returns

- Accurate submission of clinical data was regarded as essential. McGrigor introduced this on a large scale;
- Reports had to embrace every aspect of soldiers' living conditions, including diet, rations and sites of barracks, climate and prevalence of disease in various stations. The well-being of the troops was his single most important concern and he used every means at his disposal to improve their conditions;
- Accurate information on every aspect of military life relating to health was provided from every corner of the Empire from 1817 onwards;
- The statistics gathered by McGrigor were put to good use in 1835, when their full potential was demonstrated by Henry Marshall. He and

Alexander Tulloch produced a report on health in the West Indies and which is discussed in detail in Chapter 7.

Friendly Society and Army Officers' Benevolent Society

- This was established by McGrigor, and by 1840 the society's capital was £17,000;
- The first annuitant was the widow of a hospital assistant who was awarded £20 a year as financial assistance,(£1 in 1815 was the equivalent of £60 today);
- This project materially alleviated suffering.

Chairs of Military Surgery Edinburgh and Dublin

- In 1807, a Chair Military Surgery was established in Edinburgh during the Napoleonic wars. Mr John Thomson was the first Regius Professor whose only military experience was at Waterloo in 1815. His rapport with James Guthrie has already been mentioned in Chapter 4. McGrigor supported the establishment of a similar chair in Dublin.
- A Chair of Military Surgery in London was never put in place. The Crimean War prevented it and when the Army Medical School in Netley was opened as one of the post-Crimean reforms, it meant that it was never required. Similarly, the other chairs became surplus to requirement because all relevant military medical instruction was provided at Netley.

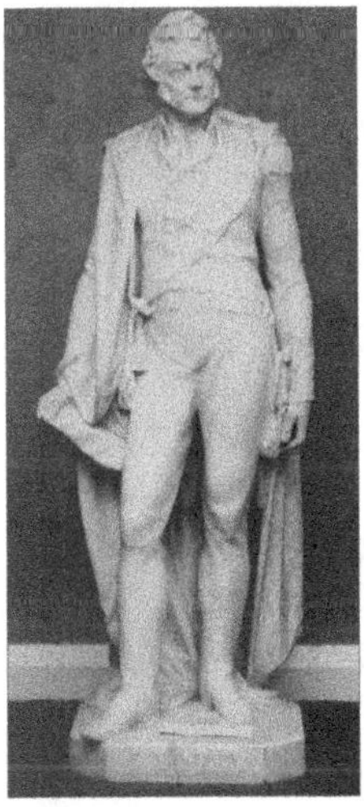

In 1831, McGrigor became a baronet and in 1850 he was invested with the Order of a Knight Commander of the Bath. He was also elected a Fellow of the Royal Society of London and was elected Lord Rector of Marischal College in Aberdeen during 1826-27 and again in 1841-43. His portrait hangs in the lecture theatre of the Aberdeen Medico-Chirurgical Society (see Chapter 2) and a small statue of McGrigor stands in the library with the full sized version being erected at the Royal Army Medical Headquarters at Millbank in London.

Figure 5.13. Statue of Sir James McGrigor in the library of Aberdeen Medico Chirurgical Society. The full-sized version was located at the Royal Army Medical College at Millbank in London. (Courtesy of the Aberdeen Medico-Chirurgical Society).

On several occasions, he felt he really ought to retire and even when he was 75 years old his old chief and friend Wellington said that there was still plenty of work left in him! He finally retired in 1851, at the age of 81, having been Director General for thirty- six years.

He died on 2 April 1858.If the reader ever walks through Duthie Park in Aberdeen, there is a commemorative obelisk to the memory of one of Aberdeen's greatest citizens who was one of the most devoted of all public servants.

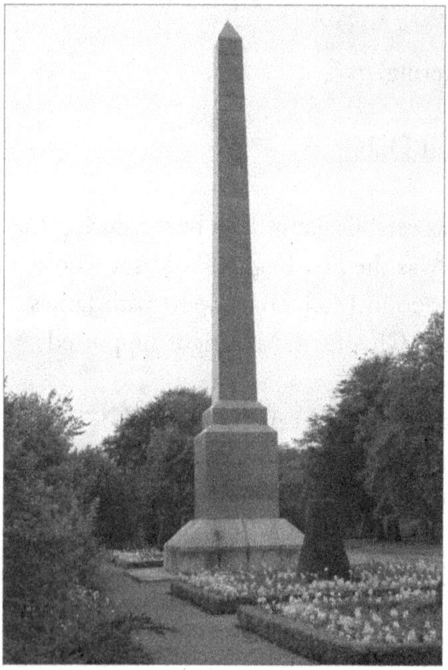

Figure 5.14. Obelisk to commemorate Sir James McGrigor in Duthie Park, Aberdeen. (Authors' photograph).

ENDNOTES

1. Hodge, W.B., "On the mortality arising from military operations". *Journal of the Statistical Society of London 1856;* 19: pp.219-271.
2. Howarth, D., *Waterloo, A Near Run Thing*. London: Collins, 1968.
3. Harvey, R., *The War of Wars. The Epic Struggle between Britain and France.* London: Constable, 2006.

4. Hodge, *op. cit.*, pp.219-271.
5. Bodart, G., *Losses of Life in Modern Wars.* Oxford: Clarendon Press, 1916, p.119.
6. Cantlie, N., *A History of the Army Medical Department.* Edinburgh: Churchill Livingston, 1974, Volume 1, pp.382-393.
7. Hennen, J., *Principles of Military Surgery* 3rd Edition. London: John Wilson, 1829.
8. Bell, C., *Letters of Sir Charles Bell.* London: John Murray, 1870, p. 227.
9. *Ibid,* p.230.
10. *Ibid.*
11. *Ibid.*
12. Guthrie, J.G., *A Treatise on Gunshot Wounds: On Inflammation, Erysipelas, and Mortification, On Injuries of Nerves.* London: Burgess and Hill, Third edition, 1827, pp.502-505.
13. *Ibid.*
14. Adam, A., J. D. Hutchison, *The Heritage of the Med-Chi. The Medico-Chirurgical Society of Aberdeen:* The Medico-Chirurgical Society of Aberdeen, Aberdeen, 2007.

6

The British Legion in Spain

HISTORICAL BACKGROUND

The Carlist Wars in Spain were civil wars in which contenders fought to establish their claims to the Spanish throne. When King Ferdinand VII of Spain died in 1833, he left two daughters, his wife Cristina having failed to provide him with a son and heir. His elder daughter was Isabella. Before his death, King Ferdinand created the Pragmatic Sanction of 1830 which he introduced to allow his daughter Isabella to accede to the throne upon his death. His widow Maria Cristina then became Regent on behalf of their infant daughter, who became Queen Isabella II.

Ferdinand VII had a brother called Carlos who rejected the notion of his niece becoming queen and accordingly he staked a claim to the throne. Carlos did not accept the validity of the Pragmatic Sanction and he became known to his followers as King Carlos V. His supporters became known as Carlists.

To make matters more complex and give some legal basis to Carlos's claim to the throne, Salic law excluded females from acceding to the throne. The country was now clearly split into two factions; the Carlists, who were the supporters of Carlos V, and the "Cristinos" or "Isabelinos", who were the supporters of Isabella. The Carlists rallied and attempted to rectify what they perceived as a great injustice, by trying to remove Isabella from the throne and installing Carlos as King Carlos V. As a result, a bitter civil war broke out in 1833.

By 1835 things were not going well for the Isabelinos and they asked their allies, Britain and France, to come to their assistance. The French sent the Foreign Legion and though Britain refused to send troops directly, in June 1835 a military volunteer corps of mercenaries was formed and paid for by the Spanish Crown. This force became known as the British Legion of Spain and the first detachments left for Spain on 10 July 1835 under the command of Sir George de Lacy Evans. By October, the force in Spain was complete.

The importance of the British Legion of Spain from a medical point of view is that it involved a relatively small force over a short period of time. The total force was 9,600 men and it remained in Spain for 23 months. All information relating to morbidity and mortality from wounds and diseases was carefully documented by Rutherford Alcock, who was the Deputy Inspector of Hospitals with the force in Spain. Alcock published his findings in 1838 in a work entitled *Notes on the Medical History and Statistics of the British Legion of Spain.*[1] All the data in the following pages is derived from Alcock's work.

By the end of October 1835, between 7,000 and 8,000 men had been put ashore on the northern coast of Spain and they congregated at Bilbao, Santander and San Sebastian, before moving inland. Alcock observed that many of these volunteers had never been medically examined before being accepted for service. He considered that approximately one eighth of the force ought never to have been enlisted. There were men with skin ulcers, varicose veins and a catalogue of what he described as "disabilities for the British Army" which should have excluded them. There were men with tuberculosis and there was even an old man with a club foot which would have made active service extremely difficult. Rather than relying on a proper medical examination to help assemble a fit and effective Legion, men were provided by recruiting agencies which were working on a commission basis. These agencies were only concerned about making a profit and not about the fitness of the men they were dealing with. Alcock estimated that most of these unfit men were destined to die without ever doing a single day's effective duty.

Alcock also noted that those men who came from a poor socio-economic background of urban poverty withstood the rigours of army life less well than their generally healthier rural counterparts in terms of susceptibility to disease. There were 3,200 English, 2,800 Irish and 1,800 Scots who made up this force. The English and Scots were recruited from the industrial areas and cities, mainly London and Glasgow and were generally poorly nourished and of low stamina. The Irish were recruited from a rural environment and were generally fitter and more resilient to all the challenges they faced. During the first winter in Vitoria (see below) 33% of the English, 20% of the Scots and 12.5% of the Irish fell ill and were admitted to the Legion's general hospitals.

At first the weather was good and the sickness rate was very low. When everything was ready, the British Legion marched inland to Vitoria on 29 October 1835, leaving a small number of sick men in general hospitals at Bilbao, Santander and San Sebastian.

The Legion arrived in Vitoria on 3 December 1835, and soon men became sick with "Vitoria Fever" which caused a very high morbidity and mortality over the winter months. Vitoria was overcrowded with troops, the winter was very severe, rations were poor and the state of hospitals was so bad that Alcock declared:

> It rendered impossible the adoption of all means which medical science indicated for the treatment of disease.[2]

MEDICAL SERVICES IN VITORIA

There were no fewer than seven general hospitals in Vitoria, mainly because the buildings used were very small. The Spanish authorities, on whom they depended to provide them with facilities, had been very uncooperative. The Inspector General of Hospitals, even with the support of the Commander in Chief General Evans, experienced great difficulty in procuring a house here, or a church or convent there to use as hospitals. Even when accommodation was finally obtained, there was a shortage of bedding and blankets. There was even a shortage of straw to lie on. Ventilation was poor and the sick lay huddled together for warmth.

The small wards soon became very overcrowded with men affected by disease and during the winter months Alcock estimated that 1,223 soldiers died in and around Vitoria. Between January and April 1836 eleven medical officers died and seventeen lay seriously ill in Vitoria. This left only 23 medical officers to look after the British Legion. Hospital sergeants, clerks and ward masters all fell ill at the same time and could not be replaced. Hospital infrastructure, such as it was, disintegrated. Approximately 1 in 5 medical officers died compared with 1 in 10 other officers.

Weather conditions were appalling and thick snow greatly restricted movement. Men frequently men lay on bare floors which were soaking wet and covered in slushy melting snow.

The medical returns of the general military hospitals during the 22 to 23 month period of service of the Legion revealed that there were 13,407 admissions and 1,588 deaths. The total number of men was 9,600, giving a death rate of one in six of the whole force. Since these figures were for general hospitals and did not include returns from the much smaller regimental hospitals, they underestimated the total number of cases treated and the number of deaths. Figure 6.1 summarises total losses from disease and wounds, where it can be clearly seen that deaths from disease greatly outnumbered those from wounds. Most of the deaths from disease over the winter months of 1835-36 were caused by "Vitoria Fever".

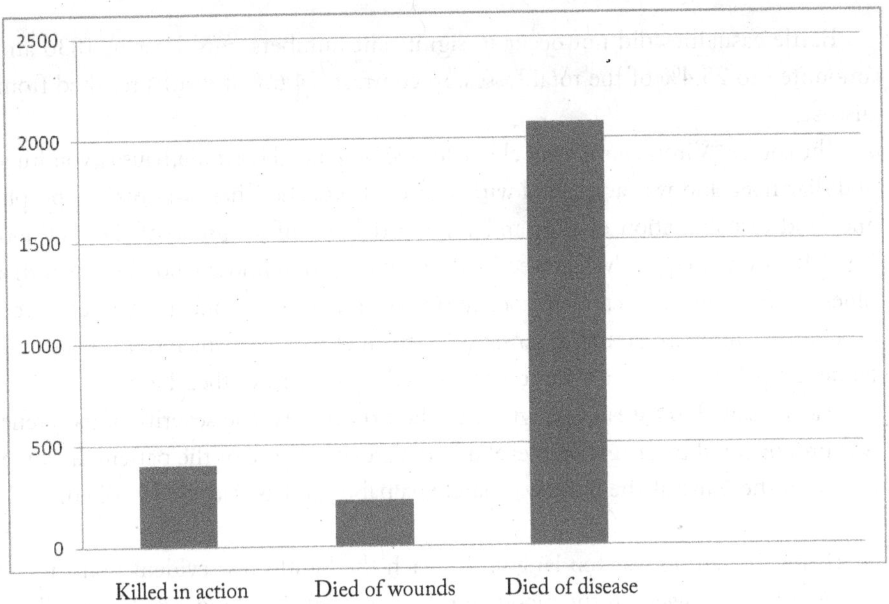

Figure 6.1. All causes of death in British Legion in Spain, 1835-1836. From Alcock, R., *Notes on the Medical History and Statistics of the British Legion of Spain.* London: John Churchill; 1838.

Table 6.1 provides a detailed breakdown of the numbers of deaths as a result of enemy action and deaths from disease. The total number of deaths was 2,479.

Table 6.1 Numbers of deaths from killed in action, died of wounds, and died from disease. The percentages are against the total number of dead.

	Officers	Other ranks	Total	% Total officers	% Total other ranks	Total
Battle Casualties Killed	20	381	401	0.8%	15.4%	16.2%
Battle Casualties Died of Wounds	16	212	228	0.60%	8.6%	9.2%
Non-Battle Casualties Died of Disease	62	1788	1,850	2.5%	72.1%	74.6%

From Alcock, R., *Notes on the Medical History and Statistics of the British Legion of Spain.* London: John Churchill, 1838.

Battle casualties did not occur in significant numbers until later in 1836 and amounted to 25.4% of the total losses. In contrast, 74.6% of deaths resulted from disease.

The course "Vitoria Fever" was characterised by general lassitude, nausea, vomiting and diarrhoea and was associated with a severe headache. There was often a purple and livid discolouration of skin and varying degrees of gangrene of the feet and legs which was frequently followed by death. Commonly those who died from this illness suffered from severe diarrhoea during its later stages. Soldiers who recovered experienced an intense burning sensation of the toes and feet, which were exquisitely tender on palpation. These symptoms persisted for the rest of their lives.

Alcock saw 300 cases of gangrene of the extremities. The severity of gangrene was proportional to the general level of circulatory collapse of the patient, in some of whom the pulse at the wrist was barely palpable, and as Alcock described:

> If the circulation was too languid to reach the hands, it is evident that the loss of vital powers in the blood vessels, to propel the blood, would be still more fatally experienced at the point furthest from the centre.[3]

In the early stages of the fever, men were treated using a variety of ineffective methods. For example they were subjected to bleeding; they were blistered round the back of the neck; they were plunged into a tub of freezing cold water; or they were given purgatives and emetics. Often they were given combinations of all these types of treatment. Success of any treatment administered was presumed in those men whose condition did not progress to the terminal stages with gangrene.

Some of the features of the disease were suggestive of typhus fever, the manifestations of which have been discussed in a previous chapter. While there may be gangrene of the fingers or toes due to poor peripheral circulatory perfusion in typhus fever, gangrenous sores on pressure points in the body are more common. There is often a pronounced rash preceding these gangrenous sores and it is interesting to note that Alcock did not mention this in his description of the disease, which perhaps makes this diagnosis less likely.

He referred to Sir James McGrigor's experience in the Peninsular War, twenty five years previously. McGrigor had to deal with a major outbreak of typhus fever in January 1812 in all the general hospitals:

> At Ciudad Rodrigo, the cases of typhus had almost universally mortification of the lower extremity, with livor, and mortification of the nose. This contagious fever soon seized on all the ward masters, nurses and orderlies.[4]

Many of the features of the disease described by Alcock would fit with a diagnosis of ergot poisoning. Ergot poisoning is caused by the presence of the fungus Claviceps Purpurea in contaminated bread. It usually affects rye, but can affect other cereals such as wheat and barley. The fungus produces alkaloids which themselves are poisonous.

These compounds may cause convulsions, painful seizures and spasms, diarrhoea, paresthesias (altered sensation in the peripheral spinal nerves) and itching. Mental effects including psychotic illness, usually accompanied by headaches, nausea and vomiting, may occur. Gangrene develops as a result of extreme vasoconstriction induced by the ergotamine-ergocristine alkaloids of the fungus. It affects the more poorly vascularised distal parts of the limbs such as the fingers and toes.

At the time of this outbreak in Vitoria, there was extreme overcrowding of dirty hospital accommodation with poor ventilation. The weather conditions were appalling and the ground was covered in thick snow, making it almost impossible to move about. The troops had very poor rations and the very poor quality of bread was singled out for special mention in Adcock's account. This supported a provisional diagnosis of ergot poisoning which would certainly explain the clinical signs and symptoms experienced by the affected men. Alcock stated:

> The bread was often made of unsound flour of the worst kind, imperfectly kneaded and baked; forming a mass of black and heavy dough, calculated to puzzle the digestion of an ostrich, incapable of affording nourishment, and well adapted, on the other hand, to produce disease. It was said the bread was intentionally mixed with deleterious matter - that it was poisoned.[5]

Alcock was of the opinion that bad bread may have had something to do with the high incidence of gangrene in those affected. Unfortunately it was not possible to apprehend and question the person responsible for providing the bread as this might have shed some light on matters and clarified the diagnosis. He had already been found guilty of corresponding and colluding with the Carlists, and of attempting to induce men to desert and certainly of poisoning their minds, if not their bodies! He had been executed along with one of the bakers.

He was garrotted in the square of Vitoria with a baker coadjutor (assistant)![6]

Unfortunately, Alcock did not elaborate on this and said nothing more on the matter.

In February 1836 a long expected supply of blankets, cooking utensils and other essential equipment finally arrived in Vitoria and medicines which had been ordered from England were also delivered. Larger convents had been obtained for hospital accommodation and conditions improved. On 12 April 1836, the Legion left Vitoria and made its way back to the coast. By May 1836, the Legion was located within the walls of San Sebastian, where it was besieged by Carlist forces. It sustained battle casualties here for the first time in significant numbers. Alcock discussed the types of wounds in detail, but first the medical arrangements in San Sebastian will be described.

MEDICAL SERVICES IN SAN SEBASTIAN

When the Legion arrived in San Sebastian, a large two-floored square building was commandeered as a fever hospital. It had two large wards, one on each floor. The large convent of San Telmo became a surgical hospital. It had two wings, a smaller wing of one floor and a main wing of four stories overlooking the sea from a rocky promontory. It was roomy and well ventilated, with sea breezes circulating round the building. One of the three floors dealt with wounds of the head, chest and abdomen; another dealt with amputations and gunshot wounds of the extremities and fractures. Each floor had a Principal Medical Officer, with assistants distributed according to the nature and number of cases. The excellent facilities in San Sebastian were in marked contrast to the crowded and squalid accommodation the Legion endured in Vitoria.

By the time this hospital was ready to receive patients on 14 May 1836 there were many wounded soldiers crowded into temporary accommodation in church halls, which were quite unsuitable for the performance of surgical procedures. Alcock referred to a large number of gunshot fractures of the femur which awaited treatment. He was in no doubt that primary amputation was the treatment of choice for compound gunshot fractures of the femur, yet circumstances dictated that the treatment of many patients was delayed till they reached the surgical hospital.

Patients were transferred to the hospital in carts designed by a Mr Cherry, twelve of which were sent to Spain with the Legion on the recommendation of George James Guthrie. Each cart could only carry four wounded sitting upright and Alcock thought that they ought to be modified to carry twelve wounded. He also thought that they should be stationed just to the rear of any action, to be able to quickly remove dangerously wounded men on stretchers and to avoid the need for up to eight and sometimes even twelve men to carry a single wounded comrade from the battle.

> I once observed, in less than an hour, a whole battalion tail off after some fifty wounded, one carrying his comrade's musket, and another his little finger.[7]

DIFFERENT TYPES OF WOUND AND THEIR PROGNOSIS

The types of wounds sustained and their outcomes can be ascertained from the statistics of those admitted into the General Military Hospital, San Telmo in San Sebastian between 14 May 1836 and 10 June 1837. Table 6.2 summarises the percentage mortality of different wounds.

All patients with compound fractures of the skull who had an associated brain injury died, whilst only 40% of those with skull fractures with no obvious underlying abnormality beneath the skull bone died. It was established during the Boer War and Great War that despite the apparently good initial status of many patients, complications arising from fractures of the skull may have serious repercussions and presumably the figure of 40% is a reflection of this phenomenon. Scalp wounds alone, without any underlying fracture of the skull bone, had a good prognosis.

Penetrating gunshot wounds of the chest and penetrating gunshot wounds of the abdomen carried a very high mortality which approached 100%. This was the result of damage to vital structures within the chest and abdominal cavities about which nothing could be done at this time. Combined thoracic and abdominal injuries were, not surprisingly, invariably fatal.

Penetrating wounds of major joints carried a 57% mortality and there were 41 such cases. Whilst Alcock did not specify, most of these were probably penetrating wounds of the knee joint. Amputation was the treatment of choice. Such wounds were associated with a poor prognosis throughout military medical history and they were still a source of great trouble during the Great War, almost a century after Alcock wrote his report. Alcock's observations were clearly in keeping with Guthrie's finding in the Peninsular War when he stated that wounded soldiers requiring an amputation were much more likely to survive if the amputation was performed early before inflammation became established.

- 22 were treated without amputation and 13 died;
- 9 underwent primary amputation (within a few hours of being wounded) and 2 died.

Table 6.2 Anatomical distribution of wounds in 1351 cases, British Legion in Spain (May 1836- June 1837). GSW – gunshot wounds; GSF –gunshot fractures.

Description of wound	Number admitted	Discharged to duty	Transferred	Invalided	Died	Remained	% Death of cases treated
GSW Cranium with brain involvement	18				18		100%
GSW Cranium with no brain involvement	10	5		1	4		40%
Abrasions pericranium	3		2		1		33%
Scalp wounds	58	52	3	2	1		
PGSW Thorax	29			2	27		93%
PGSW Thorax without lesion	1			1			
PGSW Abdomen	18				18		100%
PGSW Abdomen without lesion	1			1			
Thorax and Abdomen	3				3		100%
Penetrating wounds joints	37	2	2	11	21	1	57%
Amputations in field	15		2	8	5		33%
Spinal Injuries	2				2		100%
GSF Femur	20		2	5	12	1	60%
GSF leg	57	6	1	29	20	1	35%
GSF Arm	31	1		18	11	1	35%
GSF Forearm	52	12	7	30	3		6%

General wounds severe	403	146	131	96	45	3	11%
General wounds slight	585	548	34		3		0.5%
TOTALS	1351	774	166	208	196	7	14.5%

From Alcock, R., *Notes on the Medical History and Statistics of the British Legion of Spain.* London: John Churchill, 1838.

- 6 underwent secondary amputation (after a delay of some weeks) and all died;
- 4 primary amputations were performed in the field and one died. [8]

Gunshot fractures of the limbs were very serious wounds, particularly if they involved the femur (the thigh bone). Alcock described 32 cases of fractured femur. There were 11 fractures which Alcock described as "partial", although it is not clear what he meant by that, and 21 complete. In the partial group, there were 5 cases in which there was a fracture into the knee joint and this is referred to today as a supra-condylar fracture. There were 6 cases involving the shaft of the femur and 1 died.

There were 21 soldiers with "complete" fractures of the femur. Alcock found that these were very difficult fractures to treat with a percentage mortality of 81% (if one presumes that the one hopeless case still in hospital below died of his fracture). It is also noteworthy that primary amputation was the standard treatment for this type of wound.

	Died
• 3 were amputated in the field;	3
• 3 had primary amputation in hospital;	2
• 15 were reserved for cure or secondary amputation;	
• Of these, without amputation;	8
• In six, amputation became imperative;	3
• One remains under treatment with no hope of recovery.[9]	

Of the fifteen cases which had been "reserved for cure or secondary amputation", there were three patients who developed secondary haemorrhage for which amputation was performed in two. One died and one recovered. Secondary haemorrhage is bleeding which occurs from a major blood vessel some time after the original injury has been sustained. It is usually associated with a severe wound infection which makes the blood vessel wall more friable and therefore liable to spontaneous rupture or it may be caused by perforation of the blood vessels by sharp bone ends. In the third case, the general condition of the patient was so poor that the femoral artery was tied off. Not surprisingly, gangrene (then referred to as "sphacelus") of the foot supervened and the patient died after a further secondary haemorrhage.

Alcock confirmed that it was virtually impossible to keep the fractured ends in good juxtaposition, a problem that would not be solved until the Thomas Splint gained widespread acceptance during the Great War:

> It may be remarked, that notwithstanding the greatest care directed to them, under my own observation, and with as good means of treatment as can generally be found in military hospitals on service, several preparations have been preserves, proving abundantly the difficulty, if not impossibility of keeping the fractured portions in good juxtaposition, for the long period required by the tedious and exhausting curative process. Showing, moreover, how inadequate are even nature's vigorous efforts to repair the mischief almost invariably the result of a gun-shot fracture of the femur.[10]

There were 57 soldiers who sustained gunshot fractures of the leg (as opposed to the thigh) and 20 of these men died. Presumably these were fractures of both the tibia and fibula.[11]

There were 31 soldiers who sustained fractures of the humerus and 11 died. 22 were amputated:

- 13 had a primary amputation and 7 died;
- 9 had a secondary amputation and 2 died.[12]

By implication, 2 of the 9 not amputated died, although Alcock did not specify this. There were 52 soldiers with gunshot fractures of the hand and forearm, of whom three died. Five had an amputation; three were primary amputations with one death. The two soldiers who underwent secondary amputations both survived.

There were 17 cases of tetanus which occurred after the following wounds:

- 1 case after a primary amputation in the field;
- 1 case after flesh wound and fractured scapula;
- 1 case after fractured phalanx of big toe;

- 4 cases after compound fracture of tibia and fibula;
- 1 case after compound fracture of metacarpal bones;
- 9 cases after flesh wounds without associated fracture.

One case recovered in spite of the treatment administered, which included bleeding and the administration of opiates, calomel and opiates combined with calomel. In three cases, amputation was performed after the onset of tetanus, but by then it was too late and the patients died.

There were 12 cases of secondary haemorrhage, which was most likely due to infective erosion into large arteries causing profuse bleeding (see above). Secondary haemorrhage tended to occur in complicated wounds and this was a point which had previously been noted by James Guthrie during his experience in the Peninsular War.

- 2 occurred after secondary amputation of the thigh with haemorrhage from the femoral artery and both died;
- 3 occurred after compound fracture of the femur and two died; (see above)
- 1 occurred after a fracture of the humerus and the patient was treated by amputation and survived;
- 3 occurred in gunshot fractures of the face. The common carotid artery was secured in two cases but both died. In the third case, the haemorrhage ceased spontaneously after initial alarming and profuse bleeding;
- 1 occurred in a compound fracture of the radius involving the elbow joint but died of complications following amputation;
- 1 occurred after amputation of arm and the patient died;
- 1 occurred after compound fracture of fibula and the patient recovered.

SUMMARY

Alcock's work with a relatively small number of closely monitored soldiers accurately documented the relative proportion of deaths from disease and from wounds in the British Legion in Spain 1835-37. He recorded the surgical management and results of different wounds of the upper and lower limbs where intervention influenced the outcome. Patients with penetrating abdominal and chest wounds with associated visceral damage almost invariably died since there was nothing that could be done for these wounds. Similarly penetrating skull wounds had a very poor prognosis.

Alcock was influenced by Peninsular Surgeon George James Guthrie and frequently referred to his work and followed Guthrie's teaching closely. Guthrie's influence spanned from the Peninsular War to the Crimean War and he was the dominant surgical figure for much of that time. The sixth and final edition of his book *Commentaries on the surgery of the war in Portugal, Spain, France and the Netherlands* was published in 1862.

Alcock's *Notes on the Medical History and Statistics of the British Legion of Spain* which was published in 1838 is a remarkable documentation of military surgery of the time and provides the reader with a wonderful opportunity to understand and appreciate the operations and results which were obtained.

ENDNOTES

1. Alcock, R., *Notes on the Medical History and Statistics of the British Legion of Spain.* London: John Churchill, 1838.
2. *Ibid*, p.13.
3. *Ibid*, p.24.
4. *Ibid*, p.14.
5. *Ibid.*
6. *Ibid.*
7. *Ibid*, p.43.
8. *Ibid*, p.51.
9. *Ibid*, p.52.
10. *Ibid*, p.53.
11. *Ibid*, p.53.
12. *Ibid*, p.54.

7

Henry Marshall & the Statistics of Disease

INTRODUCTION

There were significant developments in surgery during the Peninsular War, which depended not only on a sound knowledge of anatomy but a mastery of the technical skills required to undertake surgical operations. Furthermore, surgeons had to be able to make the correct decisions and where necessary to execute these quickly and appropriately.

However, their understanding of disease processes and the pathophysiological changes underpinning these lagged far behind other advances. Surgeons of today still hold in awe the way in which men such as George James Guthrie and John Hennen developed the craft of surgery for the benefit of the wounded, although ineffective and inappropriate supportive treatments such as blistering, leeches and bleeding were not only of no use, but were frequently dangerous and often contributed to the deaths of wounded soldiers.

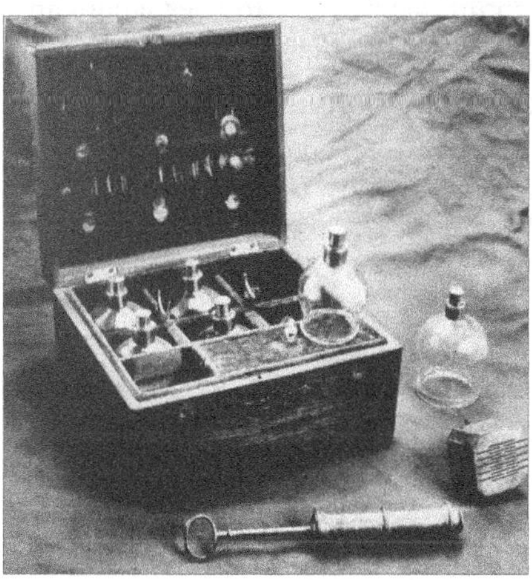

Figure 7.1. A bleeding and cupping set from the early nineteenth century. It consists of an instrument known as a scarifier, several cups and a brass syringe. The scarifier was a spring loaded, multi-barrelled instrument which was used to draw blood by plunging into the flesh to cause bleeding. The desired amount of blood was withdrawn using the cups and syringe. (Courtesy of Aberdeen Medico-Chirurgical Society).

It would need the pioneering work of Louis Pasteur to begin to recognise that bacteria and other micro-organisms were responsible for many of the diseases so prevalent amongst the troops and which were such a potent source of morbidity and mortality in the British Army throughout the nineteenth century.

PERCEIVED CAUSES OF DISEASE

The causes of diseases were extremely poorly understood and some of the common theories are highlighted below.[1]

Intemperance

Soldiers consumed large quantities of alcoholic spirits and their breakfast in the West Indies usually consisted of a tot of rum with a slice of salt boiled pork. The consumption of rum commonly continued throughout the rest of the day. Chronic intake of alcohol may progress to the medical condition of alcoholism and this is an important underlying factor in many other disease processes. For example, the ability of the immune response to respond to infections in particular may become impaired and this predisposes to an increased risk of developing wound infections. Furthermore, a person's susceptibility to a variety of diseases increases.

Alcohol is metabolised by the liver but excessive consumption may lead to liver damage. This varies in degrees from what is termed fatty change, through to inflammation and then to cirrhosis, which ultimately leads to liver failure and death. To complicate matters even further, many of the infectious disease of the time to which soldiers were exposed also caused liver inflammation and damage. Therefore, in those with pre-existing liver damage (secondary to alcohol abuse) infections were more severe with an increased risk of death.

Exposure to excesses in temperature

Exposure to heat or cold, with or without exposure to moisture in the environment, caused marked changes in the environmental temperature. This was believed to adversely affect the lungs by causing inflammation or the abdomen by predisposing to bowel diseases. Very severe wet conditions were thought to predispose to cholera.

Miasma

Miasma, or marsh vapour, was thought to be responsible for "fever" and dysentery. The solution to this was to site the camp well away from the "evil smells" emanating from marshes and other bodies of water such as tidal estuaries. This has already been discussed in Chapter 3 in the context of the Walcheren Campaign in Holland:

> All the Dutch provinces are subject to marsh distempers, but Zealand in particular, is not only low and damp like the rest, but surrounded by the mouths of the Scheldt, whose oozy beaches unite with the marshy lands, so that except the sea breeze from the westward, every wind comes laden with the pestilential vapours. The bottom of every canal that communicates with the sea is thickly covered with ooze, which, when the tide is ebbed, disperses a most offensive and noxious effluvia. The sickly season begins with June and ends with October, continuing as long as the sun has power sufficient to draw up marsh miasmata.[2]

Contagion

It was thought that disease due to contagion could occur because of uncleanliness and lack of ventilation. Such diseases included plague, typhus fever, hospital gangrene, smallpox, measles, whooping cough and scarlet fever. There was a recognition that hospitals should be well ventilated and it has already been noted in a previous chapter that they were considered as dangerous places to be. Whilst not understanding anything about the causative organisms of these conditions, doctors of that time were quite correct in appreciating the need for space and ventilation in order to create a healthier environment for the sick and wounded. They also realised that outbreaks of disease were more likely to occur in damp, overcrowded and squalid conditions which unfortunately were all too common in times of war.

FEVERS

The nomenclature of fevers in the early nineteenth century was descriptive, based solely on the pattern of the temperature changes in the person affected. The four basic types of fever were called:

- typhus;
- intermittent;
- simple continued;
- remittent.

Typhus is the same disease which we know and understand today. Intermittent fever was malaria, and simple continued and remittent fevers reflected an underlying mixture of different diseases which we cannot identify with certainty.

Sir James McGrigor meticulously documented information throughout his years in the army. Following the expedition from India to Egypt in 1801 he summarised the medical aspects of the expedition in his account *Medical Sketches of the Expedition from India to Egypt*. He was clearly very aware of the need to record data, when he said:

> Perhaps it may be thought that I have descended to a degree of minuteness: however, I conceive, that, from the facts stated, important and useful deductions may be made. I think it a matter of regret that such journals are not more frequently kept; with a little industry on the part of the profession they might always be so. Had such records been always faithfully kept, many practical points would not, as they now are, be involved in doubt and uncertainty. We should not now be so ignorant of some diseases, of the countries where we have so often made campaigns, or of which we have so long been in possession. Humble as the labours may seem, and confined as the abilities of an individual may be, were he only faithfully to relate observations made with care, to compare them with those of his contemporaries, and by them to correct the opinions of his predecessors, he would perform no mean service to his art.[3]

When he became Director General of Army Medical Services in 1815, McGrigor insisted that every medical officer, wherever he was stationed, should complete regular returns for sickness and disease amongst the troops under his care. These returns were sent initially to the Principal Medical Officer of the colony before being sent onwards to the Director General in Britain.

During his own time in the Peninsula, McGrigor kept meticulous records, many in the form of journals. In 1847 he sent that part of his collection covering the period between the beginning of his medical service until the end of the Peninsular War in 1814, to the Aberdeen Medico-Chirurgical Society. Needless to say, these documents represent the Society's most prized possession. The McGrigor Archives consist of over 60 volumes of manuscripts.

Although McGrigor collected all this data, it needed a careful analysis made by a trained statistician to unravel all of this data and to present it in a form where it could be used to understand diseases.

Henry Marshall was the son of a farmer from Kilsyth in Scotland. He was born in 1775 and attended Glasgow University before commencing his military career as a surgeon's mate in the Royal Navy in 1803. After a year he left the Navy and joined the Forfarshire Militia before joining the 89th Foot, and saw service in Cape Town, Buenos Aires and Colombo. In 1808 he was posted to Ceylon and whilst there, he began to examine diseases in his monthly returns using statistical analyses and he published accounts of his medical experience.[4] Marshall's aim was to improve the health and well being of the troops, because as well as being a statistician, he was also a military philanthropist. In 1835, Marshall used all the material meticulously collected by McGrigor and put it to practical use.

His original remit was to make enquiries regarding expenses incurred by the colonies when they had to replace soldiers who had died of disease or who had been invalided home. It became clear to Marshall that his task ought to be extended to an all-encompassing enquiry and this resulted in his ground breaking work, *Statistical report on the mortality and invaliding among the troops in the West Indies,* published in 1838.[5]

Marshall was directed by the Secretary of State for War to examine the extent and causes of sickness and mortality among the troops in the West Indies, with a view to find measures which would diminish the great loss of life experienced in these colonies.

Marshall, who was then Deputy Inspector General of Hospitals, joined forces with Captain Alexander Tulloch of the 45th Foot. Tulloch was a trained lawyer when he joined the army and while still a subaltern he had exposed various scandals concerning regimental pay and food and pension fraud within the Honourable East India Company in Burma. He was subsequently employed by the Army Recruiting Service, where his expertise in pension work led him to study mortality rates, which was when he first met Marshall.

Both men began to analyse the voluminous series of returns and reports dating back to 1816 when McGrigor first started them. They collaborated to produce the report dealing with the health of troops in the West Indies which was presented to Parliament in 1838.

Their research covered the years 1817 to 1836 and this was the first time anybody had attempted to look critically at the available data, analyse it and draw appropriate conclusions. Tulloch summarised how the information was collected from the medical officers:

> They contained the number of troops under his charge, with admissions into hospital, and deaths among them, and a specification of the diseases by which they were occasioned. The contents of the reports are condensed by the Principal Medical Officer into a single general return, and transmitted to the Medical Department where it forms a record of the state of their health for that year.[6]

Table 7.1 demonstrates the dangers presented by a posting to the West Indies. There was a very real risk that a soldier might never see home again. It shows mortalities per thousand of the troops in the Windward and Leeward Islands and in Jamaica. Mortality figures for the different civilian age groups in England are given to enable a comparison to be made. The mortality figures for civilians in England were a little lower than for soldiers of an equivalent age based in England. The mean rate of mortality amongst civilians aged between 33-40 years was 10.7 per 1,000, whilst that of soldiers in the army was 17 per 1,000 for the same age group.[7]

Table 7.1 Annual mortality figures per 1,000 of the population in various locations in Britain and West Indies.

	ANNUAL RATIO OF MORTALITY PER THOUSAND LIVING AT FOLLOWING YEARS OF AGE			
	18-25	**25-33**	**33-40**	**40-50**
In civilian life in England using Carlisle Tables	7	8.9	10.7	14.1
Troops Windward/ Leeward Islands	50	74	97	123
Troops in Jamaica	70	107	131	128

From: Marshall H., *Statistical report on the sickness, mortality, and invaliding among the troops in the West Indies.* London: W Clowes and Sons, 1838.

It is clear from Table 7.1 that the environment in the West Indies had a detrimental influence on the health of troops. It also shows that the mortality increased with an increasing age of the soldiers. The slight drop in mortality in the 40-50 years age group was because many sick men were sent home and did not stay for the full year, which was the basis of the calculation. It was a commonly held belief that Europeans gradually became acclimatised or "seasoned" to warm climates and that the mortality rates of older acclimatised soldiers was lower than younger inexperienced troops. Marshall and Tulloch in their great work *Statistical report on the mortality and invaliding among the troops in the West Indies* completely disproved this misperception:

> Soldiers are not in general liable to any greater mortality during their first year of service there than at any subsequent period.[8]

The following list summarises concepts of disease which were disproved by the statistical analyses of Marshall and Tulloch and incorporate quotes from their findings in *Statistical report on the mortality and invaliding among the troops in the West Indies.*[9]

High temperature

> The range of thermometer, for instance, in Antigua and Barbados is rather higher than in Dominica, Tobago, Jamaica or the Bahamas; yet we find that the troops in the latter stations suffer nearly three times as much as those in the former.[10]

Excess of moisture

> If the mortality of the troops depended materially on the influence of moisture, we might expect it to attain its maximum in those stations where the fall of rain was greatest, whereas the average mortality of the troops in Jamaica is at least double that which prevails in British Guiana, though the quantity of water which falls on that island is little more than half as great.[11]

The combined effects of high temperature and excess moisture

> The unhealthy character of that period of the year in which the greatest degree of heat and moisture are combined is not confined to the West

> Indies, but extends also to the East as well as over a large portion of the Western temperate zone. We advert to them to in order to guard against the error of referring to the climate of the West Indies exclusively, phenomena which are common, not only to other tropical regions, but also to those of the temperate zone.[12]

Absence of trade winds during the sickly season

> A knowledge of this fact at once overturns a plausible hypothesis which attributes the unhealthy character of the West Indies to the want of free ventilation afforded by the trade winds during the rest of the year, but which at this period either cease altogether, or become very irregular. Though these two events, the failure of the trade winds, and the increase of sickness and mortality take place at corresponding periods, the latter can never be regarded as a necessary consequence of the former, when we find in other quarters of the globe beyond the range of the trade winds, and in which ventilation is quite as perfect at that period as at any other, the unhealthy nature of these months is marked as strongly as at the West Indies.[13]

Miasma from the South American Continent

> This same fact strikes at the root of another hypothesis which attributes the sickly season in these regions to some morbific principle generated in the vast forests of the South American Continent, and wafted to these islands by the south westerly winds which generally prevail during that period. Besides, were this hypothesis correct, we might expect that British Guiana would, from its proximity to this cause of disease, be most subject to its operation, and consequently the most unhealthy; and that the colonies further to the north being least exposed to it, would enjoy the greatest degree of salubrity. The result of our investigations into the comparative mortality in each colony shows, however, that their relative salubrity is by no means affected by their proximity to, or distance from, that continent.[14]

Exhalations or emanations from the soil

Marshall and Tulloch analysed as far as possible the physical characteristics of the soil and showed that while the physical characteristics of soil might be the same in different regions, the mortality rates might be very different. They went on to say:

> It frequently happens that a station which has been remarkable for its sickly character for one or two seasons becomes without any perceptible reasons, just as remarkable for its salubrity, which could scarcely happen if the cause of sickness or mortality existed in the soil, which was constantly there to produce it.[15]

Marshes, swamps and Lagoons

> The agency, real or supposed from marshes is liable to a similar objection. That the vicinity of marshes is generally subject to fevers, both of the intermittent and remittent types, is a fact sufficiently established by multiplied experiences, both in tropical countries and in temperate zones. But that remittent, or yellow fever, may be generated when there is no such cause in operation to produce it, is sufficiently established by the fact that the sickness and mortality in British Guiana and Honduras, where swamps and marshes abound, are considerably less than at Up Park Camp, and several of the other stations in Jamaica, remote from the operation of such agencies.[16]

Marshall and Tulloch demonstrated that the commonest cause of death was yellow fever and that there were four very bad years in 1819, 1822, 1825 and 1827, when there were epidemics of yellow fever. The greatest recorded mortality amounted to 259 per 1,000 soldiers.

Table 7.2 Death rates for different fevers.

DISEASE	PERCENTAGE MORTALITY
Yellow fever	43%
Typhus fever	23%
Remittent fever	11%
Common continued Fever	4%
Intermittent fever	0.6%

From: Marshall H., *Statistical report on the sickness, mortality, and invaliding among the troops in the West Indies*. London: W Clowes and Sons, 1838.

From their statistical analysis, Marshall and Tulloch established that yellow fever was never known to occur when the location of the soldiers was at an altitude of above 2,500 feet. They also confirmed that older troops did less well than younger soldiers in surviving the rigours of a posting to the region.

Their analytical minds successfully dismissed many popular misperceptions, although they were less successful in putting forward theories as to what actually did cause disease. The two researchers concluded their statistical analysis by stating the need for further work in other regions of the world, which might shed further light on the possible causes of a variety of diseases. The work of scientists such as Louis Pasteur and Robert Koch would be needed before these causes were identified but Marshall and Tulloch made significant inroads into discovering and understanding the causes of diseases by applying themselves in a scientific way to look for answers by asking the right questions.

COMPARISON OF HEALTH IN DIFFERENT PARTS OF THE BRITISH EMPIRE

Marshall retired in 1836, and his place was taken by Assistant Surgeon Graham Balfour. Tulloch and Balfour produced a series of reports which covered all the stations in the Empire. Their work was brought to a stop by the Crimean War, after which, from 1860, Annual Reports on Army Health were instituted. Table 7.3 summarises the annual mortality figures for various parts of the Empire. This was made available thanks to the foresight of Sir James McGrigor and to the analytical skills of men like Marshall, Tulloch and Balfour.[17]

Deaths from different causes were conveniently expressed in a number per 1,000 ration strength. As can be seen from the figures, a posting to the West Indies was indeed a dangerous one, and some parts were worse than others. Gibraltar was a generally good place to be sent and Canada was almost as safe as being in billets at home. Perhaps a posting to the Cape of Good Hope would have been viewed as the equivalent of being sent to a health resort. A posting to the Gold Coast was to be avoided if at all possible because 668 out of every 1,000 soldiers who went there did not come home and special means would have to be employed to ensure that Britain's military aims would be fulfilled and these are discussed in Chapter 8.

Table 7.3 Annual Mortality figures in deaths per 1,000, in various locations round the world, ranging between 1817 and 1836.

STATION	YEAR	ANNUAL MORTALITY PER 1,000
Windward/Leeward	1817-1836	78.5
Jamaica	1817-1836	121.3
Gibraltar	1818-1836	21.4
Malta	1817-1836	16.3
Canada	1817-1836	16.1
Sierra Leone	1819-1836	483
Gold Coast	1823-1826	668
Cape of Good Hope	1818-1836	13.7
Ceylon	1817-1836	69.8
Burma	1827-1836	44.7
United Kingdom	1830-1836	14

From Cantlie, N., *A History of the Army Medical Department.* Edinburgh: Churchill Livingston, 1974, Volume 1, p.442.

SUMMARY

Henry Marshall was the first man ever in the British Army, or in any army, to apply himself to the interpretation of vital statistics. He demonstrated their practical bearing on the prevention of ill health and mortality and he made a most significant contribution to improving the efficiency of fighting units. It all began as a simple statistical compilation of relevant facts which no-one had thought of before and is an early example of evidenced based medicine as practised today.

ENDNOTES

1. Cantlie, N., *A History of the Army Medical Department.* Edinburgh: Churchill Livingston, 1974, Volume 1, pp.206-207.
2. Clarke, H., *History of the War from the commencement of the French Revolution to the present time.* London: T. Kinnersley, 1816, p.170.
3. McGrigor, J., *Medical Sketches of the Expedition from India to Egypt.* London: Murray, J., Fleet Street, 1804, pp.56-57.

4. Blanco, R.L., "Henry Marshall (1775-1851) and the health of the British Army". *Medical History:* 1970. July; 14 (3). pp.260-261.
5. Marshall, H., *Statistical report on the sickness, mortality, and invaliding among the troops in the West Indies.* London: W Clowes and Sons, 1838.
6. Marshall, *op. cit.* p.iv.
7. Chaplin, A., The Rate of Mortality in the British Army 100 years ago. *Proceedings of the Royal Society of Medicine;* 1916; p.90.
8. Marshall, *op. cit.*, p.95.
9. Marshall, H., *Statistical report on the sickness, mortality, and invaliding among the troops in the West Indies.* London: W Clowes and Sons, 1838.
10. *Ibid*, p.101.
11. *Ibid*, p.102.
12. *Ibid.*
13. *Ibid.*
14. *Ibid.*
15. *Ibid.*
16. *Ibid.*
17. Cantlie, *op. cit.*, p.442.

8

Minor Wars

INTRODUCTION

The British Empire was vast with interests spread around the globe. There were no major wars between the final defeat of Napoleon at Waterloo (1815) and the Crimean War (Great Britain's entry was 1854). However, there were often disputes and issues to be resolved elsewhere in the world which frequently required military intervention. Consequently, Great Britain was engaged in many "minor wars" throughout the nineteenth century which often resulted in battalions of British soldiers fighting alongside troops from the East India Company in a coalition army. Whilst a description of the origins, course and outcomes of these colonial conflicts is beyond the scope of this book, such engagements often highlighted important medical issues. Those minor wars occurring in the first half of the century are dealt with here.

THE WEST INDIES

In 1793, Great Britain and France fought each other in the West Indies during the French Revolutionary Wars. This was to prove extremely costly in terms of lives lost, mainly as a result of disease. The islands making up the West Indies were important because they were the main source of sugar cane and both Britain and France had colonial possessions there. The Prime Minister of the day, William Pitt the Younger, saw conflict in the West Indies as a way of militarily engaging the French during the French Revolutionary War.

In 1793, Sir Charles Grey led the first of two expeditions to the West Indies. He arrived in Barbados in January 1794 and hospitals were established in St Pierre, Tobago and Miquelon, before Grey launched operations against the French held Leeward Islands. Martinique was captured thanks to brilliant co-operation between Grey and Vice Admiral John Jervis. Jervis ordered the 'Asia', with 64 guns and the 'Zebra' sloop to storm Fort Louis, the chief defence of Fort Royal, the last French stronghold on the island. The 'Asia' was unable to reach her position and so Commander Faulkner of the 'Zebra' volunteered to attempt to capture it alone. He ran his sloop close under the walls and endured heavy fire from the fort. Faulkner jumped overboard and followed by his ship's company, stormed and captured the fort. By May 1794, Guadeloupe and St Lucia were in British hands. General hospitals were opened on the captured islands.

In July there was an outbreak of yellow fever and by the end of 1794, Grey's army had been practically wiped out by disease. Grey's force was 7,000 strong when it arrived in the West Indies in January 1793. By the end of 1794, approximately 5,000 of the original force of 7,000 had died of disease, mostly yellow fever or "yellow jack" as it was known at that time.[1] Dysentery also contributed to the high mortality. Of the officers who went with Grey's force, 27 had been killed or died of wounds, whilst 170 (86%) died of yellow fever. The Royal Navy also suffered a high mortality from disease and 46 masters and 1,100 seamen died of yellow fever. Reinforcements were sent, but they too died in their thousands and approximately 12,000 men died from disease in 1894, mostly from yellow fever.[2]

A campaign which started so successfully had become a disaster and by 1795 many of the gains from the early days of the campaign had been lost. Guadeloupe and St Lucia were back in French hands, while there was heavy fighting in Grenada and St Vincent, where British troops held on with difficulty. Men who had survived yellow fever were so demoralised that they lost the will to fight. The ships of the fleet were practically immobilised by a very high mortality amongst sailors, with the result that the Royal Navy lost control of the seas around the West Indies.

A second expedition with 18,000 men assembled under the leadership of Sir Ralph Abercromby in Portsmouth in November 1795 and a further 13,000 men led by Major General Whyte gathered in Cork. Before Whyte's force embarked from Southern Ireland for the West Indies, an epidemic of typhus and dysentery swept through his troops. 3,000 men were admitted to hospital of whom 500 died. Lawlessness, desertion and drunkenness also caused serious problems.[3] Perhaps this happened because men knew what awaited them in the West Indies.

It was decided they should land in the West Indies in November 1795, to avoid the more dangerous rainy season when diseases were known to be much more common. The rainy season coincided with the breeding season of the mosquito responsible for transmitting yellow fever (as discussed in Chapter 2). If the force arrived in November, it would give time for acclimatisation, which was mistakenly believed to protect men against fevers. When they did finally set sail, there were terrible storms and they did not reach Barbados and St Domingo until March 1796, by which time the rainy season was already well underway. The outcome was predictable. There was an outbreak of yellow fever in May 1796. James McGrigor was with Abercromby's expedition (Chapter 2) and whilst McGrigor suffered from dysentery, by good luck he avoided contracting yellow fever although many of his colleagues were not so fortunate and many medical officers died from the effects of the disease.

By the end of 1796, Abercromby's army had been reduced in strength by 50%. In the six months between April and September inclusive, there were 22,596 men sick in hospital and a further 2,428 died.[4] As a result of severe losses, there was a curtailment of operations in the West Indies by 1797.

It has been estimated that during the years 1794, 1795 and 1796, no fewer than 40,000 men died of disease and a further 40,000 were discharged as unfit for further service.[5]

Following the Battle of Trafalgar in 1805, fear of invasion of the United Kingdom faded, particularly when the Third Coalition alliance between Britain, Russia and Austria was formed to face the threat posed by Napoleon. A powerful gathering of forces in Britain heralded an impending major offensive against Napoleon. Between 1803 and 1807 there were several expeditions of a minor nature, but from 1808, all Britain's energies were concentrated on the Peninsular War, which lasted till 1814.

The military situation in the West Indies remained quiet during the Peninsular War, but even so, there were still 11,000 troops to garrison the islands and to maintain a British presence. At any one time 2,000 were in hospital suffering from a variety of diseases, although there were no significant outbreaks of yellow fever during this time.[6]

The research of Marshall and Tulloch (Chapter 7) revealed that between 1817 and 1836, when there was no fighting, there was a mortality of 121.3 per 1,000 of troops stationed in Jamaica, which constituted a huge drain on available resources, for very little in the way of perceptible gain. Marshall's *Statistical report on the sickness, mortality and invaliding among the troops in the West Indies* was published in 1838.[7]

WARS IN INDIA

There were many wars in India, and the organisation of medical services was primarily the responsibility of the Honourable East India Company (HEIC). The first British regiment to set foot in India was the 39th Foot (1st Dorsets) in 1755. With the arrival of British troops, medical officers were interchangeable between British regiments and the HEIC.

British regiments were staffed by a surgeon and two assistant surgeons and the Indian units of the HEIC had one assistant surgeon (who was European) and one Indian doctor. There were hospitals for native troops and separate garrison hospitals for British troops which were staffed by surgeons and assistant surgeons of the HEIC. [8]

THE SECOND MARATHA WAR

Throughout the 18th century, war was waged against the French in India, or against native princes who supported them and this led to wars called the Maratha Wars. The second of these (1802-1805) was notable for the decisive victory at the Battle of Assaye in September 1803. It was here that the then Major General Arthur Wellesley distinguished himself by winning his first major victory and one he later described as his finest accomplishment on the battlefield. He commanded a coalition force with the HEIC and this was the first war in which a field hospital was ever used. It was equipped with 200 beds.[9]

Administrative control of this field hospital lay entirely in the hands of a senior surgeon of the HEIC, who acted as both an administrator and consultant. He appointed a field surgeon who was chosen for his surgical expertise and there were usually several assistant surgeons, but unfortunately they were not always available. If there were no assistant surgeons, then the field surgeon would have to withdraw medical officers from their regimental hospitals to provide the necessary medical cover. This often led to delays in treating the wounded. Theft was not uncommon and a medical storekeeper was employed to safeguard the medical and surgical stores.

This fully staffed and equipped field hospital accompanied Wellesley's army. Medical supplies for three months were carried in a bullock train. Particular attention was paid to provide enough bark (for the treatment of intermittent fever) and other medicines.

As Wellesley advanced, so he established other hospitals and avoided carrying the sick and wounded on the line of his march. The Second Maratha war was prolonged and the decisive Battle of Assaye was on 23 September, 1803, when Wellesley's force of 7,000 men defeated an army of 50,000 Marathas. There were over 1,000 wounded to treat and six additional assistant surgeons were summoned to the field hospital from the regimental hospitals and extra dressers were also supplied by regimental hospitals.[10]

PINDARI WAR (1814-19)

The Third Maratha War is better known as the Pindari War, because it was directed specifically against a band of robbers and bandits based in the Maratha provinces. The Marathas had always tolerated a degree of robbery and pillage by some of their forces, even during times of peace. When it became clear the Marathas would do nothing about the problem, Lord Hastings, the Governor General, was determined to act.

The campaign against the Pindaris was elaborately planned and involved mobilising native soldiers from many surrounding provinces. The Pindaris would have to be surrounded on all sides, or they would flee into the open country and return as soon as the army withdrew. The Maratha leaders who had protected the Pindaris were forced to withdraw their support and cooperate in their destruction. Several of the most troublesome Maratha leaders were given pensions by the British as an inducement for their support.

The largest ever force on the sub-continent of India was assembled, comprising 120,000 troops and 40,000 camp followers. This war was notable because there was a serious outbreak of cholera.

Three British Army battalions were involved in this campaign and this marked the first significant British military exposure to the first Asiatic cholera pandemic, which lasted from 1817 to 1824. The deaths of a great many British soldiers drew attention to the outbreak. One regiment lost 340 men out of 800 between May and December 1818.[11] This first known pandemic originated in the Ganges river delta in India. The disease broke out near Calcutta and quickly spread through the rest of the country. By the early 1820s, colonization and trade had carried the disease to Southeast Asia, Central Asia, the Middle East, Eastern Africa and the Mediterranean coast.

Quite apart from the cholera outbreak, there was a great shortage of supplies, which led to severe friction between the regular forces of the British Army and the

HEIC, who were of course responsible for the medical arrangements. Regimental surgeons even had to supply their own instruments, medicines and equipment.

The HEIC came in for severe criticism. The official historian quoted a contemporary writer who said:

> In the field hospital there was scarcely a bit of sticking plaster for the wounded officers, and none for the men.[12]

FIRST BURMA WAR (1824)

The King of Ava was a powerful monarch who dominated Burma. He crossed the Indian frontier and invaded the adjacent territory belonging to the East India Company, which resulted in a declaration of war. This "minor" war was characterised by a very high percentage of deaths from disease amongst the soldiers. Deaths from enemy action were few, but deaths from malaria and amoebic dysentery were many. During the First Burma War, the overall annual mortality was 483 per 1,000 men. Of these, 446 per 1,000 died from disease. There were 89 cases of cholera and 48 died, a percentage mortality of 54%. [13]

There were 1,311 deaths amongst British troops in a total strength of 2,716 men. Of these deaths, 1,215 were the result of disease and 36 were from wounds, a ratio of 33:1. Deaths from enemy action were so few that they are scarcely worth mentioning.[14]

SECOND BURMA WAR (1852-3)

While some attempts were made to reduce mortality in the Second Burma War by paying stricter attention to good housing with the construction of prefabricated huts and provision of more nutritious food for the soldiers, the mortality figures were still very high. The annual death rate in 1852 was 236 per 1,000 and in 1853 it was 256 per 1,000. Most deaths were caused by dysentery. There were 785 cases of cholera, and 235, i.e. 29.9% perished.[15]

THE FIRST ASHANTI WAR (1824-1826)_

The first Ashanti War broke out because this nation of warriors threatened British trading ports on the Gold Coast.

The west coast of Africa was associated with an even higher death rate from disease than Burma. Sierra Leone, the Gold Coast and Gambia were rightly regarded as "the white man's grave." Malaria, dysentery, cholera, yellow fever and guinea worm between them ensured an annual mortality of 668 per 1,000 men from disease.[16] Soldiers from the West Indian Regiment were sent to the west coast of Africa, since it had been previously noted during fighting in the West Indies that these men were less likely to suffer such heavy losses from disease. This was because they had a certain degree of immunity to many tropical diseases disease compared with British troops who had never been exposed to them.

The mortality on the west coast of Africa was so high that between 1822 and 1825, the Royal Africa Corps was formed. This unit was formed from convicted criminals whose punishment was commuted if they agreed to join the colours and serve their country, and these men were committed to the fighting during the Ashanti War. Deaths from wounds were negligible.

Rather than employing alcohol-soaked old soldiers from the criminal fraternity, a policy was then introduced to use young and healthy recruits. Within a short time, from a ration strength of a group of 108 young soldiers, 48 were dead, 21 invalided, 29 unfit from fever and only 10 fit for duty. [17]

In 1830, the war office finally stopped sending soldiers to the west coast of Africa, recognising that to do so would result in almost certain death.

FIRST AFGHAN WAR (1839-42)

The First Anglo-Afghan War was also known as Auckland's Folly [18], since as Governor General of India he decided to invade Afghanistan. This war was fought between British India and Afghanistan. It was one of the first major conflicts during the "Great Game", which was the term used to describe the 19th century competition for power and influence in Central Asia between Great Britain and Russia.

The war marked one of the worst setbacks inflicted on British power in the region since the consolidation of the British Raj by the East India Company and is considered to be one of Britain's worst nineteenth century disasters in Asia.

The invading force of the HEIC comprised a Bengal Division (5,000 men) and a Bombay Division (5,000 men) with thousands of camp followers who set off to invade Afghanistan. There were also four British infantry regiments, two cavalry regiments and 6,000 Indian auxiliaries. The total strength of the force was approximately 16,000 men.[19]

They marched into Afghanistan through extremely hostile country in baking heat and many suffered from heat stroke. After occupying Quetta, the divisions moved on to Kandahar, where there were supply problems leading to shortages of water and food. Many camp followers were killed en route by Afghan tribesmen. Lines of communication were precarious and most horses and 20,000 camels died. There were outbreaks of dysentery and cholera. From Kandahar, the next goal was Kabul, which was eventually reached, whereupon the Bombay Division left, and set off to return to India. By the time it departed, there were 1,500 men left of the original 5,000. The others had died or were too weak to travel. Cholera spread rapidly through the remnants of this division, and the road was strewn with emaciated corpses.

The occupation of Kabul continued for two and a half years but was difficult to maintain. Afghan tribesmen were bribed into peaceful co-operation, but the more money they were given, the more they wanted. By November 1841, matters had become critical with the Afghans everywhere in open revolt. In January 1842, Kabul was evacuated after assurances of a safe passage back to India had been given. The long march from Kabul to India began and the troops passed through dangerous mountain passes in the middle of winter.

Afghan tribesmen attacked and killed the weary travellers on a daily basis and when food supplies ran out, numbers soon dwindled away and only one man survived the journey back to Jalalabad. He was a medical officer called Dr William Brydon and he was badly wounded, with part of his skull sheared off by an Afghan sword. He had only survived because he had insulated himself against the cold by putting a copy of *Blackwood's Magazine* into his hat in order to reduce the heat loss from his head. This was indeed a lucky move; the magazine had absorbed most of the blow of the sword and saved the doctor's life!

THE FIRST CHINA WAR (1839-1842)

This was also known as the Opium War and was started by the HEIC. India sold huge quantities of opium to the Chinese market and this had become a very lucrative trade. The Chinese authorities wanted to ban it because of the usage of opium and the detrimental effect it was having on the nation's health. Chinese drug addicts yearned for opium and British merchants wanted the profits from its sale. As a consequence, the merchants were expelled by the Chinese authorities but Lord Auckland, the Governor General of India, was ordered to uphold Britain's right to trade.

This resulted in an invasion of China by the East India Company and an outbreak of diseases amongst the troops. On this occasion, dysentery, malaria and typhoid fever were the main causes of death. The sole supply of drinking water came from irrigation channels in fields which were usually contaminated by dead animals and decaying vegetable matter. The most notable feature of this expedition was that it was regarded as a most unsanitary and disgraceful debacle. A force of 2,500 British soldiers had 3,239 hospital admissions and 445 deaths giving a death rate of 178 per 1,000 ration strength.[20] The Chinese, however, were beaten, and Hong Kong was acquired as compensation.

Hong Kong proved to be a poisoned chalice since it was as unhealthy as most other places in the Far East. In July and August 1847, stricken with malaria, men of the 95th Foot stationed there buried so many of their regimental comrades on a daily basis that the remnants of the regiment moved offshore into billets on board ships in an attempt to escape from almost certain death.[21] This did not help, since the tiny but deadly anopheles mosquito blew gently in the offshore breeze to the ships at anchor in the bay.

FIRST SIKH WAR (1845-1846)

The First Anglo-Sikh War was fought between the Sikh Empire and the East India Company between 1845 and 1846.

This conflict was marked by the woefully deficient medical resources put in place by the HEIC. It will be remembered that a field hospital was first introduced by the East India Company in 1802. On this occasion, the Company failed to provide any field hospitals at all and the regimental hospitals had to bear the entire brunt of sick and wounded. Many severely wounded soldiers lay on a battlefield all night whilst there was complete chaos in the provision of medical care resulting from a lack of medical leadership. A letter was written by a regimental surgeon to surgeon George James Guthrie, who took up the cause and publicly denounced the medical arrangements that had been put in place by the HEIC.

Sir James McGrigor emphasised the fundamental need for the provision of medical facilities to permit primary amputations of severely wounded limbs, and

Guthrie added to the debate by commenting strongly about the loss of life which must have resulted from having no field hospitals to provide adequate surgical care.

Regimental surgeons had been torn between conflicting responsibilities, although Sir James McGrigor was in no doubt as to where the responsibilities of regimental surgeons lay:

> The duty of the regimental surgeon is to be with the wounded, no matter whether they be in the field or at a depot near at hand, until all capital operations are performed.[22]

Many commanding officers however retained the regimental surgeon at headquarters, leaving surgery to less skilled assistants.[23]

McGrigor decided that since the HEIC had failed to provide efficient treatment, a senior Army Medical Department (AMD) officer should be present at any future engagement to look after the interests of the British forces in any joint enterprise with the HEIC.

SECOND SIKH WAR (1848-1849)

Medical arrangements were better and there was adequate provision of field hospitals after the medical disorganisation that had characterised the First Sikh War. At least the lessons of the First Sikh War had been learned and had been acted upon to improve the quality of care that was provided to the wounded.

SCINDE (1842-1843)

This involved the conquest of Scinde in India by Sir Charles Napier. There were two principal battles at Miani and Hyderabad. Subsequently, malaria was a major problem as usual, but then cholera broke out in Karachi in 1846. In the course of a single week, the 86th regiment (2nd Royal Ulster Rifles) lost 208 men and over seven months there were 1,838 admissions and 918 deaths from cholera in a community numbering 8,566.[24]

Doctors were powerless to mitigate the effects of Asiatic cholera. All patients were bled by venesection procedures, removing variable quantities of blood in the early stage of the disease. This was the standard treatment of the day and in addition, equally ineffective remedies such as calomel (a mercury based purgative), croton oil (a powerful purgative) and diacetate of lead were employed with no success.

During this outbreak, cholera sent many thousands of British troops and their families to their deaths throughout the entire length and breadth of India.

General Sir Charles Napier, who was the British Army's Commander in Chief in India, did his best to improve housing, sanitation and ventilation. He laid down directions for a minimum requirement for housing space for each soldier in a barracks and tried to cut down on the consumption of alcohol in an effort to improve the general health of the troops. Any deaths from wounds in this location were inconsequential, when compared with the morbidity and mortality due to disease.

CHOLERA

This brief account of "minor engagements" clearly illustrates that Asiatic cholera had well and truly arrived. The second pandemic (1829-1849) started in India and reached Russia by 1830 before continuing into Finland and Poland. A two-year outbreak began in Britain in October 1831 and claimed 22,000 lives. Irish immigrants, fleeing poverty and the potato famine, carried the disease from Europe to North America. On their arrival in the summer of 1832, 1,220 died in Montreal and another 1,000 across the state of Quebec. The disease then entered the United States through Detroit and New York and reached Latin America by 1833. Another outbreak across England and Wales began in 1848, killing 52,000 over two years.

There were six Asiatic cholera pandemics in the nineteenth century [25] and their dates are outlined below but they all began in India.

- First Pandemic 1817-1823;
- Second Pandemic 1829-1849;
- Third Pandemic 1852-1859;
- Fourth Pandemic 1863-1879;
- Fifth Pandemic 1881-1896;
- Sixth pandemic 1899-1923.

Cholera is caused by the contamination of food and drink by strains of the bacteria vibrio cholerae. Robert Koch isolated the organism in 1883 and is generally credited with having discovered the causative organism. In fact, Italian scientist Filipo Pacini described the vibrio cholerae when cholera came to Florence in 1854. Unfortunately he did not appreciate the full global implication of what he had observed and his discovery remained in obscurity.[26]

In an outbreak of cholera in London in 1848-1849 during the third pandemic, physician John Snow noted that people who lived in the upper Thames area were healthier that in the lower Thames, where sewage from the upper Thames contaminated the drinking water. He was the first person to make the association between contaminated water and cholera.[27]

In 1855, he developed his hypothesis, when he studied a locality where there was a large cluster of cholera cases. He focused on the now famous Broad Street pump in Soho, where he confirmed that cholera was water borne. He also conducted a larger, although inconclusive study, on how the municipal water supply of London was associated with the disease pattern.

The cholera vibrio multiplies in the lumen of the small bowel and does not invade the bowel wall. The bacterium secretes a very powerful toxin which stimulates the bowel to produce massive amounts of fluid. Even although the absorptive ability of the bowel is unimpaired, there is so much fluid produced that severe dehydration quickly supervenes with electrolyte loss and fluid imbalances and severe and profuse diarrhoea. Renal failure may quickly follow and death from circulatory failure commonly occurs within a few hours without the adequate treatment that may now be available.[28]

While this is a description of the very worst type of case, in many instances the disease is less severe and the patient survives. In areas where the disease is endemic, cholera is maintained by very mild infections in a population with considerable resistance.

Prevention of spread of disease requires strict personal hygiene and water for drinking must come from a cleaned, piped supply, or else it must be boiled. Transmission by flies and their contamination of food is also a common mechanism whereby the disease is passed on to people.

SUMMARY

This brief outline of minor colonial wars is not a history of these conflicts and anyone interested in the origins and outcomes of these minor wars must obtain further information elsewhere. However, it is clear that losses from wounds were of very little consequence compared with the preponderance of deaths from a variety of diseases. Dysentery, malaria and typhus fever were forever present in crowded and squalid conditions, whilst epidemics of yellow fever in the West Indies accounted for approximately 160,000 losses between 1793 and 1798 and exerted a major adverse influence on Britain's ability to wage war.

The Asiatic cholera pandemics in the nineteenth century ensured that the disease would encircle the globe, thanks to a large extent to the movements of British troops going from one outpost of the Empire to another. These pandemics raised the profile of cholera well above the level of military loss, to a truly massive and global level.

ENDNOTES

1. Cantlie, N., *A History of the Army Medical Department.* Edinburgh: Churchill Livingston, 1974, Volume 1, pp.235-6.
2. *Ibid,* p.236.
3. *Ibid,* p.240.
4. *Ibid,* p.244.
5. *Ibid,* p.249.
6. *Ibid,* p.283.
7. Marshall, H., *Statistical report on the sickness, mortality, and invaliding among the troops in the West Indies.* London: W. Clowes and Sons, 1838.
8. Cantlie, N., *A History of the Army Medical Department.* Edinburgh: Churchill Livingston, 1974, Volume 1, p.412.
9. *Ibid,* p.412.
10. *Ibid,* p 414.
11. *Ibid,* p.416.
12. *Ibid.*
13. *Ibid,* p.459.
14. *Ibid.*
15. *Ibid,* p.492.
16. *Ibid,* pp.459-462.
17. *Ibid,* pp.459-462.
18. Hopkirk, P., *The Great Game.* London: John Murray Publishers, 1990, pp.189-192.
19. Cantlie, *op. cit.*, p.468-477.
20. *Ibid,* p.478.
21. *Ibid,* p.481.
22. *Ibid,* p.485.

23. *Ibid*, pp.484-5.
24. *Ibid*, p.488.
25. Colwell, R.R., "Global Climate and Infectious Disease; the Cholera Paradigm". *Science:* Volume. 274, No 5295 (Dec 20, 1996) pp.2025-2031.
26. Echenberg, M., *Africa in the Time of Cholera. A History of the Pandemics from 1817 to the Present.* Cambridge: Cambridge University Press, 2011, p.33.
27. Smith, G.D., "Commentary: Behind the Broad Street pump; aetiology, epidemiology and .prevention of cholera in mid-19th Century Britain". *International Journal of Epidemiology,* 2002:31; pp.920-932.
28. MacLeod, J., *Davidson's Principles and Practice of Medicine.* 13th Edition. Edinburgh: Churchill Livingstone, 1981, p.830.

9

Development of Military Anaesthesia in the 19th Century

> "The pain endured by the bleeding sailor or soldier, wounded in fighting battles of his country, is deeply deplored by every feeling mind; and a discovery that can prevent so much of it, as depends on the operations necessary to save his life, must be hailed as a great blessing..."
>
> John Snow Lecture to Military Medical Officers
> 12th May 1847[1]

British military surgery in the first half of the nineteenth century depended on sound anatomical knowledge, speed and accuracy. Surgeons George James Guthrie and John Hennen knew the importance of speed, because patients were awake and aware of what was happening during a surgical procedure. Perhaps recently wounded soldiers undergoing an amputation while still in a heightened emotional state felt less pain than those enduring surgery days or even weeks later, when every slice of the knife, and cut of the saw through bone would be too agonizing to contemplate and to endure.

The experience of performing operations on conscious patients who were in terrible pain, had such an adverse effect on many surgeons, that John Thomson, Professor of Military Surgery at the University of Edinburgh, felt moved to say that many surgeons felt so overwhelmed by the sight of such misery, that it rendered them indifferent to life.[2]

By the outbreak of the Crimean War in 1853, Britain's first major campaign since the Peninsular War, all that was changing. General anaesthesia had been invented.

The eighteenth century had become known as "The Age of Enlightenment" or "The Age of Reason" during which time superstition and belief gave way to scientific reasoning. Scientific progress, which began in the sixteenth century, gathered speed in the seventeenth century and made rapid progress in the eighteenth century. It led to many improvements in everyday life but advances in the practice of medicine were virtually non-existent.

In 1628, Harvey established the circulation, or flow of blood around the human body. Prior to that date, blood was thought to be manufactured in the liver and transported to different parts of the body to provide nourishment and needed to be continually renewed. Harvey measured the capacity of the heart and worked out how much blood was being pumped into the arteries each minute. He estimated that the heart pumped out 260 litres an hour and although inaccurate, he realised that such a volume, amounting to three times the weight of a man, could not be continually manufactured and distributed. This was a much more scientific way in which to approach a medical problem and echoed scientific reasoning used by the great astronomers Kepler and Galileo.

During the seventeenth century a number of brilliant individuals working in isolation, namely Robert Hooke, Edmond Halley and Isaac Newton took scientific research to new levels. They had at their disposal the first scientific instruments, including telescopes and microscopes, to test their ideas. The realization that the physical world was governed by scientific laws then spread to the biological sciences and with it an appreciation that the workings of the human body might be subject to similar scientific reasoning. The vision of man's place at the centre of the Universe was diminishing.[3]

The end of the eighteenth century saw the development of the new gas chemistry. Joseph Priestley, originally a minister, experimented with what he called "different kinds of airs". Priestley went on to identify a number of gases including ammonia, hydrogen chloride, nitrous oxide and his greatest discovery, oxygen.

Priestley was one of a group of learned men called the Lunar Society, who met monthly in order to find their way home by moonlight. They wished to improve society by scientific advancement.[4] Advancements in medicine were crucial to improving everyday life but in essence, with one or two exceptions, such as Peruvian bark for the treatment of intermittent fever and digitalis for heart failure doctors had almost no medicines that were of any use. The idea that these new airs or gases might be beneficial in curing disease was seized upon by Thomas Beddoes, one member of the group.

Beddoes was a doctor, but he had also studied chemistry. He hoped that breathing these gases might cure tuberculosis and with financial help from members of the Lunar Society, he set up his pneumatic institute in Bristol in 1799. He asked James Watt, famous for his design of steam engines, to develop an apparatus to produce oxygen and hired the young Humphry Davy as an assistant. Davy began to experiment with nitrous oxide.[5] He found that after breathing this gas, he felt unusually light and pleasurable and after acquainting a number of colleagues with the effect, it became known as "laughing gas". Davy also noticed that it helped with the pain from a troublesome wisdom tooth, but he didn't capitalize on the observation. There were no therapeutic breakthroughs at the Pneumatic Institute but Davy had shown that breathing a gas could change behaviour. Nitrous oxide would only be used as entertainment at exhibitions for a number of decades and to enhance the frivolity at parties. It would be many years before its anaesthetic properties would be appreciated.

PAIN RELIEF PRIOR TO GENERAL ANAESTHESIA

During the Napoleonic Wars, physicians and surgeons of all nationalities had only one pain reliever at their disposal, namely morphine. The human race had co-existed with suffering since the beginning of time and the inevitable association of pain with surgery didn't halt progress. Surgeons sought to save lives and if possible limbs, while advancing the art of surgery, despite the lack of suitable pain killers.

Morphine was certainly included in the panniers of drugs and dressings advised by Hennen for each surgeon in his book, *Principles of Military Surgery* published in 1825. He also advocated the use of alcohol to surgeons stating that:

> I would strenuously recommend that he never omits a canteen of good wine or spirits diluted. Many men sink beyond recovery for want of a timely cordial before, during and after operations and many of the primary operations would be rendered much more favourable in their results by the administration of a single glass of wine.[6]

Dominique Larrey, surgeon to Napoleon's army had noticed that during the retreat from Moscow in 1812, soldiers whose legs had become frozen stiff felt almost no pain during amputation. Furthermore if he packed the stumps in ice after amputation then the post- amputation pain was much reduced.[7] This effect was due to the abolition of function in the sensory nerve endings of peripheral spinal nerves and a similar effect may be obtained today by injecting these nerves with local anaesthetic agents to abolish pain.

Surgery without anaesthesia was a truly terrifying prospect and the concept of somehow rendering a person unconscious for the purpose of surgery and then bringing them back to life again was of course unimagined for these early surgeons.

MESMERISM

In 1775, Mesmer (who gave his name to a process involving hypnotism) discovered that he could alter the conscious state of a person perhaps achieving a medical cure and in 1830, James Esdaile, a Scottish surgeon appointed to the East India Company, claimed to have carried out 1000 operations under this hypnotic state.[8] However, this was the age of science and such a method was considered a sham, since it didn't stand up to scientific reasoning.

EARLY USE OF GASES IN AN ATTEMPT TO PRODUCE PAIN RELIEF

The idea of some kind of unconscious state being procured for the benefit of surgery was the brainchild of Henry Hill Hickman, a surgeon living and working in the town of Tenbury. It is impossible to know what promoted his ideas but around 1823 he began experimenting with carbon dioxide to produce unconsciousness in dogs. He enclosed puppies in an atmosphere of carbon dioxide and waited for them to be unconscious. He then cut off part of their ear without causing pain and reintroduced them to air whereupon they appeared to come back to life again.

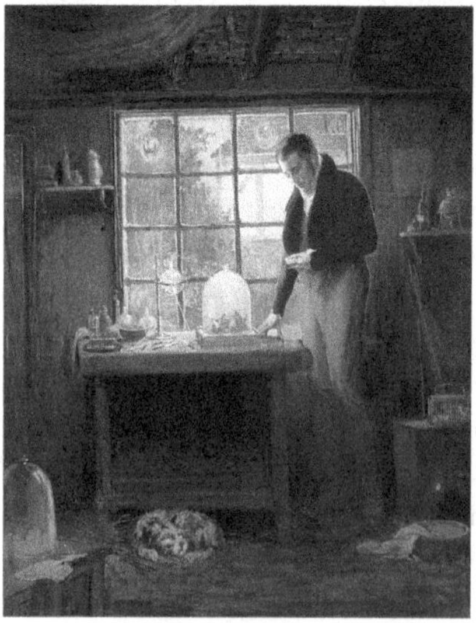

Figure 9.1. Henry Hill Hickman performing experiments on suspended animation. (Courtesy of Wellcome Library, London).

In 1824 he wrote a letter to one of the presidents of the Royal Society on *Suspended Animation and its probable utility in surgical operations on the human subject.*

Hickman was of course asphyxiating the dogs dangerously close to death by denying them oxygen and in Britain his ideas failed to gain support. So convinced was he as to the value of his technique that in 1828 he travelled to France. He wrote to the king, Charles X, and his letter was passed to the Academie Royale de Medecine. He wished to carry out an experiment on a human subject before the surgeons of Paris. His letter was treated with contempt by all but Baron

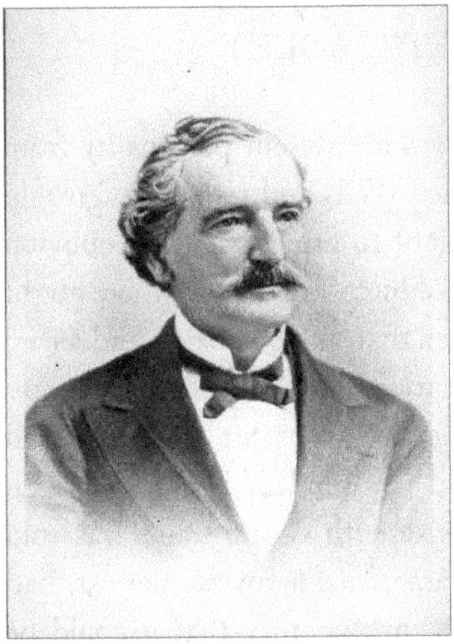

Figure 9.2. Gardner Quincy Colton. (Courtesy of the Wood Library-Museum of Anesthesiology, Park Ridge, IL).

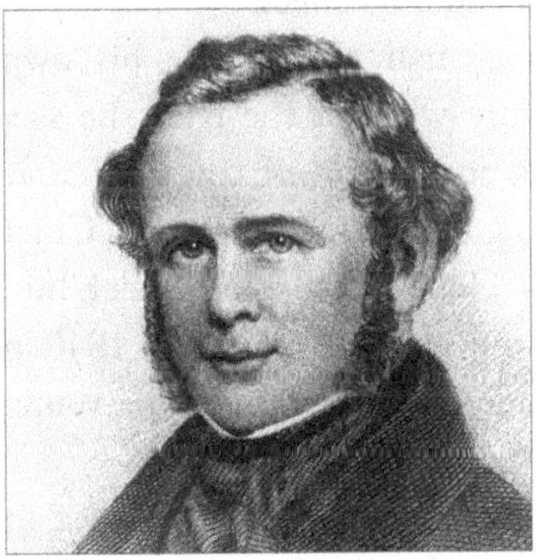

Figure 9.3. Horace Wells. (Courtesy of the Wood Library-Museum of Anaesthesiology, Park Ridge, IL).

Dominique Larrey. However, despite a stay in Paris of six months or so, his ideas were still not accepted and he returned to England a very disappointed man. He died in 1830 when only 30, possibly having committed suicide.[9]

Meanwhile nitrous oxide was still used at demonstrations for the entertainment of the public. Gardner Quincy Colton, an American, gave up his study of medicine and dentistry when he realized that he could earn more by demonstrating nitrous oxide.

In December 1844, one of these demonstrations was attended by Horace Wells, a local dentist and by all accounts a compassionate man who disliked inflicting pain on his patients.

Wells noticed that one young man who breathed the gas appeared to bruise his legs without pain and seeing the potential of the effect, offered to have a tooth removed whilst breathing nitrous oxide. The procedure was done successfully without pain. Wells tried it out on a number of patients himself before deciding at the end of 1846 to attempt a public demonstration. On 9 December, spurred on by his associate William Morton, he attempted such a feat.

Unfortunately it turned into a public humiliation. Wells was no performer and his nerves got the better of him. The gas was withdrawn too soon and the patient was heard to cry out and although he stated later that he felt no pain, it was declared a humbug. Wells wasn't given a second chance.[10]

FIRST USE OF ETHER AS AN ANAESTHETIC AGENT

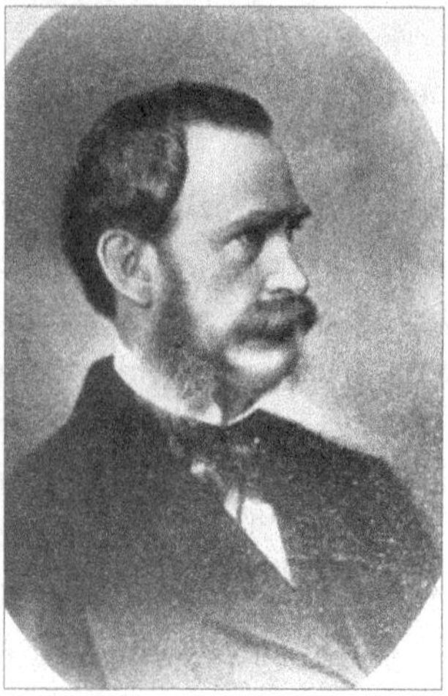

Figure 9.4. William Morton. (Courtesy of the Wood Library-Museum of Anesthesiology, Park Ridge, IL).

William Morton was a different personality from his colleague Horace Wells and refused to give up the quest for an agent to provide reliable oblivion during surgical procedures. He thought there might be something better than nitrous oxide and asked fellow dentist Charles Jackson for suggestions. Jackson had used ether drops for toothache and knew that it could be inhaled. Ether had been around since the sixteenth century and was sold as oil of vitriol. Paracelsus, a Swiss chemist, had noticed in the sixteenth century that it could be used to stun chickens which then "came back to life" but nothing was tried until Crawford Long, a doctor working alone in the Southern State of Georgia in the early 1840s, carried out a number of small operations under its effect.

Long was not a man to promote his own ideas and was unsure whether the effect he saw was real or imagined by the patient. Morton was not so self-effacing, and after demonstrating its effect he waited for a moment to go public. He persuaded Chief Surgeon John Collins Warren at Massachusetts General Hospital to let him demonstrate the remarkable substance and on the morning of 16 October 1846 in front of an audience of surgeons he removed a tumour from the neck of a young man after rendering him unconscious with ether.

A new era in surgery was born that morning and Morton was determined to capitalize on his success. He and Jackson applied for, and were granted, a patent for ether, despite the medical profession at large declaring that this was too important a discovery to be patented.[11]

THE RAPID SPREAD OF ETHER AS AN ANAESTHETIC AGENT - ITS FIRST USE IN THE UK

The news spread swiftly across the Atlantic. A letter was sent from Jacob Bigelow to Francis Boott in London, on the SS *Acadia*, which reached Glasgow on 16 December 1846. Bigelow's son Henry was a surgeon who had observed Morton's

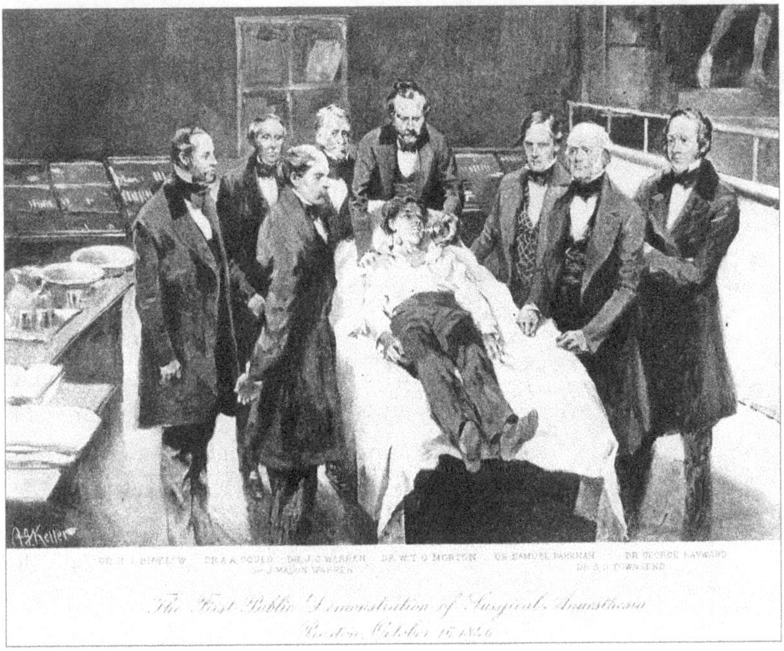

Figure 9.5. First Demonstration of Surgical Anaesthesia, 16th October 1846. (Courtesy of Wellcome Library, London).

demonstration and Boott and Bigelow were both botanists. Whilst Bigelow became Professor of Materia Medica at Harvard, Boott had settled in London. Appreciating the importance of the discovery Boott wrote to Robert Liston, surgeon at University College London, to the *Lancet* and to a dentist by the name of Robinson, who lived in the same street as Boott. Robinson was a fiery character who had been instrumental in setting up dentistry as a profession rather than a trade. He demonstrated the use of ether for tooth extraction, perhaps using apparatus made for them by Hooper of Pall Mall and on 21st December 1846, a successful demonstration was given at University College Hospital, London with Robert Liston the surgeon involved declaring that "this Yankee dodge beats mesmerism hollow"(see Chapter 4).

However, attempts to recreate the event met with varying degrees of success and the use of ether might have remained patchy had it not been for the work of John Snow, whose work on proving that cholera is a waterborne infection was discussed in Chapter 8.

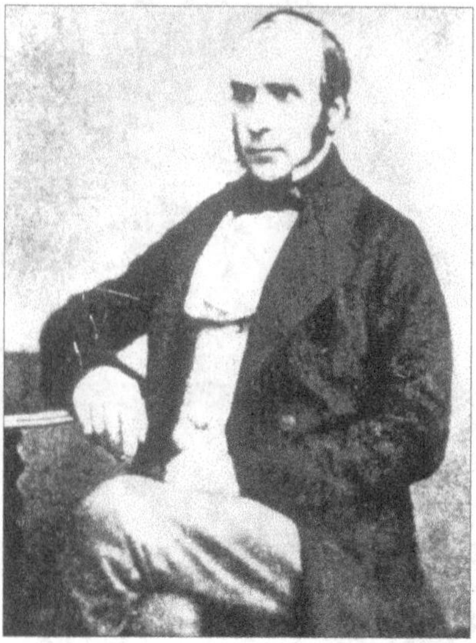

Figure 9.6. John Snow. (Reproduced by kind permission of the Association of Anaesthetists of Great Britain & Ireland).

The son of a Yorkshire labourer, Snow must have looked somewhat out of place in fashionable London. Snow recognized the importance of approaching this new application of ether in a scientific way. He experimented until he found a way of ensuring that he could produce a regular amount and he invented an inhaler. He managed to convince Liston, who was on the point of giving up, that it was a valuable tool and Liston, who was impressed by Snow's calm unassuming manner, ensured that Snow would develop a successful etherizing practice in London. Unfortunately in March 1847 disaster struck and a young woman failed to regain consciousness after inhaling ether for the removal of a tumour on her leg. Some doctors began to question the wisdom of anaesthesia. Perhaps this new technique of abolishing pain was bad for patients. Was pain a necessary aid to recovery? Had the patient's nervous system had been irreversibly depressed? However Snow continued to give ether successfully and the public's demand for painless surgery was unremitting.[12]

FIRST USE OF ANAESTHESIA IN WARFARE

Whilst Morton was carrying out the first demonstration of ether in Massachusetts, America was fighting Mexico for possession of Texas and other North Mexican territories. The first use of anaesthesia in time of war is thought to have occurred in the spring of 1847 during these hostilities. Edward H. Barton, surgeon of the 3rd Dragoons, Cavalry Brigade and a graduate of the University of Pennsylvania, wrote to the US Surgeon General, Thomas Lawson on 16 December 1846, urging the use of ether for the relief of surgical pain in wounded soldiers.

In the spring of 1847, he arrived in Vera Cruz where the church of San Francisco was being used as a hospital. A German teamster had arrived with terrible destruction of both legs due to the accidental discharge of a musket. One of his legs had already been amputated by the time Barton arrived with an apparatus for administering ether used by Morton and called The Letheon. Ether was given to the man successfully and his leg was amputated painlessly.[13] Unfortunately John B. Porter, who was probably the surgeon who carried out the amputation, held ether responsible for excessive haemorrhage that occurred during surgery and for infection, impaired wound healing and haemoptysis (coughing up blood) that occurred post-operatively. He later stated that ether was "unnecessary for gunshot wounds and universally injurious". Thus its use was never fully exploited by the Americans and ether was abandoned at the hospital in Vera Cruz.[14] This was also perhaps the first recorded instance of a surgeon blaming his anaesthetist for things going wrong during and after an operation!

On the Mexican side, Pedro van der Linden, Chief Surgeon to the Mexican Army was able to demonstrate the successful use of ether for leg amputations.

It is possible that Porter's bad experiences with ether might have been due to the high altitude and warm weather which would have created conditions in which ether was much more rapidly vapourized than in the cold of a Boston winter.

USE OF ETHER IN MALTA BY A NAVAL SURGEON

Also practicing military anaesthesia at the time of Morton's demonstration was Horace Spencer Wells, who was serving as assistant surgeon at the Malta Naval Hospital in Bighi. Another testimony as to how quickly the news of ether was spreading is to be found in the Malta Times where the first 200 applications by Morton were reported on 22 December 1846. Wells and two other surgeons were quick to take up the idea and on 9 March 1847 the *Malta Times* reported that Wells had administered ether from a homemade apparatus for partial amputation of a patient's hand. He then sent for a Hooper Inhaler which had been manufactured at the request of Robinson and Bigelow in London and subsequently successfully used ether on a number of occasions. Although Wells presented his work to the *Societa Medica d'Incorragiamento* in Malta there was never an official documentation of his ether usage by the Royal Navy.[15]

EXPERIMENTATION IN RUSSIA WITH RECTAL ETHER, AND GROWING EXPERIENCE IN MILITARY SURGERY

Over on the other side of Europe Nikolai Ivanovich Pirogoff, Professor of Surgery at St Petersburg, started investigating ether on 14 February 1847. Using primitive equipment he administered ether to 50 patients and 40 volunteers. He also experimented on dogs. He tried applying ether directly to nerves and the brain and then injecting it intravenously before finally giving it rectally (through the back passage). He designed an apparatus for administering it this way and claimed it as superior to inhalation as there was no excitement.

When ether is used as an inhalation patients go through a period of excitement when they struggle and might have to be forcibly restrained before surgical anaesthesia is achieved. With rectal ether, anaesthesia was induced rapidly and it lasted longer. He wrote a book *Recherché pratiques et physiologiques sur l'etherisation* which was published at the end of May 1847. Furthermore around this time he had the chance to try out anaesthesia in a military setting. In the beginning of spring 1847 mountain tribes in the Caucasus area rebelled against the Russian Government and Pirogoff was sent there to treat the wounded. He appears to have taken a number of anaesthetic masks with him; so many, if not all, of the anaesthetics must have been given by inhalation. The war only lasted for two months but in 1849 he published *Report medical d'un voyage Caucase.* A whole chapter was devoted to the use of ether in war. Having given it to 100 wounded soldiers his experience could not have been more different to Porter's and he concluded that it had no adverse influence on surgical results.[16]

JAMES YOUNG SIMPSON AND CHLOROFORM

There was no doubt that ether was having an effect on surgery both in war and peace within six months of its introduction into Europe. It must have been welcomed by soldier and civilian alike. However in civilian practice it seemed less than ideal. It had a very pungent smell and irritated patient's lungs and the excitable stage that patients passed through on their way to surgical anaesthesia could prove difficult to manage. In Scotland, James Young Simpson, Professor of Midwifery at the University of Edinburgh felt that there must be better agents that could be used, and set about investigating them.

Simpson began using ether in 1847 to relieve the pain of childbirth but was dissatisfied with some of ether's drawbacks, such as its disagreeable smell, the large quantities required and the lung irritation it caused. Ether was also explosive, which was a problem for doctors who often worked by candlelight in rooms heated by fireplaces! On the evening of 4 November 1847, Simpson and two doctor friends inhaled some chloroform and after feeling very happy and talkative, promptly passed out.

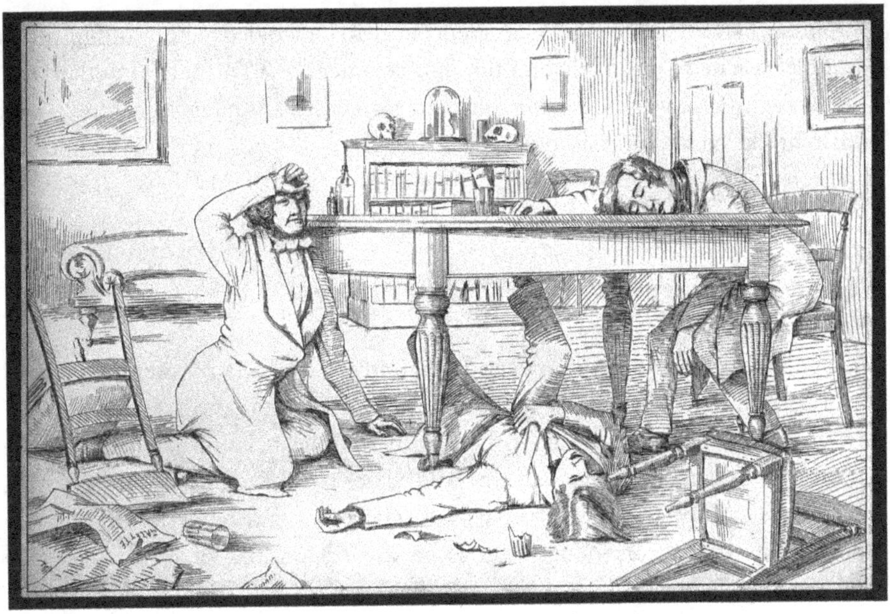

Figure 9.7. Simpson, Duncan & Keith recovering from the effects of the inhalation of chloroform. (Courtesy of Wellcome Library, London).

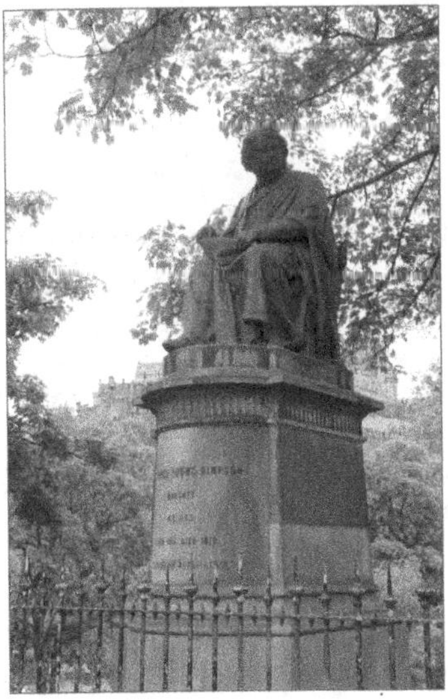

Figure 9.8. James Young Simpson. Statue in Princes Street Gardens, Edinburgh. (Photograph by James Robertson).

One of Simpson's companions was James Matthews Duncan, who was born in Aberdeen in 1826 and was the son of a shipping merchant. He was educated at the Grammar School and at Marischal College in Aberdeen where he took a Master of Arts degree. Medical studies followed in Aberdeen, Edinburgh and Paris, and in 1846 at the age of 20 he obtained an Aberdeen doctorate of medicine. Impressed with chloroform's potency and rapid effects, Simpson immediately knew that a new anaesthetic agent had been discovered.[17]

Simpson announced the discovery to the Medical and Chirurgical Society of Edinburgh on 10 November and he produced a pamphlet explaining its properties. Snow started to use chloroform as soon as he heard of its success. He warned however that it would need to be given more carefully than ether if accidents were to be avoided. A copy of Simpson's pamphlet reached Queen Victoria through her friend the Duchess of Sutherland. The new substance was much more pleasant than ether, less pungent without smell and it produced anaesthesia quickly and required nothing more than a pocket handkerchief for its administration.

A MAJOR DRAWBACK TO USE OF CHLOROFORM

Disaster struck on the 28th January 1848, and whilst having a toenail removed under its influence, Hannah Greener died. Hope turned to fear.

Discussions about what caused her death were heated and inconclusive. The pathologist said that the doctors involved weren't to blame. Simpson said that the doctors suffocated her whilst trying to revive her and Snow felt that giving chloroform without controlling the dosage was responsible. It proved to be the first of many deaths and the debate about the safety of chloroform versus ether began and went on for the rest of the century. Eventually in America, doctors reverted to using ether. "A good trial for manslaughter by a New England Jury would bring British doctors to a quickened sense of responsibility," commented the *Boston Medical and Surgical Journal* in 1870.[18]

CHLOROFORM IN WARFARE

Chloroform seems to have been used for casualties first of all in the Paris riots of 1848. Velpeau, a highly respected surgeon in Paris, cautioned against the use of chloroform in gunshot wounds because:

> Chloroform evidently depresses the nervous system and as great prostration always exists in patients who have received gunshot wounds it is advisable to refrain from any anaesthetic means.[19]

During the British war in the Punjab in India in 1848 and 1849 it was argued by J.J. Cole, military surgeon, that the stimulating effect of pain was necessary for the survival of soldiers with gunshot wounds.[20]

However, chloroform was used with success in two further campaigns before the outbreak of the Crimean War. In the Danish-Prussian War of 1850-51, all operations performed by surgeons from Schleswig-Holstein were undertaken using chloroform but this work wasn't published in a form that reached British doctors.[21] Furthermore the *Lancet* published a letter in 1851 from W.B. M'Egan, assistant surgeon to His Highness the Nizam's 2nd Regiment of Cavalry in India. He administered chloroform to 49 wounded enemy soldiers including 18 undergoing amputations, of whom only 3 succumbed. Why this report was overlooked is not known. Perhaps it was because the surgeon was unknown, or because it was thought that Indians would react differently to British soldiers.[22]

CHLOROFORM IN THE CRIMEAN WAR

Whatever the reason, there seemed to be a concern that chloroform would do more harm than good, and at the outbreak of the Crimean War the Principal Medical Officer of the British Army, John Hall, about whom much will be said in Chapter 10, cautioned against its use:

> However barbarous it may appear, the smart of the knife is a powerful stimulant and it is much better to hear a man bawl lustily than see him sink silently into the grave.[23]

James Syme, Professor of Clinical Surgery at Edinburgh wrote a quick reply to Hall's recommendations in which he stated:

> Pain, instead of being a powerful stimulant, most injuriously expends the nervous energy of weak patients, and therefore as far as the safety of the operation may be in question, chloroform proves useful directly in proportion to the severity of the injury, the disease, the danger and the degree of exhaustion or shock.[24]

Although by this time it was already obvious that ether was a much safer agent than chloroform the latter would always be the agent of choice for military anaesthesia on account of its ease of administration, speed of onset, the much smaller amount that was required to be transported and the fact that it wasn't explosive.

USE OF EXTREME COLD AS A MEANS OF PRODUCING ANAESTHESIA

In 1854 James Arnott published an article on *Instructions for using benumbing cold in operations*. He described at length a method for producing numbness of such intensity that operations including amputations could be carried out.[25] He was, of course, looking backwards to Larrey's observations during the retreat from Moscow that the limbs of soldiers made extremely cold by bad weather could be painlessly removed, and forward to the time when local anaesthesia would produce the same effect chemically. The patient remained conscious, thus adding to safety and there was a reduction in postoperative inflammation. Unfortunately despite these advantages, the time taken to use this technique would render it useless in war and so chloroform was perceived as being the only viable option.

The safety of chloroform was debated at length at various meetings of the Crimean Medical and Surgical Society for the duration of the war but it was never suggested that ether should be used instead unless in combination with other agents.

That surgeons ignored Hall's directive and proceeded to use chloroform is evident from the writings of the time. It wasn't always available in the quantities that were needed and recent research has shown, by analyzing ship and hospital store records, that during certain times the lack of availability of chloroform curtailed its use considerably.[26]

Another problem might have been lack of personnel to deliver chloroform. In answer to criticisms from the medical press that chloroform wasn't being used enough one surgeon wrote after the Battle of Inkerman:

> I hear there is a great cry against our not using chloroform; but the more I see the more I am strongly convinced that it is not of much value in the field; it reduces the number of medical men available for duty. It would be simply murder to leave the administration of it to any but educated hands and seldom can you get more than one doctor to assist at an operation.[27]

In the hospitals at Scutari chloroform seems to have been used in most cases despite the lack of "educated hands". The Rev. Osborne writing in his book *Scutari and its Hospitals* stated:

> Chloroform was always used and it appeared to me with the greatest of success; which I attribute a good deal, to the practice of using it on a

> handkerchief held lightly to the face, instead of the plan I have seen elsewhere of using some instrument, which whilst it secured the inhalation of the anaesthetic, excluded too much of the atmospheric air. I assisted at one very painful case........I am afraid to say the length of time the patient was under the influence of chloroform; his head was on my knee the greater part of the time, and I had to keep up the administration of this inestimable agent......I was then left with one of the surgeons, to try and recover him from the torpor under which he had, without pain, borne a most severe application of the knife etc. Our only hope from the quantity of blood he had lost, was, to get some stimulant taken as soon as we could; in vain we tried every means of rousing him; the pulsation of the heart was so weak, his whole appearance such, I had begun to despair. As a last resort, I found out his name, and had him sharply spoken to, so strong was the force of habit, that he made just sufficient effort to waken, to enable us to order him to drink the wine we gave him, keeping up the same sharp military tone of voice, we got more and more swallowed and he soon recovered![28]

For some surgeons the use of chloroform seemed to enable the patient to withstand the stress of a major operation better and they promoted its use. In 1856 James McGowan serving with HM's 55th Regiment stated:

> I need hardly add that all the capital operations were performed, the patients being first put under the influence of chloroform; indeed the amputation through the neck of the femur could not have been performed without anaesthesia with any prospect of the patient surviving the shock.[29]

Others found that it added to the stress and they concurred with Hall's idea. At the meeting of the Military Medical and Surgical Society on 10 July1856, Dr Mouat C.B., Deputy Inspector General, put the cat among the pigeons with an address which started as follows:

> The subject of the administration of chloroform in the well-known shock or depression following severe gunshot injuries is. ...... a fit and proper one for discussion in this Society. The profession at home naturally looks to the medical officers of the army to contribute their mite of practical experience towards the settlement of this important and disputed question; but I much fear they will be somewhat disappointed in the results and conclusions arrived at. Great and grave doubts are beginning to arise in the minds of

> some unprejudiced surgeons and thinking observers at home and abroad as to the indiscriminate use of this powerful anaesthetic, so tempting to the sufferer, yet at times so fraught with danger ....[30]

He felt that Hall's order given at the outbreak of war was:

> a wise and humane caution from an old and experienced officer in the field to his younger professional brethren.[31]

He reached the conclusion that it was unwise to risk the consequences of chloroform when the operation was relatively small such as a finger or toe amputation and dangerous to employ it when the injuries were extensive.

The use of chloroform during the Crimean War enabled many wounded soldiers to endure the pain of surgery and survive desperate operations but an equally large number would be so close to death at the point of being anaesthetized that the effect of chloroform, which is a cardiac depressant, would be disastrous. There is little evidence that any attention was paid to what we would call "care of the airway". When a patient is rendered unconscious, the tongue falls back and the breathing becomes obstructed unless manipulation of the jaw is carried out to prevent this happening. These effects of chloroform were probably short lived in most subjects and this didn't become an issue, but it must surely have had a deleterious effect on a significant minority of patients.

This truth about chloroform was perhaps best summed up by the comments of Richard Mackenzie, a young Edinburgh surgeon who distinguished himself at the Battle of Alma by performing 27 amputations in 24 hours only to succumb to cholera two days later. In a letter home he wrote:

> There is some truth in the use of chloroform being attended with risk in gunshot wounds. But surely the surgeons of the army have sufficient sense not to give it when a man is in a state of collapse bordering on death. Dr Hall's order is intended to discourage the use of it altogether. No one I should think will take any notice of it.[32]

The French also seem to have been shy of the use of chloroform at the beginning of the war, despite experience with it in the Algerian Wars. Perhaps the experiences of Velpeau with gunshot wounds had made an impression. However it was eventually used in nearly all cases. M. Mounier, chief medical officer of the hospital of Dolmar-Bagtche at Constantinople employed it in several thousand cases before 1855. He dispensed with complicated apparatus and used a simple cone made of paper with the apex cut off to allow the passage of air. The wider base was placed over the patient's nose and mouth and lint soaked in 20 to 30 drops of chloroform was added at the top. The cone was brought into contact with the patient for a few seconds and then lifted and replaced with greater frequency whilst the patient became used to the idea. He believed that there was no necessity to take the patient to the depths of anaesthesia where movement was completely abolished. The patient was to be horizontal and an assistant employed to watch the pulse and respiration. There is much to recommend M. Mounier's method and if given carefully as he recommended, the danger of chloroform would be greatly reduced. He felt that familiarizing native students of medicine in Constantinople with the safe use of chloroform was a useful benefit to have conferred on the local society.[33]

By the time of the 1855 meeting of the Academie des Sciences, chloroform had been used in 25,000 cases. The French employed it in three particular ways: *chloroformisation de prudence* to allow examination of patients, *chloroformisation de charite* to abolish severe pain in hopeless cases and *chloroformisation de necessite* for amputations and other painful procedures.

The Russians were perhaps the most enthusiastic users of chloroform under the direction of their medical leader, Pirogoff, who had pioneered rectal anaesthesia. In October 1854, Pirigoff was sent to Sevastopol, where he stayed until the war was over in 1856. He wanted chloroform used in all cases including dressings and examinations and it was reported by the French that wounded Russian soldiers would beg by signs to be given chloroform.

The vast experience of anaesthesia during the Crimea must have contributed to its establishment as a requirement in all forms of surgery. However there seems to have been little written about the effects of anaesthesia on the development of surgery. It was a significant boost to a soldier's morale not to hear the cries of their fellows suffering surgery without anaesthesia but surgical advances attributable to the availability of anaesthesia were minimal.

THE AMERICAN CIVIL WAR

Despite the early warnings from North America that British surgeons should revert to the safety of ether, when it came to the American Civil War, chloroform was used in abundance. The war began in 1861 when 11 Southern States declared themselves a confederacy in opposition to an anti- slave republican leader of the

Union States of the North. In the fourteen or so years since the discovery of ether and chloroform as anaesthetic agents, considerable knowledge had been amassed about them and experience gained in their delivery. Various pieces of apparatus had been devised for regulating the amount of anaesthetic used but free delivery of air was a problem and many practitioners preferred to use a towel shaped into a mask placed over the nose and mouth onto which chloroform or ether could be dripped. The American surgeon Valentine Mott, who wrote an essay on anaesthetics in 1862, stated:

> It was better to employ no special apparatus for inhalation. All that is needed is a common linen handkerchief on which the liquid is poured. This should be held loosely in the hands of the operator, as in the folded condition it might interfere too much with respiration.[34]

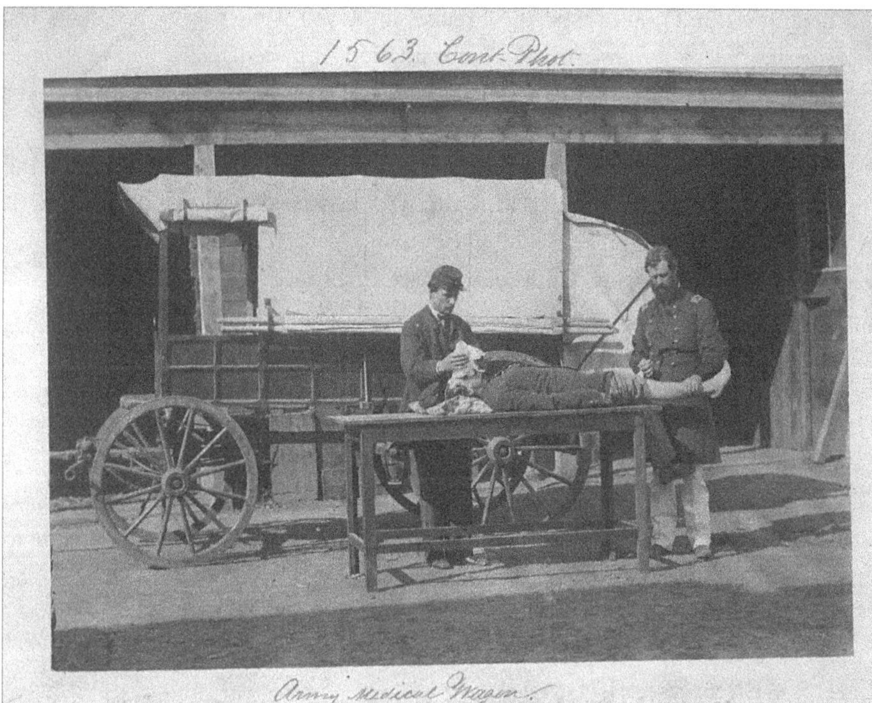

Figure 9.9. Staging of an amputation. The surgeon examines the leg while an assistant gives the anaesthetic on a sponge inside a cloth or towel held over the patient's face. In the background is a medicine wagon containing medicines, surgical supplies and instruments. (Courtesy of Otis Historical Archives. National Museum of Health and Medicine).

On the battlefield, inflammability, a rapid induction and the smaller volume required, made chloroform the preferred drug, whereas in the fixed base hospitals, ether was used.

Anaesthetic agents were mainly manufactured in the Northern States or imported from abroad. Mott was in the habit of using the chloroform made in Scotland by Duncan & Flockhart in Edinburgh, but Dr Squibb of Brooklyn was also able to manufacture the drug. Chloroform could therefore easily be obtained by Union forces in the North, but blockades of the ports made it much more difficult for Confederate forces to obtain adequate supplies. They did this by blockade running on the seas and capturing the supplies of the Union armies. There were also reports of smuggling of the drug in rag dolls. Eventually they developed manufacturing plants themselves.[35]

Much of the information about the extent of the use of anaesthetics in the American Civil War comes from the second volume of the third part of the *Medical and Surgical History of the War of the Rebellion* published in 1883,[36] which contains information about 80,000 cases treated under anaesthesia including 8,900 major operations. Chloroform was used in over 75% of cases.

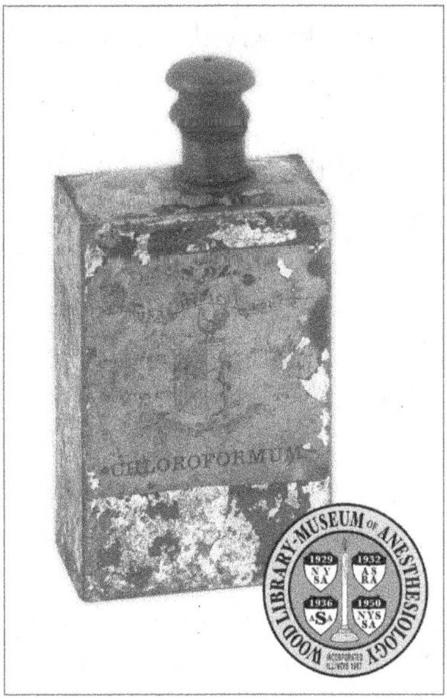

Figure 9.10. Tin of Chloroform. (Courtesy of the Wood Library-Museum of Anesthesiology, Park Ridge, IL).

ETHER AND ETHER/CHLOROFORM DURING AMERICAN CIVIL WAR - EARLY RESUSCITATION METHODS

The remaining cases were anaesthetized using either ether or a mixture of chloroform and ether. The deaths that occurred were all listed and to some extent analyzed. Two cases are recorded where "suspended animation was restored by energetic and prompt interference" and provide information on early resuscitation methods. They refer to the use of Marshall Hall's "ready method". Marshall Hall was an English physiologist who cast scorn on older methods of resuscitation and perhaps obviously to a 21st century mind advocated artificial respiration when breathing had stopped. This involved turning the patient on their front so that the tongue moved forward and didn't occlude the windpipe. Then the patient was turned on their side and alternately (about 15 times per minute) turned prone and back again to their side in order to expand the lungs. Initially drowning was the main indication for employing the technique, but it was also used to resuscitate the newborn, and then when life was ebbing away, after surgery or trauma. It was successful in the two cases described, although both men succumbed a number of days later.

Estimates of the use of anaesthesia during the Civil War amounted to some 125,000 cases. That it wasn't used in every case is shown in the writings of Louisa M. Alcott famous later for her "Little Women" books. She served as a volunteer nurse in the Union hospital at Georgetown and wrote:

> The amputations were reserved till the morrow and the merciful magic of ether was not thought necessary that day so the poor souls had to bear their pains as best they might.[37]

PIONEERING PRACTITIONERS IN UNION AND CONFEDERATE ARMIES

Two figures helped to promote the use of anaesthesia. In the Southern States, John Chisholm realized that the knowledge of military anaesthesia was scanty and produced a manual of military surgery which went through three editions. He was a strong advocate of the use of chloroform and it was claimed that he didn't have a single death in more than 10,000 cases, a remarkable achievement if true. As chloroform was difficult to come by in the South, he devised an inhaler that conserved its use. It consisted of a rectangular hollow portion with two metal

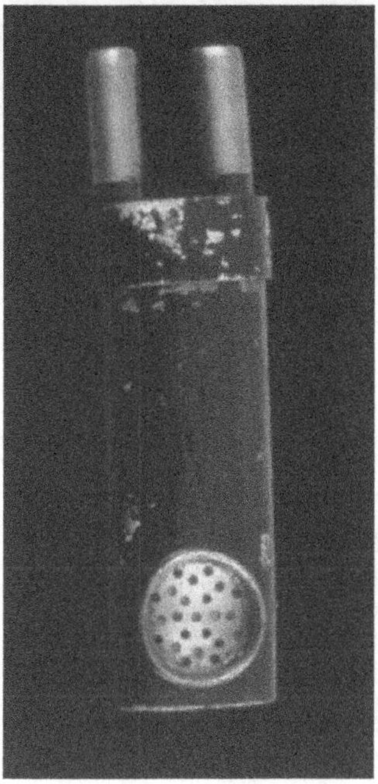

Figure 9.11. Chisholm Inhaler. (Courtesy of Otis Historical Archives. National Museum of Health and Medicine).

prongs which were inserted into the nostrils. The hollow part was filled with absorbent cotton, and a grid allowed chloroform to be poured onto the cotton. The inhaler was small enough to be carried in the pocket with the two prongs being pushed into the main body.[38]

In the north, Thomas Green Morton, who had successfully demonstrated the use of ether at the Massachusetts General Hospital in 1846 and who was a dentist by profession, probably became the first full time military anaesthetist. His experiences began at the Battle of Fredericksburg in 1862 and he was notified before the Battle of the Wilderness in 1864 that his services would be required. His original paper on the *Use of ether as an anaesthetic at the Battle of the Wilderness in the Civil War* commenced thus:

> On previous occasions it had been my privilege to visit battlefields and there to administer the pain destroying agent which it pleased God to make me the human agent to introduce for the benefit of suffering humanity. How little did I think, however, when originally experimenting with the properties of sulphuric ether on my own person, that I should ever successfully administer it to hundreds in one day and thus prevent an amount of agony fearful to contemplate.[39]

His paper described the terrible journey that soldiers had to endure on mule carts across unmade roads. Many had traumatic amputations and were begging pitifully for water. "It is the most sickening sight of war" he stated, "this tide of the wounded flowing back."

Mansions and churches were used as hospitals and he described the Baptist Church where the tank intended for immersion was used as a bath and operations were performed in the pastor's study at the back of the pulpit.

When the Battle of Spotsylvania Court House broke out a number of days later, Morton started a tour of the field hospitals to produce anaesthesia where capital (major) operations were to be performed:

> On the arrival of a train of ambulances at a field hospital the wounds were hastily examined and those who could bear the journey were sent to Fredericksburg. The nature of the operations to be performed was then decided on and noted on a piece of paper pinned to the pillow or roll of blanket under each patient's head. When this had been done I prepared the patient for the knife producing perfect anaesthesia in an average time of three minutes..........It was surprising to see with what dexterity and rapidity surgical operations were performed by scores in the same time really taken up by one case in peaceful regions.[40]

Morton was full of praise for the bravery of soldiers and the care they received at the hospitals around Washington once they could be evacuated.

It is difficult to know if the war had any effect on the subsequent practice of civilian anaesthesia, as the figures concerning its use were published so long afterwards, but it was certainly welcomed by all wounded soldiers. General "Stonewall" Jackson of the Confederacy, so named because of his refusal to allow the enemy to overcome his lines at the First Battle of Bull Run, was wounded by his own men through mistaken identity on 2 May 1863. On the way to the field infirmary he was described as having cold hands, clammy skin and bloodless lips. Quite clearly, he was suffering the effects of wound shock from loss of blood.

During the ambulance journey he was given whiskey and morphia, the former to revive him and the latter to provide pain relief. When, after arrival at the hospital, an amputation of the arm was considered necessary, he was given chloroform. As his conscious level fell he exclaimed "What an infinite blessing" and continued to repeat the word blessing until he became insensible. He lived for a few days after this, but the wound to his shoulder eventually proved fatal.[41]

THE FIRST MILITARY BLOOD TRANSFUSION IN THE AMERICAN CIVIL WAR

At the beginning of the nineteenth century wounded soldiers who had most likely already lost a considerable amount of blood were bled as part of their treatment. As discussed in Chapter 4, the amount of blood withdrawn was proportional to the severity of the initial wound. In many cases, this procedure must have contributed to their deaths.

While bloodletting was still held on to as a treatment for some decades, a few doctors began to realize that civilian patients and wounded soldiers were dying from blood loss. James Blundell, a London obstetrician carried out the first person to person transfusion in 1812 to save the life of a woman dying from a post partum haemorrhage. He was an Edinburgh graduate and may have been influenced by the work of John Leacock, another Edinburgh graduate who eventually practiced in Barbados. In 1816 he wrote *On the transfusion of blood in extreme cases of haemorrhage.* He argued against transfusion of blood between different species which had been attempted before Blundell's successful case and wrote:

> The consequences of haemorrhage where the functions are not dangerously affected do not of course require transfusion since other remedies will suffice. But when the danger is imminent and the common means are ineffectual as when a parturient woman trembles on the brink of the grave from uterine haemorrhage or when a soldier is at the point of death from loss of blood, what reason can be alleged for not having recourse to this last hope, and for not attempting the recruit from exhausted frame and turning the ebb of life.[42]

The first two military blood transfusions were carried out on patients during the American Civil War, one of whom survived and the other died. Both transfusions took place after the patients had suffered a secondary haemorrhage, which is often the result of infection destroying the blood vessels several days after the initial wounding. Both patients had been transferred to general hospitals. The blood was extracted from a donor with a syringe and injected directly into the recipient. The first patient received 16 ounces, the second just 2 but both showed an improvement with a stronger pulse. However whilst the first died some ten days later the second patient survived his wounds and yet it would be extraordinary to think that as little as 2 ounces of blood had saved his life.[43]

The Civil War lasted for four years but these two transfusions took place within days of each other in Union hospitals many miles apart. Perhaps it is puzzling that the technique wasn't practiced more widely but it seems fortuitous that in both cases the blood must have come from a compatible donor as haemolysis (destruction of red blood cells when blood is incompatible) didn't take place. The other problems that had to be overcome before transfusion was acceptable were transmission of infection and the tendency of the blood to clot when outside the body. The initial experimentation with blood replacement during the American Civil War was inexorably linked with the state known today as hypovolaemic shock, secondary to blood loss, although examination of various observations made during the nineteenth century reveals a very rudimentary understanding of the condition.

SHOCK

The state of hypovolaemic shock is characterized by a pale, cold and clammy patient with a weak pulse who lies largely unresponsive to his surroundings. The term is thought to come from a mistranslation of the word choc used by a French surgeon Henri Francois leDran (1685-1770) in a *Treatise of Reflections drawn from Gunshot Wounds* (1731) where it indicated a severe impact or jolt often leading to death.[44]

Peninsular surgeon George James Guthrie (Chapter 4) was the first person to use the term to describe the physiological instability seen after wounding, but he used it also to describe the effect on the nervous system of being involved in severe trauma. Indeed for the remainder of the century doctors would confuse the roles of the nervous and cardiovascular systems in producing the state of shock. It is the nervous system that controls the heart and blood vessels and puts the compensatory mechanisms in place. By constricting the peripheral blood vessels in the skin, it ensures that blood is directed to the vital organs such as the brain, thus rendering the skin cold and pale.

In severe trauma blood loss is the main problem, although soldiers were often dehydrated as well and would lose tissue fluid into severely injured parts. In certain climates, cold also played a part. One of the basic first aid measures to combat shock is to remove all wet clothing and provide warm blankets and a source of heat to bring the core body temperature to normal and in so doing, to improve the general condition of the wounded individual.

Even although there was a poor understanding of shock, it was written about by many of the surgeons involved in the American Civil War. Therapies recommended include stimulants such as alcohol, ammonia, hartshorn (ammonium carbonate) and turpentine. Mustard plasters and poultices of hot clay were also advised and Chisholm himself recommended that the combat surgeon treat casualties suffering from internal haemorrhage by performing urgent venotomy to bleed the patient and "save him from immediate death". To a 21st century mind it is extraordinary that the belief in bloodletting continued for so long when the transfusion of blood had already been introduced in an attempt to save lives. However, it would not be until 1917, during the Great War, that blood transfusion would become firmly established as a recognized and important weapon to be used in the treatment of shock, when stored blood was used for the first time at the Battle of Cambrai.

Between 1890 and the beginning of the Great War, work by George Washington Crile, an American surgeon who operated on trauma victims in Ohio, would lay the foundations for the work carried out on wound shock during that war. He appreciated that measuring blood pressure gave a clinical indication of the degree of shock and was one of those who pioneered the use of intravenous fluids and blood transfusion. He was able to put some of his knowledge into practice when he arrived at the American Hospital in Paris in 1914. However it would be later on in the Great War when the British put together a team of surgeons and physiologists to investigate shock that real progress was made.[45]

RE-EMERGENCE OF NITROUS OXIDE AS AN ANAESTHETIC

The possibility that nitrous oxide could be a useful anaesthetic did not re-emerge until 1862 when Gardner Quincy Colton, who was still performing his demonstrations of "laughing gas" in Paris whilst the rest of his countrymen were fighting a war, was asked by a lady if she could have a tooth extracted under its effects. With Colton giving the gas, a dentist successfully extracted a tooth without the patient feeling pain. Colton soon realised that he could earn a substantial living using nitrous oxide for dentistry. Spragues of Boston invented an apparatus for manufacturing it and methods for administering it were devised.

In 1867 Colton demonstrated his apparatus at the fourth international exhibition in Paris, where also the First International Congress of Medicine was being held. Colton had by this time used nitrous oxide in 24,000 cases.[46] Some doctors claimed that it was an asphyxiating agent and to a certain extent they were correct but it also has pain killing properties. In order to produce an anaesthetic state it is necessary to breathe the gas at almost 100% concentration, thus denying the patient an adequate supply of oxygen. This of course can only be carried out without harm if it is done for a limited period of time thereby enabling the extraction of a tooth.

The Spragues apparatus was costly and cumbersome and could only be installed by the most prosperous dentists. In July 1869 nitrous oxide could be compressed into cylinders and was produced on a commercial scale. Shortly afterwards Coxeter & Sons of London managed to do the same and also provided gasometers for dental surgeries into which the gas could be decanted. In 1870, spurred on by work in France, Coxeter managed to store the compressed gas in liquid form in cylinders.

THE FRANCO-PRUSSIAN WAR

Prior to the Franco-Prussian War of 1870-71 antisepsis as advocated by Lister (Chapter13) had been introduced into European practice and was the concern of every civilian operating surgeon. Perhaps the inevitable concentration of the mind towards this aspect of practice, led to the possibility that anaesthetic developments could have been overshadowed.

An International Committee for the Relief of Wounded and Combatants (later to be the Red Cross) had been established in Geneva in 1863 but it wasn't until August 1870 that a similar committee was convened in Britain (Chapter 13). This committee initially sent out a number of surgeons and nurses to France to serve in equal proportions in French and Prussian armies. Large sums of money were collected and stores and equipment procured including surgical instruments and chloroform.

On 27 September, soon after the fall of Strasbourg, some British Red Cross workers entered the city "where blood and iron, passion and hatred had done their worst". They arrived with chloroform and this was "probably the first instance of such mitigation of the horrors of a siege".

The British surgeons and nurses seemed to have played quite a substantial role in the hospitals. Sir William MacCormac became surgeon-in-chief to the Anglo-American Ambulance and he stressed the need for early examination of gunshot wounds before inflammation had a chance to arise, the cautious use of bullet extraction forceps, early primary amputation and the use of chloroform and carbolic lotion.[47]

BLOOD TRANSFUSION IN FRANCO-PRUSSIAN WAR

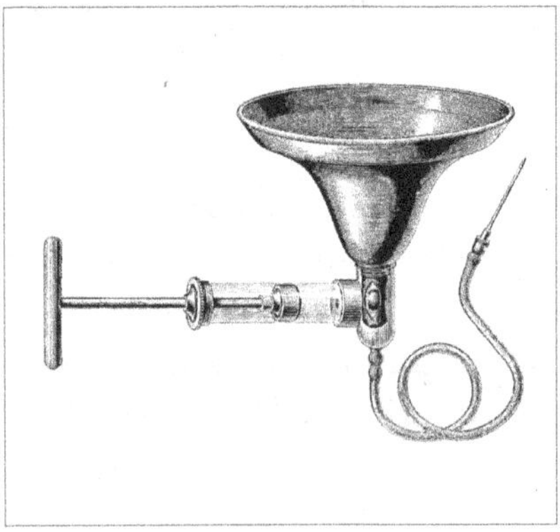

Figure 9.12. Collins Transfuser. (From Esmarch, F., (translated Clutton, H. H.,). *The Surgeon's Handbook on the Treatment of the Wounded in War.* New York: L. W. Schmidt, 1878.

Reports of blood transfusion being carried out during the Franco- Prussian War are difficult to find although we know from indirect sources that it was used to some extent. In 1864 Dr J. Roussel of Geneva devised an apparatus to allow direct transfusion from one individual to another. Previously, methods of removing fibrin (clots) from blood were devised known as defibrinators but Roussel's apparatus served to extract the blood from the donor by a syringe and immediately inject it into a recipient's vein before clotting could occur.48 Writing about it later he deplored the fact that it hadn't really been used to good effect during the Franco-Prussian War and it was 1876 before it was demonstrated to the Medical Society of London.[49]

However on the German side blood transfusion is believed to have been used more extensively and perhaps even on the battlefield. Friedrich von Esmarch was appointed surgeon general to the Prussian Army in 1870 and produced a handbook of military surgery after the war.[50] In it he ascribed several pages to the transfusion of blood and the mechanism by which it should be given. Blood was defibrinated by twirling it with a spatula and then sieving it through linen into a glass vessel where it was kept until needed. He advocated a Collins transfuser apparatus for transfusion and said that this has been introduced into the French Army.

A MISSED OPPORTUNITY

An opportunity to discover the benefits of nitrous oxide in warfare was lost at this time.

Dr J.L.W. Thudichum, a German living in England and director of a newly formed chemico-pathological laboratory at St Thomas's Hospital, appealed in the press for the use of nitrous oxide in military surgery. The nitrous oxide fund reached £184 10s, and Coxeter forwarded 3,000 gallons of the compressed gas to Dr Thudichum and 2,000 gallons to Paris. There was no evidence that it was ever used.[51]

It was not until the Great War that nitrous oxide came into its own when it was recognized that it was the only safe agent in wounded soldiers who were close to death from shock. A quick whiff of nitrous oxide and oxygen, although insufficient to produce anaesthesia in the healthy and robust, would allow amputation of a limb and the arrest of haemorrhage in the badly wounded who might succumb if given chloroform or ether. Had doctors made use of the substantial amounts of nitrous oxide made available during the Franco-Prussian War, they would probably have discovered its useful properties and become aware of its relative safety for use with badly wounded soldiers.

THE DANGER OF CHLOROFORM

Deaths from chloroform anaesthesia were regularly reported in the medical press and this prompted the formation of seven committees and commissions over the course of the second half of the nineteenth century and the beginning of the twentieth century to investigate the cause and to make recommendations.[52]

Most of the deaths occurred in young and healthy subjects undergoing minor procedures and this was of concern to medical men, despite living in an age when death from incurable disease, surgery and trauma was a daily occurrence.

Chloroform committees and commissions

- 1864 Royal Medico-Chirurgical Society;
- 1877 The Glasgow Committee;
- 1888 First Hyderabad Commission;
- 1889 Second Hyderabad Commission;
- 1891 BMA Anaesthetics Committee;
- 1893 *Lancet* Questionnaire;
- 1901 BMA Special Chloroform Committee.

Both of the first two committees reported that chloroform had a deleterious effect on the heart. The first suggested using chloroform in a mixture with ether and alcohol and the second using a new agent ethidene which they considered to occupy an intermediate position between ether and chloroform. In other words, they sought to mitigate the deleterious effects of chloroform whilst preserving its advantages in terms of speed of onset.

The first Hyderabad Commission of 1888 was somewhat different. Surgeon-Major Lawrie of the Bengal Medical Service and Principal of the Hyderabad Medical School carried out a series of experiments on dogs in which he stated that in no way did the heart become dangerously affected until after the breathing had stopped. He said that in 40 or 50 thousand cases he had never seen the heart affected and that deaths would continue to occur until the London schools ignored the heart altogether or confined themselves to giving ether which they knew how to manage!

This prompted the sending of a physiologist, T. Lauder Brunton, paid for by the Nizam of Hyderabad, to repeat the experiments. Four hundred and ninety animals were subjected to the effects of chloroform and Brunton concurred with Lawrie, that respiration was affected before the heart stopped. The report was published over many months in the *Lancet*, and in 1893 this publication sent out a questionnaire to every hospital in Great Britain and a number abroad. Chloroform was most commonly given from a handkerchief or sponge and showed that clinically death appeared to occur from heart failure. This was in complete opposition to the results from Hyderabad.

The committee set up by the British Medical Association in 1891 showed that chloroform was the commonest anaesthetic used and that it had a higher death rate.

These committees therefore never really solved the controversy, but they did result in research being directed to a more physiological level.

There was no doubt that the ease and speed of giving chloroform was preferred by many people especially those trained in Edinburgh and they sought to argue against the known safety of ether in a way that to our safety conscious society would seem at best ill guided. It was not until 1911, sixty-four years after its introduction that Goodman Levy, a physiologist, demonstrated that chloroform could produce fibrillation of the heart muscle, which is an uncontrolled quivering which renders the heart useless as a pump. Furthermore, if circulating adrenaline was high as in the case of an anxious patient, particularly if lightly anaesthetized, then the effect was compounded. The cause of Hannah Greener's death was finally known.

SECOND BOER WAR (1899-1902)

Anaesthesia receives little mention in accounts of the Second Boer War of 1899-1902 and the Surgeon General's report of the war stated:

> The proper anaesthetic for the field and the only one desirable in hot climates is chloroform.[53]

Doctors on horseback were provided with a saddle bag containing a bottle of chloroform and base hospitals were supplied with ten pounds of chloroform and five pounds of ether. The only reference to a change might be the indication by a British surgeon that he used ethyl chloride. This substance was originally used as a spray to obtain local anaesthesia but its general anaesthetic properties were recognized in the 1890s and it enjoyed some usage for about twenty years.

At the siege of Ladysmith (Chapter 15) anaesthetics were given by junior surgeons. On arrival at a field hospital a soldier requiring an operation might be given Bovril or brandy as pre-medication along with morphine if necessary.[54] There was of course no monitoring of the patient's condition in terms of blood pressure. Perhaps a finger was kept on the pulse and some regard paid to colour and respiration but this is only conjecture. Cardiovascular collapse was treated with strychnine and brandy and sometimes musk derived from the glands of musk deer found in India which stimulated the part of the brain controlling respiration. If the patient was shocked, that is cold, grey and clammy from blood loss then their legs were elevated and they were given subcutaneous ether, strychnine and sometimes rectal saline. Hewitt had, in his 1893 book *Anaesthetics and their Administration*, suggested the use of intravenous saline as a method of raising the blood pressure but there was little interest in this idea and rectal saline remained an accepted practice up to and including the Great War.

EARLY TRAINING OF ANAESTHETISTS

The early pioneers of anaesthesia learned their profession by experience and to some extent by trial and error. Anaesthetic agents were new drugs and the inhalational route was a new way of giving a drug. There was nothing before 1847 that would prepare these men for their careers and a vision of what the future might be in surgical practice was unimaginable. For the most part it was sufficient that surgical pain could be abolished. However the development of the speciality has always relied on men willing to devote time and energy to the subject. John Snow and Joseph Clover are notable early examples of this but the death of Joseph Clover in 1882 deprived anaesthesia of a figurehead to drive the speciality forward. Despite his legacy he didn't leave a manual of practice that could be followed. This led to a number of untrained and infrequent practitioners administering anaesthesia.

However, by 1890 two anaesthetists arrived on the scene who tried to change this practice. They were Dudley Buxton of University College Hospital and Frederick Hewitt of the London and Charing Cross Hospitals. Both men produced manuals of anaesthetics which set out methodically the principles involved in administering anaesthesia. In 1892 Frederick Silk, assistant anaesthetist to Guys Medical School advocated that training should be systematic and included in every medical student's curriculum.[55] However it would be 1912 before the General Medical Council, largely as a result of the lobbying of these three individuals, would include anaesthetics as the last of 16 subjects to be included in the undergraduate curriculum of all medical schools.

DEVELOPMENT OF ARMY MEDICAL SERVICES

One of Hewitt's colleagues at the London Hospital was the surgeon Frederick Treves (the two of them would be called upon to operate on the appendix abscess of Edward VII in 1902.) Treves had volunteered to lead a civilian surgical team to assist in the South African War in 1899. He wrote an account of his time there called *The Tale of a Field Hospital* but his only mention of anaesthesia is to state that:

> There is little room in the tent for other than the surgeon, his assistant, the anaesthetist and a couple of orderlies.[56]

Treves is supposed to have written a paper about chloroform but no trace can be found of it. Although supportive of the army medical services at the time Treves was critical of their organization and training after the war. Many of his observations were incorporated into army medical regulations and the revised RAMC Training Book published in 1911. This army training manual makes no mention of anaesthesia other than to say "that a small table is made available for the anaesthetist's use".

In 1908 general hospital units were formed within the newly formed Territorial Army. Treves wrote to the British Medical Journal asking members for feedback regarding the interests that should be available in these hospitals. This led to correspondence with Robert James Probyn-Williams, Senior Consulting Anaesthetist and Instructor in Anaesthetics at the London Hospital and the then President of the London Society of Anaesthetists. Treves sent the following reply:

> Dear Dr Williams
>
> There is no such post as Anaesthetist in the Army Medical Service nor does an Anaesthetist figure among the staff of a General Hospital.
>
> This applies to the Regular Service. In the Territorial Force there will be four General Hospitals in London and there can be no doubt whatever but that Anaesthetists will be required for these hospitals and that their services will be very highly appreciated. The Territorial Force is being mobilized on the lines of the Regular Army and therefore no such post as Anaesthetist appears.

> I think you would do well to join one of the General Hospitals as a Physician or Surgeon it being understood that in the event of an invasion you would act in your usual capacity as Anaesthetist..........
>
> Yours very truly
> Frederick Treves.[57]

It would seem from this letter that although Treves acknowledged the value and necessity of anaesthetists he did not intend to influence the army, either regular or territorial, to adopt the role officially. This was a huge opportunity lost and led to anaesthesia at the outbreak of the Great War being given by a largely untrained work force. In particular there was no one to lead and steer its practice and when casualties streamed into casualty clearing stations requiring immediate and definitive surgery a few career anaesthetists and many more junior doctors did the best they could. It would be 1917 before Geoffrey Marshall carried out his work defining the best anaesthetics for particular situations.

At the beginning of the nineteenth century a wounded soldier or seaman could hope for little more than a tot of brandy to help him through the trauma of surgery but by the time Queen Victoria's reign ended anaesthesia was a firmly established routine and all battle wounded could expect oblivion for an operative procedure.

Advances in physiology which enabled doctors to understand how the cardiovascular and respiratory systems functioned in health and disease, along with instruments to monitor and measure what was happening, would be required before real progress was made during the Great War.

ENDNOTES

1. Snow, J.," On the Inhalation of Vapour of Ether in Surgical Operations", *The Lancet* 1847; (i): pp.551-554.
2. Stanley, P., *For Fear of Pain - British Surgery, 1790-1850,* Amsterdam-New York: Editions Rodopi B.V, 2003.
3. Gribbin, J., *Science: A History.* London: The Penguin Press, 2002.
4. Uglow, J., *The Lunar Men.* London: Faber and Faber Ltd, 2002.
5. Lamont-Brown, R., *Humphrey Davy: Life Beyond the Lamp:* Gloucestershire: Sutton Publishing Ltd., 2004.
6. Hennen, J., *Principles of Military Surgery.* London: John Wilson, 1829.

7. Yudin, S.S., "Refrigeration Anesthesia for Amputations", *Anaesthesia and Analgesia* 1945; pp.216-219.
8. Snow, Stephanie J., *Blessed days of anaesthesia,* New York: Oxford University Press, 2008, p.22.
9. Smith, W.D.A., *Henry Hill Hickman.* Sheffield: J.W. Northend Limited, 2005.
10. Snow, *op.cit,* p.21.
11. *Ibid.*
12. *Ibid.*
13. Aldrete, J.A., G.M. Marron, A.J.Wright, "The first administration of anaesthesia in military surgery: on occasion of the Mexican-American War", *Anesthesiology* 1984; 61: pp.585-8.
14. Porter, J.B., "Medical and Surgical Notes of Campaigns in the war with Mexico, during the years 1845, 1846, 1847 & 1848", *The American Journal of the Medical Sciences* 1852; 45: pp.13-37.
15. Glew, P.A., "The Naval Career of Thomas Spencer Wells", *Proceedings of the History of Anaesthesia Society* 1996; 19: pp.31-37.
16. Secher, O., "Nikolai Ivanovich Pirogoff", *Anaesthesia* 1986; 41: pp.829-837.
17. Snow, *Op.cit,* p.44.
18. Snow, *Op.cit,* p.51.
19. Velpeau, M., "Gravity and Treatment of Gunshot Wounds", *The Lancet* 1848; (i): pp.3-5.
20. Connor, H., "The Use of Military Anaesthesia in the 19th century", In: Drury, P.M.E. (Editor): *Proceedings of the Sixth International Symposium on the History of Anaesthesia.* Reading: Conservatree, 2007.
21. Metcalfe, N.H., " The influence of the military on civilian uncertainty about modern anaesthesia between its origins in 1846 and the end of the Crimean War in 1856", *Anaesthesia*, 2005; 60: pp.549-601.
22. McEgan, W.B., "Chloroform in India", *The Lancet* 1851; (ii): p.1851.
23. Snow, *Op.cit,* p.99.
24. Shepherd, J A., "The Smart of the Knife – Early Anesthesia in the services", *Journal of the Royal Army Medical Corps* 1985; 131: pp.109-115.
25. Arnott, J., "Instructions for using benumbing cold in operations", *Med. Times and Gaz.* 1854; ii: pp.488-90.
26. Connor, H., "The Use of Chloroform by British Army Surgeons during the Crimean War", *Medical History,* 1998; 42: pp.161-193.
27. Shepherd, J.A., *Op.cit.*
28. Osborne, S G., *Scutari and its Hospitals.* London: Dickinson Brothers, 1855.

29. McGowan, J. H., "An Account of the Wounded of H.M.'s Fifty-Fifth Regiment", *Med. Times & Gaz.*, 1856; pp.205-206.
30. Mouat, A., "Observations on some points connected with the use of chloroform in military practice". *The Lancet* 1856; ii: pp.78-81.
31. (Memoir of Mackenzie) *Monthly Journal of Medical Science* 1854; 19: pp.474-478.
32. *Ibid.*
33. Mounier, M., "On the employment of chloroform in the Army of the East", *Medical Times & Gazette* 1855; 1: p.605.
34. Mott, V. *Pain and Anaesthetics an Essay.* Washington: Government Printing Office, 1862.
35. Wilbur, C.K., *Civil War Medicine.* Guildford, Connecticut: The Globe Pequot Press, 1998.
36. United States Surgeon General's Office. *Medical and Surgical History of the War of the Rebellion.* Washington, 1883; 2 (iii): pp.887-898.
37. Alcott, L.M., *Hospital sketches and Camp and Fireside Stories.* Boston: Roberts Brothers, 1869.
38. Worthington, W.C., "Confederates, Chloroform and Cataracts: Julian John Chisholm (1830-1903)", *Southern Medical Journal,* 1986; 79: pp.748-752.
39. Morton, W.T.G., "The Use of Ether as an anesthetic at the Battle of the Wilderness", Chicago: Reprint. *Journal of the American Medical Association.* April 23, 1904.
40. *Ibid.*
41. Aldin, M.S., "The Use of Anesthetics during the Civil War, 1861-1865", *Bulletin of Anesthesia History*, 2001; 19: pp.1-11.
42. Learoyd, P., *A Short History of Blood Transfusion.* Published by the National Blood Service.
43. Kuhns, W.J., "Historic Milestones Blood Transfusion in the Civil War", *Transfusion* 1965; 5: pp.92-94.
44. Millham, F H., " A brief History of Shock", *Surgery* 2010; 148: pp.1026-1037.
45. Boulton, T.B., "The Role of George Washington Crile in the development of anaesthesia", *Proceedings of the History of Anaesthesia Society* 1991; 9B: pp.54-59.
46. Duncum, B., *The Development of Inhalational Anaesthesia.* London: Oxford University Press 1947.
47. Swain, A.J.V., "Franco-Prussian War 1870-71: Voluntary Aid for the Wounded and Sick", *British Medical Journal* 1970; 3: pp.514-517.

48. Lefrere, J.J. & Danic, B., "Pictorial Representation of transfusion over the years", *Transfusion* 2009; 49: pp.1007-1017.
49. Royal Medical and Chirurgical Society Oct 28 1876. *The Lancet*; 108: pp.608-609.
50. Esmarch, F., (translated Clutton, H. H.,). *The Surgeons Handbook on the treatment of the Wounded in War.* New York: L. W. Schmidt, 1878.
51. Gray, T Cecil., "Mitchiner Memorial Lecture 'Another Side of Mars", *Journal of the Royal Army Medical Corps* 1984; 130: pp.3-11.
52. Thomas, K B., "Chloroform: Commissions and Omissions", *Proceedings of the Royal Society of Medicine* 1974; 67: pp.723-730.
53. Metcalfe, N H., " Military influence upon the development of anaesthesia from the American Civil War (1861-1865) to the outbreak of the First World War", *Anaesthesia* 2005; 60: pp.1213-1217.
54. Hovell, B., "Anaesthesia and the Siege of Ladysmith", *Proceedings of the History of Anaesthesia Society* 1994; 15: pp.55-59.
55. Silk, J.F.W., "Anaesthetics a necessary part of the curriculum", *The Lancet* 1891; 139: pp.1178-1180.
56. Treves, F., The *Tale of a Field Hospital.* London, Paris, New York & Melbourne: Cassell and Company Ltd., 1900.
57. Bennett, J. A., "War of Ideas", *Proceedings of the History of Anaesthesia Society* 1994; 15: pp.59-65.

10

The Crimea

BACKGROUND

The Crimean War (1853-56) was fought between the Russian Empire and a strategic alliance comprising the British Empire, France, the Ottoman Empire and Sardinia.

Following the treaty of Vienna on 25 March 1815, (also known as "Treaty of General Alliance") Austria, Britain, Prussia and Russia agreed to put 150,000 men in the field against Napoleon Bonaparte following his escape from Elba. The War of the Seventh Coalition culminated with the defeat of Napoleon at Waterloo. Russia subsequently assumed the role of the "policeman of Europe" with the intention of maintaining a balance of power within Europe and preventing further conflicts. In turn, Russia expected other European countries to allow it to resolve its own problems with the declining Ottoman Empire, referred to as the "Sick man of Europe" without any opposition or intervention. The Sultan of the Ottoman Empire was unable to control his vast Empire effectively and all the European powers were aware of this. The potential breakup of the Empire might lead to some taking advantage of the situation and they all watched each other very carefully.

Russia was keen to develop and extend its own influence in the Balkans and to take control of the straits between the Mediterranean and the Black Sea from the Ottoman Empire. The International Straits Commission of 1841 resulted in the closure of the Bosphorus and the Dardanelles to warships of all nationalities and this included Russia. As a result, the Russian naval fleet was confined to the Black Sea. Other European nations were concerned by Russia's desire to extend its interest into the Balkans and even to Constantiople, which was of strategic importance in controlling trade between Europe and Asia.

These predisposing factors and rising tensions were important in setting the course for war and a further key event occurred in 1851, when Napoleon III made it known that he wanted France to assume the sovereign role in the Holy Land. This was of major significance because an earlier treaty (Kuchuk Kainarji, 1774) had established Russia as the protector of Orthodox Christianity within the Ottoman Empire. France initially moved along diplomatic lines, but soon added to diplomacy with a show of naval strength when it sent one of its warships, "Charlemagne", into the Black Sea. As a result, Sultan Abdulmecid I agreed to a new treaty, which established the Roman Catholic Church and France as the authority in the Holy Land with concomitant control over the key Christian sites.

This was a provocation to Russia and Tsar Nicholas I responded by positioning his 4th and 5th armies along the River Danube while he continued to pursue a diplomatic course with Britain and France. A key aspect of Russia's policy was to avoid involvement of Britain or France should a military conflict arise between Russia and the Ottoman Empire. Despite a series of diplomatic manoeuvres, some aggressive negotiating by a Russian diplomat, Prince Menshikov, caused tensions to rise further. In February 1853, Menshikov arrived on a Russian naval ship for further discussions in Constantinople. He made a series of demands on the Ottoman Empire and requested an international conference to negotiate a new treaty which would establish Russia with the same role for Orthodox Christians, as had been granted to France for Catholics.

Russia's demand was rejected by the Ottoman Empire in which it was supported by the new British envoy, Lord Stratford, representing Lord Aberdeen's government and war moved ever closer. Russia used the Ottoman rejection as a reason, one might even say an excuse, to provide protection for Orthodox Christians and Russian armies moved into the Ottoman–ruled Principalities of Moldavia and Wallachia (along the River Danube) on 2 July 1853, over which they had a previously agreed right to protect Orthodox Christians. In response to this threat of Russian expansionism, both Britain and France sent fleets into the Dardanelles and whilst still hoping that a diplomatic solution to the crisis might occur, further negotiations failed.

On 23 October 1853, the Ottoman Empire declared war on Russia and both land and sea battles ensued. The Ottoman fleet was destroyed at the Battle of Sinope on 30 November 1853. Fighting continued along the Danube in the occupied Principalities and by the spring of 1854 Russian forces crossed the River Danube and occupied Bulgaria, a Turkish province. By doing so they hoped to encourage Serbs and Bulgarians living under Ottoman rule to rebel but they showed little interest in doing so. There was fierce fighting on both banks of the river.

An Anglo-French ultimatum was issued to Russia to withdraw from the Danubian Principalities by 28 March 1854 which was ignored and Britain and France declared war on Russia.

Russian forces finally began to pull back from the Danube in June 1854 when they came under increasing pressure from Austria which felt threatened by the Russian presence. Tsar Nicholas 1 completed the withdrawal of his armies from the Danubian Principalities in July 1854 and by doing so he effectively removed the cause for the war with Britain and France.

However Britain and France persevered. They saw this as an opportunity to put a stop to Russian expansionism into the states of the weakened and crumbling Ottoman Empire. In June 1854 British and French ships landed an allied expeditionary force at Varna on the Bulgarian coast and at Constantinople. The troops in Varna were intended to support the Ottoman forces on the Danube; they remained at their base and made no move inland towards the Russian armies.

In September 1854 the Allies landed at Eupatoria to the north of Sevastopol on the Crimean Peninsula. Their objective was to besiege the Russian Black Sea naval base at Sevastopol where there were 24,400 Russian troops. Allied forces

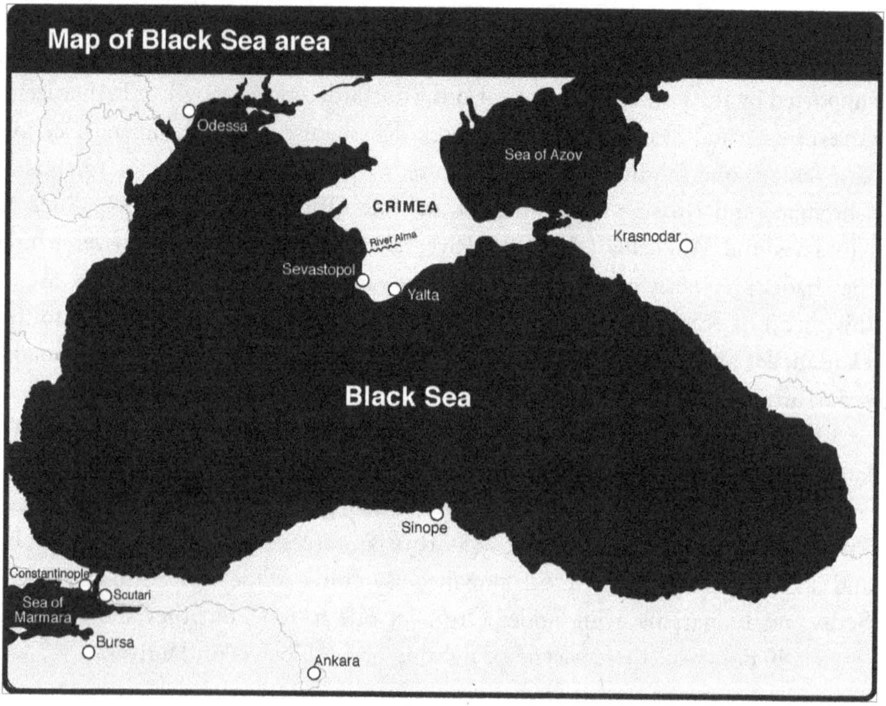

Figure 10.1. Map of the Crimea showing the situation in general.

numbered 23,000 British, 33,000 French and 7,000 Turks. They planned to destroy the base and fleet before it could become a threat elsewhere.

The allies thought that victory would be achieved within 3 months but they miscalculated badly and it required three major battles over a period of 12 months to achieve their objective.

The Battle of the River Alma was on 20 September 1854 and this was followed by the Battle of Balaclava on 25 October 1854, when the Russians attacked an allied supply base. While the Russian attack at Balaclava was defeated, it was here that the infamous Charge of the Light Brigade, led by the Earl of Cardigan took place. Of the 700 men taking part in this cavalry charge, approximately 200 survived unscathed. This action led to the award of the first Victoria Cross to a medical officer, surgeon James Mouat. Mouat was born in 1815 in Chatham, England. He was the son of a surgeon also called James Mouat. After studying medicine at University College Hospital, London he qualified in 1837. He joined the army and served in various places including India before his time in the Crimea. Mouat won his Victoria Cross by saving the life of Acting Lieutenant Colonel Morris of the 17th Lancers, who had been severely wounded in the skull and arm, by stopping life-threatening bleeding whilst under severe enemy fire[1]. He survived the Crimean War and went on to serve in New Zealand, before becoming Inspector General. He was knighted in 1894.

The Battle of Inkerman was on 5 November 1854. Russian forces tried to create a diversion to relieve the siege of Sevastopol by attacking the allies at the nearby town of Inkerman, but without success.

The allies had dug in around Sevastopol and the Russians endured sustained attacks, but severe winter weather brought a close to operations until April 1855, when attacks resumed until the city fell on 9 September 1855.

Fighting continued, not just in the Crimea but also in the Baltic, White Sea and in the Far East around the Kamchatka Peninsula and the Islands of Sakhalin and Urup.

Peace negotiations at the Congress of Paris began on 1 February 1856 where all the great European powers were represented and by 30 March 1856 the Treaty of Paris was signed to end the war. All powers agreed to maintain "the integrity of the Ottoman Empire" and to ensure that Turkey remained independent. The borders of Russia and Turkey were realigned to where they had been before the war. Russia gave up its claim to be the protector of Orthodox Christians and Moldavia, Wallachia and Serbia became self-governing principalities under the protection of other European powers. The Black Sea and River Danube would be open to all nations but warships would not be allowed into the Black Sea. By the

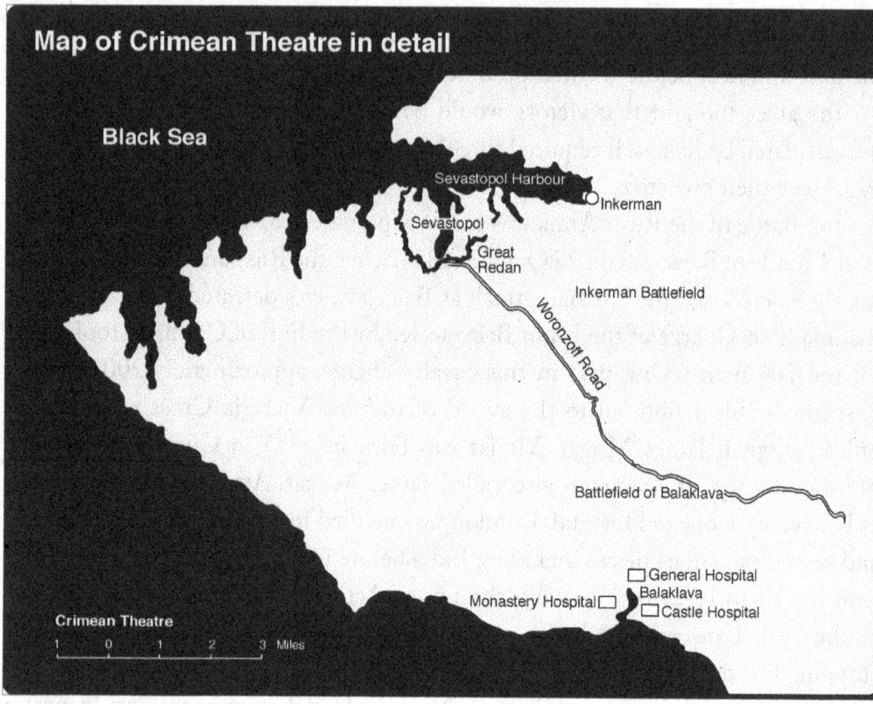

Figure 10.2. Map of the Crimea focusing on the Crimean Peninsula.

end of the war Russia had sustained 450,000 casualties, Britain 22,000 and France approximately 95,000. A more detailed breakdown of casualties is given in Table 10.1.[2]

Table 10.1 Mortality for the British and French armies 1854-1856.

	BRITISH	FRENCH
Number of troops	97,964	309,268
Deaths from all causes (% of troops)	21,827 (22.3%)	72,415 (23%)
Died from wounds/killed in action (% of all deaths)	4,602 (21%)	12,604 (17%)
Died from infections/disease (% of all deaths)	17,225 (79%)	59.815 (83%)

From Gill, C.J., G.C.Gill, "Nightingale in Scutari: her legacy re-examined". *Clinical Infectious Diseases 2005*, 40: pp. 1799-1805.

THE MEDICAL SERVICES DURING THE LEAD UP TO WAR

The Director General of the Army Medical Department was Dr Andrew Smith, the son of a Scottish crofter. The medical services were ill-prepared for war in 1854. Smith was informed that he must provide medical support for an army in response to the Russian threat only twelve days before troops were due to embark. Smith had little idea of the likely medical requirements although he tried to get some idea from existing documentation of the Peninsular War. He alone was left to plan the medical support and to decide what equipment and personnel would be required.[3] There was no existing plan on which to base the requirements for a European war.

Smith was informed that a force of 10,000 would be despatched to Malta and that it might be expected to support Turkish soldiers fighting against the Russians. He was to supply medical personnel together with all the necessary medicines and supplies. He sent three surgeons to anticipated areas of conflict to get some idea of medical requirements. They were sent to the Black Sea, the Balkans, to Constantinople, Gallipoli and Belgrade.

Smith was greatly hindered by bureaucracy. He was accountable to many different departments and worked within a difficult, cumbersome and time-consuming framework with some examples below:[4]

- Matters of policy – in all matters relating to finance, equipment, supplies and promotions he was accountable to the military secretary to the Commander-in-Chief at the Horse Guards and to the Secretary of State for War;
- All medical matters concerning the Artillery – he was accountable to the Master General of the Ordnance;
- Equipment and hospital stores – he was accountable to the Board of the Ordnance through the Military Secretary.

The Army Medical Department was a civilian department which was given no respect and received none of the priority given to other military departments. Doctors were considered neither officers nor gentlemen! As a result, the Army Medical Department either never received or was slow in getting important information that would have been helpful in making appropriate arrangements.

Regimental Delivery of Care

It has already been noted in Chapter 4 which deals with the Peninsular War, that it suited James McGrigor to develop the regimental hospital system. This meant that sick and wounded soldiers could reach there quickly, avoiding long and arduous journeys on bullock cart or on the backs of mules to distant base hospitals.

During the Crimean War, medical care was still delivered at the regimental level, although as will be seen, there were serious deficiencies with this system. Each regiment had its own medical officer whose duty was to care for the sick and wounded in that regiment. He wore the uniform of the regiment to which he was attached. Each regiment had a hospital, but the administrative responsibility for this hospital lay not with the medical officer, but with the commanding officer of the regiment. The delivery of clinical care was the responsibility of the surgeon, who was accountable to inspecting medical officers who made annual or six monthly visits.[5]

Regimental hospitals were small, with only 12 beds within a tent marquee as a ward, and the surgeon had his own tent. Supplies included bedding, a six-month supply of medicines and a range of dressings. An assistant surgeon provided medical support and there was a hospital sergeant, a small number of orderlies (all taken from the regiment) and bandsmen, who became the stretcher bearers when necessary. The hospital was mobile and could be packed away into two horse-drawn carts which were supplied by the Army Medical Department or regiment. The medicine chest was so large that it was often left behind when the troops moved into the field, resulting in shortages when they were needed most.

Medical officers had to provide, and pay for, their own surgical instruments and books! Texts that the surgeon might have taken along included *Commentaries on surgery of war in Portugal, Spain, France and the Netherlands* written by surgeon George James Guthrie and based on his experience in these wars[6] or Ballingall's military surgery text.[7] The surgery undertaken was frequently amputation and debridement of wounds.

In time of war, up to four general hospitals would be established, staffed by non-regimental medical officers and recruited specifically for these posts. Their dress regulation was less clear than that of the regimental medical officers and some wore civilian suits. One medical officer, Patrick Heron Watson from Edinburgh, recommended that any officer coming to the Crimea should bring with him two suits of common tweed.[8] Furthermore, for the summer heat, Watson equipped himself with a waistcoat and trousers made from grey, blue and brown linen cloth by a civilian tailor from Scutari.[9] The medical officers often lived in private accommodation away from the hospital and hired local servants.

The Director General's plan for medical support

Smith began to make the necessary preparations, knowing that no provisions or supplies had been set aside in case of war. One of the many problems facing him was that the Purveyor's department, responsible for obtaining hospital equipment and the Apothecary's department for supplying medicines, had both been closed down to make financial savings. In spite of the difficulties, Smith made his plans:[10]

- He ordered 5,000 beds. It was accepted practice to provide for 25% of the 10,000 troops being sent. Smith added a further 25% for additional requirement that might be predicted to occur. Purveyors from the Peninsular War had to come out of retirement;
- He ordered hospital furniture needed to equip a general hospital;
- He ordered 12 ambulance carts, 6 ambulance wagons and 300 stretchers to evacuate the wounded from the battlefield and to transport them to medical facilities.

Smith was responsible for the provision of medical staff and while subordinate staff would be obtained by negotiation and agreement of the military commander in the region where the hospital was situated, Smith decided on the following medical structure:

- One Deputy Inspector General as Principal Medical Officer;
- Three staff surgeons to lead departments;
- 3 further staff surgeons;
- 6 assistant staff surgeons;
- 1 assistant staff surgeon to have the responsibility for medical stores; dressings and medicines to be obtained from the Apothecaries Hall.

Smith decided that additional medical officers should be available for further duties, such as accompanying the wounded when they were transported between medical units.

There had been no major conflict since the Peninsular War and no new hospitals had been built in the United Kingdom. There was a chronic shortage of men to work as orderlies in general hospitals and Smith tried to address this shortage by suggesting the formation of a "Hospital Corps". Although this was agreed to, attempts to recruit enough men from those serving overseas failed. The Army's solution was to employ men who had retired from the army (aged 40 to 45 years) and more than 350 men were drafted in to work as hospital orderlies or as ambulance drivers. Smith declared that many of these men could hardly carry themselves let alone care for the sick and wounded.[11] He obtained approval to recruit local Turkish men.

Smith requested the Admiralty to supply hospital ships, but the Admiralty later denied it had ever been asked. This had consequences which will be discussed later.

Smith sent Dr David Dumbreck and two other doctors to visit the areas of likely conflict. Dumbreck was born in Kincardine O'Neil, Aberdeenshire in 1805 and was an Edinburgh graduate. He travelled through Serbia, Bulgaria and the Balkans on his fact finding mission. This was a potentially very important exercise which was largely ignored and certainly not acted upon by the British Army. Dumbreck studied the geography of the area, the climate, the people and the diseases that were prevalent and ascertained available possible food sources. Some of the important points and advice he gave are listed below.[12, 13]

- The severity of the winter climate would require better clothing than the army currently had available;
- For hot weather different uniforms of different materials and alternative head gear would be essential for the men to fight effectively in the heat;
- Adequate bedding would be required;
- Adequate food would be needed to maintain the health of the soldiers (the normal daily ration contained fresh or salted meat, bread or biscuit, coffee, sugar and rice);
- Dumbreck noted the swampy areas and poor hygiene, and expressed concern about the risks of malaria, dysentery, typhus and typhoid;
- He recommended malaria prophylaxis in the form of quinine taken in the morning and evening;
- He recommended removal of refuse, waste, stagnant water and filtration of water supplies when troops were stationed in built up areas;
- He recommended that enough operating tables should be taken as the houses there did not contain tables.

Based on the information he obtained from Dumbreck, Smith made the necessary requests through appropriate channels. Nothing happened. It was impractical for soldiers to be supplied with two uniforms; there was a shortage of transport and lack of time to make the necessary preparations.[14]

Requirements for more medical support

As the political tensions across Europe continued to rise, the British Government increased the numbers of troops who would be sent to Malta to 25,000 men, organised into divisions.[15] Medical requirements increased proportionately and the Director General asked for more staff. The medical officer in overall charge of the campaign was the Inspector General, also called the "Principal Medical Officer." Each division had a Deputy Inspector General or Principal Medical Officer for a division.

The total staff required to provide medical care for the four divisions resulted in the provision of 174 medical officers and is detailed as follows:[16]

- 1 Principal Medical Officer for the Crimea (Inspector General);
- 1 Principal Medical Officer for each Division (Deputy Inspector General);
- 12 Senior Staff Surgeons who would be the senior medical officers for each Brigade;
- 70 Assistant Staff Surgeons to be deployed in the hospitals;
- 4 apothecaries.

The Senior Medical Officer in Malta, where the army was assembling was Surgeon William Burrell, Deputy Inspector General. Smith decided that since the numbers of troops and medical staff assembling there had increased substantially a more senior person would now be required. He chose John Hall for this task.

Hall was born in Westmoreland in 1795, the son of a local landowner. He began his medical studies at Guys and St Thomas' Hospitals in London, but qualified in medicine at St Andrews, gaining an MD. He joined the army just after the Battle of Waterloo and after a series of postings (including Belgium, Spain, and the West Indies) he became Deputy Inspector General in 1847. He served during the Frontier Wars in 1847 and 1850-1851. In 1854 he was in India when he was recalled by the Director General. Hall was appointed Inspector General for the Crimean campaign on 28 March 1854.

Hall was fully aware of the difficulties which lay ahead, of the economies that had been made and of the lack of support experienced by medical staff. It is reported that he said to friends in India, that whilst acknowledging what an honour this appointment was, he would willingly forfeit a year's pay if he could avoid having to do it.[17]

He travelled back from India via Bombay and Suez and arrived at Constantinople on 17 June 1854 to take up his position with the British Army under the command of Lord Raglan. Burrell considered that the post to which Hall had been appointed was rightfully his and when he was offered Hall's position in India he refused, resigned and returned to England.[18]

When Hall arrived in Constantinople, the strength of the army included the four divisions of Infantry together with a further division of cavalry (the medical officer being in charge was a 1st Class Staff Surgeon Mitchell and not a Deputy Inspector General). In terms of troop distribution, the Light Division was in the fortified Bulgarian port of Varna on the Black Sea Coast, the First and Second Divisions of Infantry sailed out to Varna a few days later and the Third Division was in Gallipoli but then also moved to Varna. The sick from the Third Division who were unable to transfer to Varna were treated in hospital in Gallipoli, while the sick from the other Divisions were transferred from their Regimental Hospitals, (which numbered 30), to the General Hospital in Scutari (a district in Constantinople) which was opened for this purpose. The divisions remained relatively inactive in Varna for approximately three months. On 7 September 1854, a force of some 57,000 allied troops set sail from Varna, and landed at Eupatoria to begin their march to take up positions and besiege Sevastopol by the end of September 1854.

THE VARNA AND SCUTARI HOSPITALS

By the end of June 1854, David Dumbreck had established a 350 bed hospital at Varna in an old broken down Turkish army barracks, which was shared with French medical services. It was filthy and not fit for purpose. Dumbreck lacked support to improve the site, but did the best he could. The French, in contrast, had adequate help and support to make their part of the hospital up to a reasonable standard. Despite a shortage of men, orderlies and transport, Dumbreck filled up the hospital with 200 sick men almost as soon as it opened its doors.

Large numbers of men were billeted in camps where living conditions were deteriorating. It was too hot, there were food shortages and the water was dirty and contaminated. It was not uncommon for animals to drink from the same supposedly fresh water sources, for clothes to be washed in it and for butchers to discard animal waste into it.[19] Many soldiers consumed too much alcohol. Admissions to the regimental hospitals and the Varna general hospitals began to rapidly increase, predominantly with soldiers suffering from fevers, cholera and dysentery and this was paralleled by increasing numbers of deaths. Although it could be difficult to differentiate cholera from dysentery it is recorded that by the end of July there were 459 cases of cholera with 285 deaths and all regiments were affected. The epidemic continued in Varna and the numbers affected from June to August are shown below in Table 10.2.[20]

Table 10.2 Deaths from cholera where British troops were stationed at the beginning of the war.

MONTH	NUMBER OF CASES	NUMBER OF DEATHS (%)
June	3	1 (33%)
July	449	285 (63%)
August	938	611 (65%)

From Cantlie, N., *A History of the Army Medical Department.* Edinburgh and London: Churchill Livingstone, 1974, Volume 2.

Almost 900 soldiers died from disease before the war began, which was bad for morale. A further 4,000 soldiers suffered from malaria, typhus, typhoid and sand fly fever with an approximate overall 5% mortality. There were a further 5,677cases of diarrhoea over these three months which resulted in significant reductions in the number of men fit for duty.[21]

Hall agreed that the Scutari hospitals should be the main base for the Crimea. The principal hospitals were the General, the Barrack and the Koulali. The first two were established ahead of the Koulali which did not become fully operational until January 1855.The 5,000 beds that the Director General had requested in his preparations for war only became available by the end of 1854.

Dr Duncan Menzies was in administrative medical charge of the Scutari hospitals between June 1854 and the beginning of January 1855 and posed a significant problem in a situation which was getting out of control. He was introduced to the Reverend Sydney Osborne from England, a friend of Sidney Herbert, Secretary of State for War. Osborne had travelled to the Crimea with a letter of introduction to see if there was anything he could do to help. He met Menzies on 8 November 1954 and after being shown the facilities at the General Hospital, recorded that he asked Menzies what help he needed, offering to give money from his own to help the sick and wounded, or to obtain funds from England.

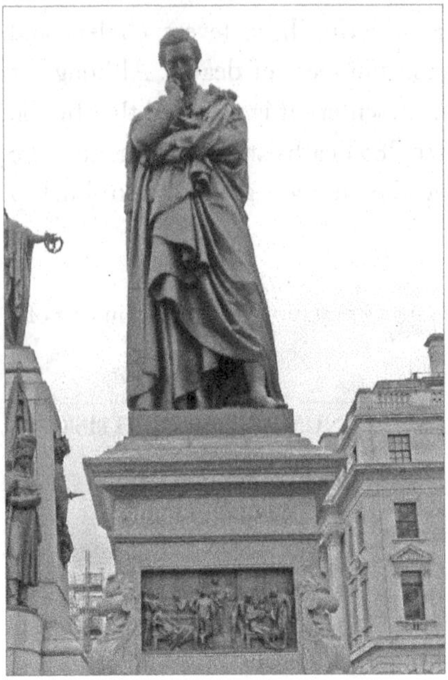

Figure 10.3. Sculpture of Sidney Herbert by John Henry Foley, London. (Authors' photograph).

Menzies replied that "they had everything – nothing was wanted". This was a wasted opportunity since Lord Ratcliffe, Minister of Foreign Affairs, was prepared to ensure that the sick and wounded received all they required, hence the reason for Osborne's question. Osborne expressed sympathy for the British Government and observed that the most senior medical officer was "deluded" and was unable to articulate what the services lacked and required urgently. Florence Nightingale arrived with her nurses at approximately the same time and faced the same problem. This will be discussed in more detail later.

Menzies' health broke down and he became increasingly ineffective and was brought home. He had diagnosed himself with bronchitis and renal complaints. He was succeeded by Dr John Forrest in December 1854. Forrest was born in Stirling and was an Edinburgh graduate, but had a rather dubious background. He had been convicted of grave-robbing whilst a medical student and outlawed from Scotland (Cases decided in the Court of Session – Patrick Shaw & Alex Dunlop (Vol II 12th Nov 1822 – 11th Mar 1824) No.99 p.103), before having his conviction quashed. This practice provided the corpses necessary for surgeons to learn anatomy since it wasn't possible to obtain sufficient cadavers by legitimate means.

James McGrigor, a pivotal figure discussed in previous chapters, put his signature to a letter in 1794, which was addressed to the Aberdeen Medical Society, urging them to pursue the practice of dissection of the human body. The students in Aberdeen followed his advice and they became "resurrectionists". Trips out to the Deeside area during the night (after getting a bit of information here and there from grave-diggers who were financially rewarded for the information they provided) became normal practice and could be very rewarding for the students!

Relatives of the newly deceased were aware of this macabre pastime and went to great lengths to prevent it. Figure 10.4 shows the heavy metal coffin (called a mort safe) which was placed over the deceased's coffin to foil the grave robbers because its weight made the corpse effectively inaccessible. It was left in place till the rotting remains were no longer of interest to the resurrectionists. An earlier version of the mort safe was a heavy granite slab placed over the coffin. This did not foil the resurrectionists who dug down, opened the coffin from the top end, put a rope round the neck of the corpse and dragged it out. The aim of the exercise was to obtain raw material for acquiring knowledge of anatomy and Figure 10.5 shows an anatomical dissection from Aberdeen around 1820 and is courtesy of the Aberdeen Medico-Chirurgical Society.

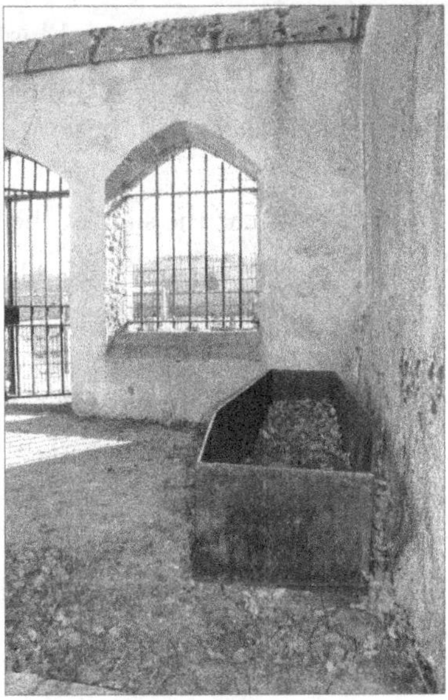

Figure 10.4. A heavy metal coffin used to surround the deceased's own coffin to prevent the Resurrectionists stealing the body. (Authors' photograph).

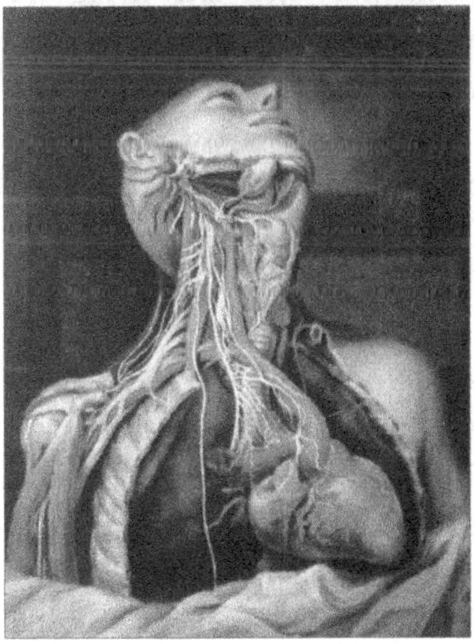

Figure 10.5. An anatomical dissection from Aberdeen in approximately 1820. (Courtesy of the Aberdeen Medico-Chirurgical Society)

Forrest joined the army after resuming his studies and qualified in medicine. He served in the military from 1825 and gained experience in many locations including the West Indies and Africa. He found the conditions in the Crimea too difficult to cope with and wrote to Sir John Hall stating "I feel confident I shall break down" (Hall/Forrest letters 4.1.85). After only 2 weeks in charge he resigned and returned to England with a dubious diagnosis of "inflammation of the liver"!

After Forrest's departure there continued to be a lack of command and control. Two doctors, called Lawson and Cruikshank were in charge for a time, but the precise details of the part they played were unclear both at the time and after the war. There was considerable confusion since military doctors ignored the chains of command and indulged in petty jealousies. Senior medical figures such as the Deputy Inspectors-General criticised each other and resorted to derogatory personal remarks about each other. Lawson was under a cloud with respect to his professional performance earlier in his career and his appointment by Sir John Hall was controversial, as will be explained later in this chapter. Miss Nightingale wrote back to her friends in high places with her own views of the performances of senior doctors in the Crimea.

This dysfunctional state was not confined to senior doctors. At the start of the war, the senior hospital administrator was Major Sillery, who showed no leadership qualities, being inexperienced in hospital matters. Others, including the more senior General William Paulett, contributed little to the administrative efforts to run the hospitals. Purveyors did not obtain the equipment needed by the medical staff and the apothecary employed an outdated operating system which only improved after his death in November 1854. All of these factors conspired against efficient and effective medical services which were completely unable to cope with what they were being asked to do. Not only was the volume of work too great but the organisation of the services was not fit for the purposes required.

TRANSPORT FROM BALACLAVA TO SCUTARI

The first hospital treatment for the wounded was provided by regimental hospitals. Wounded soldiers were collected from the battlefield, often after lying for prolonged periods. In some cases more than 50 hours might have elapsed between sustaining a wound and receiving the first medical attention. As the war progressed in addition to the surgeons in the hospital there were up to 12 assistant surgeons. Truces would be declared and under the protection of white flags, both sides would retrieve their wounded, while officers from both sides exchanged cordial greetings before hostilities were resumed.[22]

After their wounds had been treated, casualties were transferred from the regimental hospital tent to the port of Balaclava, from where they were sent in groups of up to 200 men by ship to base hospitals in Scutari. The British Army relied on French mule litters to get to Balaclava because there were no ambulance trains. Surgeon Edward Wrench provided a vivid account of how this happened.[23] On one particular occasion he was sitting on the hospital mule, with a bottle of rum in each holster and with instructions that he should not let any of the 300 sick die during the journey to Balaclava – some 7 miles over snow-covered, frozen ground. Soldiers were ill-equipped for the journey and often they had no boots and no warm clothing. Those who were too ill to sit were laid flat in ammunition wagons. The horses pulling the wagons were sick and several died. One man with a bullet wound through his chest was thrown out of the wagon:

...and crimsoned the snow from his reopened wound...

Wrench described how he was:

....encouraging the sick and supplying those who looked faint and likely to die with a suck from the rum bottle.[24]

Frequently, ambulance drivers were either sick themselves or were so drunk that there were recorded episodes of wounded driving the ambulance, since the drivers were in no fit condition to work.

The sick were left at Balaclava harbour and because of a shortage of ships to take them to Scutari they often lay for hours on an exposed pier with no protection from the elements. They were filthy and were surrounded by dead and rotting animal carcases, while in the water of the adjacent harbour, animal offal, the remnants of destroyed ships, and human bodies or body parts floated in the water.[25]

Available British resources for transporting the wounded were woefully inadequate. When the British army arrived in the Crimea each regiment had one pony and 10 canvas stretchers. The Principle Medical Officer had requested a total of 42 wagons, 336 canvas stretchers and 672 men for the Hospital Corps. Instead, he was given 2 wagons without horses or drivers.[26] The French helped after the Battle of the Alma by lending mules and litters to transport the wounded (with long delays of up to 2 days). The same thing happened after the Battle of Inkerman, when the French lent 500 mules to the British, thus ensuring that on this occasion at least, the casualties reached hospital on that same day.[27]

Available ships to transport the sick and wounded from Balaclava were often not designed for the purpose, and up to 10% of wounded men died in transit and were thrown overboard into a sea grave.[28] There was overcrowding, lack of bedding and shortage of food and water. Often the weakest men, who had the most severe wounds, or who had perhaps had a recent amputation, suffered the most. The only sustenance available was salt meat and a hard biscuit and occasionally rice. The journey took up to 3 weeks and was termed "the middle passage." At either end of the journey the embarkation and disembarkation procedures lacked structure and organisation which added to the discomfort of the sick and wounded.

There were some hospital ships available which had better facilities and were provided with medical officers and orderlies. Infectious diseases such as dysentery and cholera spread very easily on board all vessels.

If the sick and wounded survived the sea journey, they were taken to one of the Scutari hospitals and this was often a major ordeal. There was a shortage of stretcher bearers, who were often unfit. The wounded struggled up the hill themselves, or were dragged up by less severely wounded comrades. Even when the wounded reached hospital, it was often the wrong one, or there were no beds and they were left lying in the courtyards unattended for long periods.[29]

It is worth pausing to consider what it was actually like in the hospitals in Scutari. This is the Reverend Osborne's account as he ministered to the sick and it provides a vivid description of the scenes in the wards and corridors of these hospitals at that time:

> It has been my lot in life to minister at the death beds of many who I have seen die surrounded with everything money could obtain, and affectionate kindness suggest, to make less painful the severe trial of that moment. It has been my privilege to see what at such a time a true Christian faith can do to console and support; I saw men, after years spent in their country's service, now far from the land of those they loved, worn out by the privations of war, endured too, under all the aggravations of pestilence and neglect; lying on the clothes, they had not changed for months, in wards presenting every feature to depress and to annoy, but made more depressing and distressing by the dreadful death-scenes of each day and night; yet, listening with every symptom of grateful delight to the invitations, the promises of Him, who left his home in heaven to contend to death, for every penitent who would trust his soul to Him".[30]

The hospital buildings were of poor quality, with inadequate drainage. Sewage, filth and vermin were everywhere. There was overcrowding and the windows wouldn't open to supply much needed ventilation. There were shortages of essentials such as bedsteads, bed clothes (which were of canvas), eating utensils, soap, towels and materials for cleaning.

Hospitals were overwhelmed by the sick and wounded and during the Battle of the Alma in September 1854 more than 3,000 men were admitted during one week, of whom 1,000 had been wounded. The commander of the British Army forces in the Crimea, Lord Raglan, was blamed both by the government and the newspapers. Just prior to the Crimean winter there were only 9,000 men fit for duty and 23,000 men unfit because of sickness.[31]

Raglan tried to establish what was wrong with the medical services, acutely aware that ultimately it was his responsibility. It was clear that the Inspector-General of Hospitals, Dr John Hall, was not being helpful and at worst, he was a positive obstruction. Hall focused on minor issues of little importance, whilst trying to assure Raglan that there were no problems in his department.[32] When Hall was sent to Scutari to examine the base hospitals, he reported that they lacked for nothing, and were "on a creditable footing". The reality was quite the opposite as reported by others, including Florence Nightingale.

Other incidents led to rising tensions. The Principal Medical Officer at Balaclava (Dr Lawson) had been dismissed by Raglan because he neglected wounded men left lying on the deck of a transport ship in Balaclava Harbour for two weeks with little protection against the elements and very little medical care. Hall appointed Lawson to be the Senior Medical Officer at the Barrack Hospital at Scutari despite his poor track record providing clear evidence that he was a quite unsuitable candidate for the position. Naturally this was not to Raglan's liking, who even went as far "naming and shaming" Hall and his deputy. However very little changed, and the provision of care to the sick and wounded remained inadequate and unacceptable.

It is not surprising therefore, that there was a growing concern in Britain at the way in which the war was being prosecuted, particularly as the first Crimean winter was rapidly approaching. Both Raglan and the government of the day were held responsible and came under severe and increasing pressure. *The Times* newspaper reporters William Howard Russell in the Crimea and Thomas Chenery in Constantinople applied much of that pressure. These journalists were particularly vociferous in their criticism. They often compared the standard of care delivered by the British with that given by the French to their soldiers.

Russell was born in Ireland and entered Trinity College Dublin but failed to obtain a degree. He moved to London where he tried to join the army. He was unsuccessful and became a teacher of mathematics. While working in Kensington Grammar School, he wrote articles for *The Times*. He was a friend of Charles Dickens and led an active social life in London, especially at the Garrick Club where he established useful connections. Russell was sent to cover the Crimean War by the editor of *The Times*, John Delane, at the beginning of 1854 and he did so for almost 2 years.

Russell had a difficult relationship with Raglan and his frank reports caused considerable discomfort in Britain. Both Queen Victoria and Prince Albert expressed the view that he was not supporting his country and at times the information he was providing might well have been helpful to the enemy. Nevertheless Russell continued to send his reports home undeterred.

On 15 September and 22 September 1854, in articles dealing with inadequate standards of nursing care in the Crimea, he wrote:

> Are there no devoted women among us, able and willing to go forth and minister to the sick and suffering soldiers of the East in the hospitals of Scutari? Are none of the daughters of England, at this extreme hour of need, ready for such work of mercy? Must we fall so far below the French in self-sacrifice and devotedness?

On October 13 1854 Cheney wrote:

> The worn-out pensioners who were brought out as an ambulance corps are totally useless, and not only are surgeons not to be had, but there are no dressers or nurses to carry out the surgeon's directions and to attend on the sick during intervals between his visits. Here the French are greatly our superiors. Their medical arrangements are extremely good, their surgeons more numerous, and they have also the help of the Sisters of Charity, who have accompanied the expedition in incredible numbers. These devoted women are excellent nurses.

The call was answered by Florence Nightingale who volunteered on 4 October 1854 in a letter to Elizabeth Herbert, the wife of her friend the Secretary of State for War, Sidney Herbert. At almost the same time, Sidney Herbert wrote a letter to Florence Nightingale on 15 October 1854, asking for her help.[33] Herbert stated that it had not been possible to use female nurses before, because it had been considered inappropriate to deploy them in regimental hospitals. Now that the hospitals in Scutari were static it would be quite acceptable.

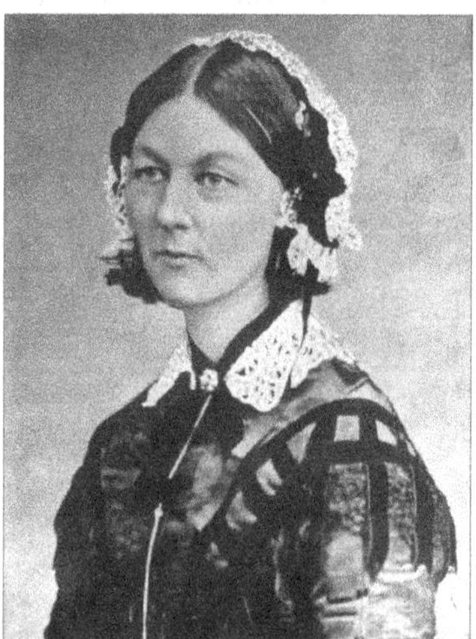

Figure 10.6. Florence Nightingale. (Public Domain).

Herbert declared that although female nurses had approached him offering their services, he believed that they were unsuitable as they were not aware of the nature of the task. He also stated that Lady Maria Forrester, daughter of Lord Roden, had volunteered to go with or send a female nursing team but, "Lady Maria Forrester has not tested the willingness of the trained nurses to go and is incapable of directing or ruling them".

Herbert considered that Nightingale was the one person he knew who could lead a team of female nurses and could provide the care that was required because of her previous administrative experience and capability. He set out in his persuasive letter the framework within which she would be working, should she chose to accept the challenge, which of course she did:

> You would of course, have plenary authority over all the nurses and I think I could secure the fullest assistance and cooperation from the medical staff and you would also have an unlimited power drawing on the Government for whatever you think requisite for the success of your Mission.

But the key to providing her with what she needed to succeed came at the end of his letter:

> Deriving your authority from the Government your position would ensure respect and consideration of everyone, especially in a service where official rank carries so much weight. This would secure you any attention or comfort on your way out there, together with a complete submission to your orders.

Herbert's wife sent a separate letter on the same day exhorting her to undertake this task and also asking at what time Nightingale would be able to meet her husband the following day. Within a week, on 21 October 1854, Nightingale departed for the Crimea accompanied by her team of nurses.

Herbert then wrote to the editor of the newspaper, the *Morning Chronicle* on that day, 21 October 1854, explaining that although some women might have volunteered, those who were going to the Crimea had to be fully aware of the conditions there and to have the necessary skills. He publicly stated the Government's support for Nightingale and the way in which she would work:

> ...to appoint someone on whose energy, experience and direction they can rely, who should be the one authority to select, to superintend, and direct, in the British General Hospitals of Turkey, a staff of female nurses, herself acting under the immediate orders of the medical authorities........ and that she will act in the strictest subordination to the chief medical officer of the hospital.[34]

Medical staff were made aware of Miss Nightingale's arrival and Menzies was instructed by the Government to ensure that she had all the help necessary and that there should be cooperation between the doctors and nurses.

But why did Herbert have such confidence in Nightingale, and why were things so easy for her when they had been so difficult for the Director General?

NIGHTINGALE'S BACKGROUND AND SUITABILITY FOR THE CRIMEA

Florence Nightingale was born in Florence in Italy in 1820, the daughter of William Edward Shore who himself was the son of a banker from Sheffield. He took the new family name of "Nightingale" from his mother's uncle's surname and he inherited estates in Derbyshire and Hampshire at the age of 21. Her parents went on a 2 year honeymoon touring Europe and they all returned to England the following year and lived on the estates in Derbyshire and Hampshire.

Her childhood was not typical for a girl of the time; she studied mathematics, history, philosophy and languages and was able to write and understand the classics. She spoke French and German and her father was an important figure in supporting her education.[35] She had strong religious convictions and from the age of 16 she believed that she had been chosen to play an important role in relieving human suffering. The family was well connected and both Florence and her sister were presented to Queen Victoria and had a place in British society but she didn't conform, she declined suitors and steered clear of social events, preferring to study with a focus on helping others.[36]

Lord Palmerston, Prime Minister for much of the Crimean War, was a close family friend; their respective family estates in Hampshire were close together. Sidney Herbert, Minister for War, was also a close friend as were others within *The Times*. She first met Sidney Herbert and his wife, Elizabeth, in Rome in 1846 and they became great friends. Nightingale often went to the Herberts' house in Wiltshire and supported Elizabeth during one of her confinements.

Over a period of more than 10 years she visited many hospitals, particularly in London but also in various English towns. She considered that nursing might be a suitable way in which she could help the sick. Her family were not in favour since nursing was generally held in low esteem and required little education and no qualifications.

It was perhaps during a visit to friends in Egypt in 1849-1850 that her mind was made up. She met the St Vincent de Paul sisters and understood that their discipline and excellent organisation gave them a huge advantage in the provision of care for the sick. She then sought appropriate training and underwent two short periods of instruction (1850 and 1851) at the Institute of Protestant Deaconesses at Kaiserswerth in Germany.

She was appointed Superintendent of the Hospital for Invalid Gentlewomen in Harley Street, London, in 1853 at the age of 33 and was well supported by Mrs Herbert. There had also been the option of a senior post in King's College London.[37] She was able to demonstrate her effectiveness in administrative duties by improving the working environment and the way in which care was delivered. She developed skills to deal with doctors and ensured that they co-operated with her! A biography written by Sir Edward Cook highlighted her effective characteristics: "it was the combination of masterful powers of organisation with womanly gentleness and sympathy"[38] and in addition she had "great tact and diplomacy, and a capacity for wire-pulling".[39] However, was that really the case, and why did she dismiss virtually all the staff she had chosen for this institution?[40]

NIGHTINGALE'S ARRIVAL AT SCUTARI

Nightingale arrived at Scutari on 4 November 1854, 10 days after the Battle of Balaclava and the day before the Battle of Inkerman. She was accompanied by 38 female nurses coming from a range of difference backgrounds:

- 10 Roman Catholic sisters;
- 6 nurses from St John's Institute;
- 8 Anglican Sisters of Mercy;
- 14 nurses from other hospitals.

Unfortunately there were concerns about the nurses' competence and Nightingale herself had worries about 22 of them. It was reported that some were stout middle aged females whose motivates were geared towards financial gain and who were promiscuous, were often intoxicated with alcohol and did not always attend to the needs of their patients.[41] Those with a religious background were often more interested in the souls of their patients than the physical needs dictated by their wounds.

Nightingale and her team dealt with more than 2,000 wounded soldiers from the Battle of Inkerman: a baptism of fire. On one occasion, 500 arrived at the same time. Although there was initial reluctance to utilise the nurses' skills, they soon settled in and started work. Matters were not helped when an investigating party of three civilians came to the hospital. Mr Augustus Stafford MP, the Reverend

Osborne and Mr MacDonald from *The Times* arrived to make an inspection. Since medical staff had not been informed of their arrival and their purpose, it is not surprising that relationships were strained.

Nightingale experienced problems when she tried to obtain necessary supplies from the purveyor, as indeed had medical staff before. The original purveyor was Mr Ward, a 67 year old for whom the job proved too much and who was clearly not competent. In October he was succeeded by Mr Wreford as Purveyor-in-Chief and whilst there had been some improvement, Wreford was said to be "obstructive and unimaginative and was wedded to the concept that it was his duty to save money".[42] She wrote to her friend Herbert, bypassing Menzies and asked that the purveyor's department be improved and completely reformed if necessary. Menzies was not able to address problems in his own hospitals and Nightingale perceived him as being unfit to command.

She wanted a younger member of staff appointed to the position of Purveyor-in-Chief, but instead another official, a Mr Milton, was sent from England to supervise Wreford. This also met with little success in a department staffed by men with little or no training and an incomplete understanding of what they were expected to do. Osborne felt the situation was intolerable and complained constantly and whilst there is no doubt there were occasions when supplies were inadequate, perhaps things were not quite as bad as he claimed.

The number of nurses increased with the arrival of Miss Stanley and her group. Stanley was the daughter of the Bishop of Norwich, sister of the Dean of Westminster and friend of Nightingale and of the Herberts'. She had helped Nightingale to select the first nurses to go. Stanley was keen to provide religious comfort to the sick and was herself a devout Catholic. Herbert authorised her to go to the Crimea with 46 nurses, 15 of whom were nuns from the Sisters of Mercy order. Nightingale opposed Herbert's decision and wrote to him saying he should not have permitted Stanley to go without prior consultation. Nightingale firmly believed that nursing success would only come about as a result of clear management and authority. Stanley's Catholic nurses only acknowledged their own nun in charge and Stanley herself only answered to her bishop! As a result, when Stanley and her nurses arrived, they were not made welcome by Nightingale, who wouldn't work with them.[43]

Stanley's nurses remained on their transport ship until the British Ambassador provided accommodation for them in Therapia. Stanley and Nightingale continued to be at odds as each tried to outmanoeuvre the other.

Agreements and compromises had to be reached and eventually Mary Stanley and her nurses were placed in the convalescent hospital at Koulali which then

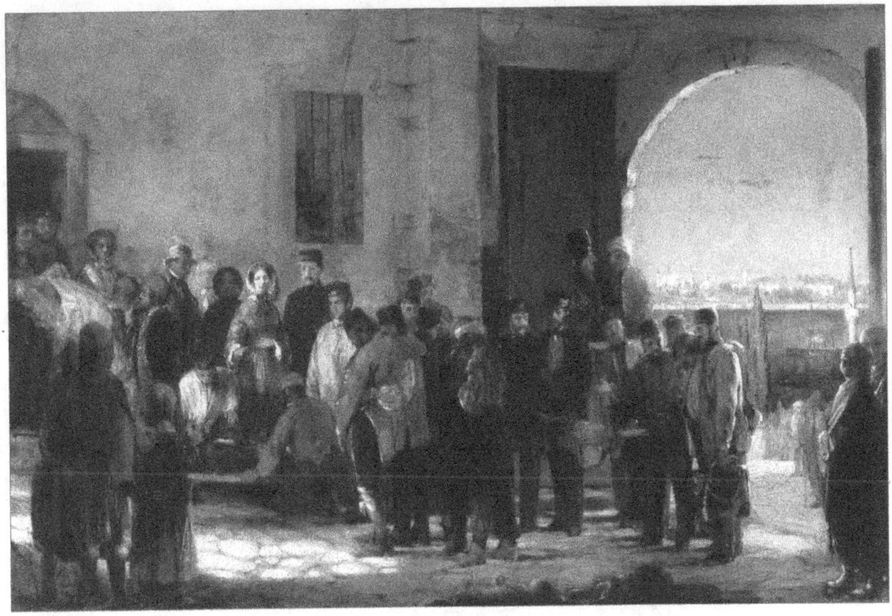

Figure 10.7. 'The Mission of Mercy: Florence Nightingale receiving the Wounded at Scutari' by Jerry Barret about 1856. This painting also included Sir William Linton, Alexis Benoît Soyer and Sir Henry Knight Storks. (With permission of the National Portrait Gallery, London).

changed to become a general hospital administered by Stanley on 24 January 1855. She did not succeed and within a week requested further nursing help. Nightingale attributed Stanley's failure to her inability to manage effectively, referring to her endeavour as "a spiritual flirtation between the ladies and soldiers."[44] The situation and conditions in Koulali deteriorated over the next few months and Stanley returned home in May 1855, leaving no effective functioning hospital in Koulali.[45]

Nightingale initially considered that the high death rate from disease was due to poor nutrition and exhaustion of the soldiers and she rejected the notion of contagion[46] even although there was a recognisable association between the deaths of the sick and wounded in hospital and the filthy conditions, the air that was breathed and the water and food that was consumed. She did not recognise poor hygiene as a direct cause of death! On that subject she received unwelcome assistance from Dr James M. Barry in formulating a plan of action. Their difficult relationship is discussed later in the Chapter, together with the role and recommendations of the Sanitary Commission. Although the existence of bacteria was not known at this time and it would be ten years before Louis Pasteur proposed the germ

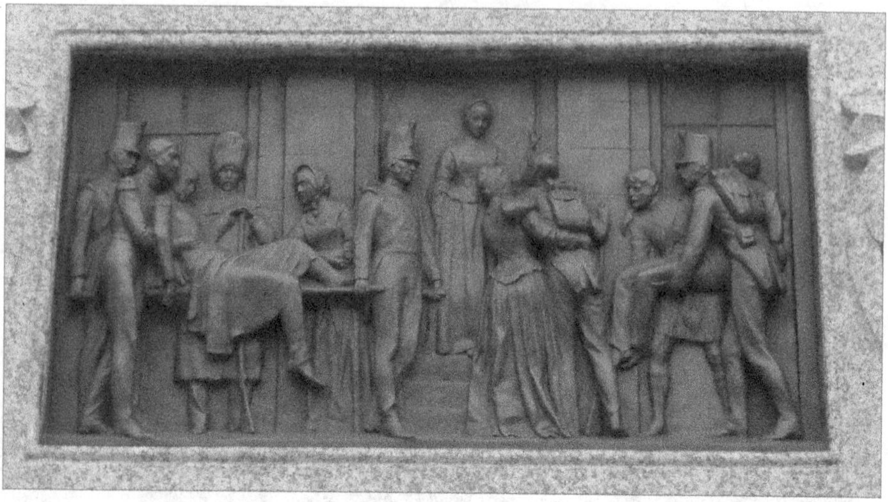

Figure 10.8. Plaque at the base of the statue of Florence Nightingale on the Crimean War Memorial, London, which shows her receiving the wounded. (Authors' photograph).

theory of disease (see Chapter 13), nevertheless the following areas were going to be targeted: [47]

- Cleaning the wounded casualties on arrival by removing contaminated clothing and cleaning their wounds;
- Cleanliness in the wards;
- Cleanliness of the patients, clean clothing, new clothing, clean bed-linen;
- Boiling clothes and linen to destroy infesting lice;
- Each soldier had their own cloth to use when washing;
- Ensuring that food and supplies were available (often funded from other sources; a relief fund organised by *The Times* was put at her disposal), which were commonly stolen and sold elsewhere;
- Ensuring that patients received adequate nutrition, properly prepared and cooked;
- Ensuring that wards had adequate ventilation and windows which opened.

There were now more nurses and they were attached to specific surgeons and wards. Even so there was still a shortage, since the nurse/patient ratio in one instance was 1,000 patients for a single nurse. While many duties were carried out some of the key ones are outlined below: [48]

- Nurses were central to providing patients' diets (see Table 10.3) which were prescribed on a daily basis by their surgeon. Nurses were responsible particularly for patients on "spoon" diets, who were amongst the sickest. Meat was frequently of poor quality and was badly prepared, but very importantly the nurses recognised the dangers of the water, and ensured that it was boiled before it was drunk;
- Nurses tried to ensure that there was clean bed linen and shirts for the patients, although their supply was inadequate and it was common for patients to be left in bedding that had not been changed for weeks and both the bedding and the clothes could be infested with lice;
- Nurses taught hospital orderlies who were of varying capabilities and interest, in the provision of adequate care for the sick and wounded.

Nurses did not usually carry out specialised tasks as they would do now, e.g. dressing of wounds, but they provided a level of care and support that would otherwise not have been given. They lived in poor, rat-infested quarters, suffered infectious diseases and some died. They certainly worked hard, though often displayed limited capabilities, which Nightingale frequently commented on in her

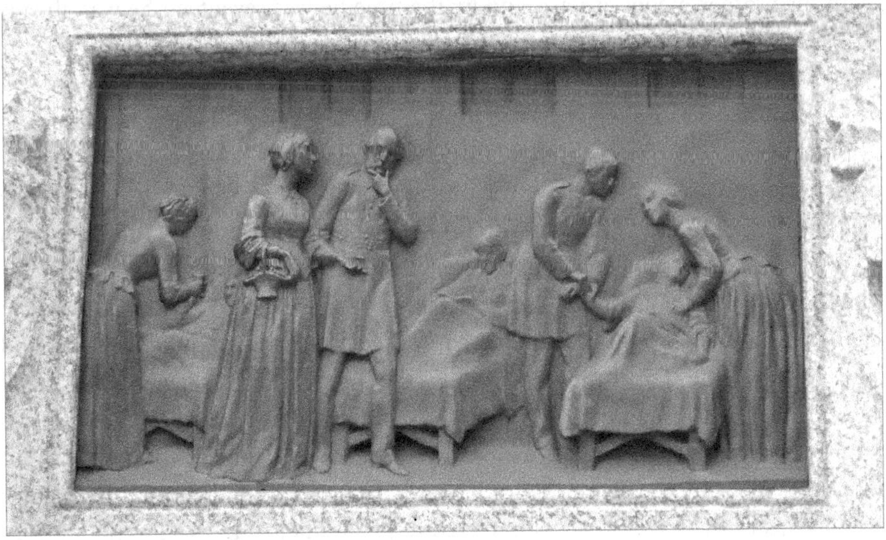

Figure 10.9. Plaque at the base of the statue of Florence Nightingale on the Crimean War Memorial, London, which shows her on the ward with the medical officer and the wounded. (Authors' photograph).

letters to Herbert. Some of the nurses were sent home as a result of drunkenness or sexual misdemeanours. The supply of port wine for the patients was not infrequently stolen and resulted in the intoxication of nurses and orderlies.

Table 10. 3 Hospital diet for the wounded.

TYPE OF DIET	CONSTITUENTS
Full	1lb meat, 1lb bread, 1lb potatoes, 2 pints of tea, ½ pint of porter
Half diet	Half of the above quantities
Quarter diet	One quarter of the above
Spoon diet	1lb of bread and 2 pints of tea

Celebrity Chef in the Crimea

One of the improvements made was the provision of better diets for the sick and wounded. Alexis Soyer was born in Meaux-en-Brie, France, in 1810 into a family which had fallen on difficult times. At the age of nine he went to work with his brother, a chef in Paris and by the time he was seventeen he was already a well-known culinary expert with 12 other chefs working under his instruction. He married the artist Elizabeth Emma Jones in 1837 and the following year was appointed head chef at the Reform Club in London. He even redesigned the kitchens. He pioneered the use of gas-powered temperature controlled ovens, which was certainly advanced for the time. In 1847 Soyer was given leave from the Reform Club to go to Dublin to help bring relief to those who were suffering from malnutrition during the potato famine and he developed the first "soup kitchen" for the Government, which served up to 5,000 people per day. When he returned to London, he set up several similar kitchens for the poor in different locations around the city. His fame spread and he toured England promoting his new cookery book and his so-called "Magic Stove" which allowed food to be cooked on the table.

He was reported to be a womaniser, a bigamist, an alcoholic and was without doubt a colourful and flamboyant character! Spurred on by reports of the poor conditions in the Crimea, he volunteered to go and help. He was given authority to do so by Lord Panmure and before he left invented the "Soyer's Field Stove" powered by gas which was used by the British Army for more than 100 years.

When he arrived at Scutari, he set about his task with enthusiasm and dealt with issues at Barrack Hospital first. There was a shortage of working boilers, food was improperly cooked, there were large wastages and utensils were dirty. He ordered the boilers to be repaired, installed new ovens and ensured that meat was now properly prepared.

Based on his experience in Ireland, he knew the nutritious value of the stock in which the meat was cooked and instructed cooks how to use this to make soups. These measures were adopted by other hospitals and Soyer continued to give advice and to supervise cooking. He taught Highland regiments how to cook and could perhaps justifiably be called the first Celebrity Chef. It was reported in *The Morning Chronicle* that, "he saved as many lives through his kitchens as Florence Nightingale did through her wards."[49]. He returned to England in 1857 and died the following year, his death being described by Nightingale as "a disaster for the nation".

Nightingale and conflicts with Dr James M Barry

Nightingale believed that the high death rates were due to poor nutrition and exhaustion of the soldiers and this viewpoint brought her into conflict with another strong-willed and uncompromising figure, Dr James M. Barry, a graduate of the University of Edinburgh. Barry had a special interest in the importance of nutrition, exercise, hygiene and sanitation in the maintenance of good health. In 1820 he performed one of the first caesarean sections in South Africa (both mother and child survived) and was clearly a very skilled surgeon. He was controversial, opinionated and argumentative and displayed lack of respect for military regulation and authority. He spoke with a high pitched voice and was "effeminate", seeking confrontation with his military superiors and although frequently reprimanded, continued with his work regardless.

At the start of war, Barry was posted to Corfu, where many of the wounded were treated. Barry's method of nursing sick and wounded soldiers evacuated from the Crimea was so successful that his recovery rate was the highest for the whole Crimean campaign. When he heard what was happening in Scutari, Barry applied to go but he was turned down. He decided to go anyway and this brought him into conflict with Nightingale. They had a public confrontation. Barry believed that disease was caused by poor hospital sanitation and bad ventilation and left Florence Nightingale in no doubt that poor hygiene was the cause of disease and that she had not addressed the problem. Barry scolded Nightingale for her unclean practices. She responded strongly, and in her words, Barry was "a brute" and "the most hardened creature I ever met throughout the army" and many years later after Barry's death in 1865, she said:

> As Mr. Whitehead wants remarks, I will mention that I never had such a blackguard rating in all my life - I who have had more than any woman than from this Barrie sitting on (her) horse, while I was crossing the Hospital Square, with only my cap on, in the sun. (He) kept me standing in the midst of quite a crowd of soldiers, commissariat servants, camp followers, etc., etc., everyone of whom behaved like a gentleman during the scolding I received, while (she) behaved like a brute. After (she) was dead, I was told (he) was a woman.[50]

It was unfortunate that two such single-minded individuals as James Barry and Florence Nightingale did not see "eye to eye". They were both determined to improve matters, and although they held different views as to the cause of the high mortality amongst troops they were both on the right lines for tackling the problem from their respective approaches. Had they combined their skills, instead of being in conflict with each other, the outcome for many soldiers might have been more favourable.

After the Crimean War they both returned to England but there was a twist in the tale. Nightingale received praise and was recognised for the remarkable reduction in deaths due to infectious disease and she continued to work tirelessly for health reforms. Such praise and fame probably had an element of "Victorian spin," focussing public attention on the "lady with the lamp," while at the same time diverting the nation's focus away from the awful reality of the Crimean War. By way of contrast Barry was forced to retire from the army against his will in 1859. He died six years later from influenza, with very little money and in relative obscurity. After his death, despite having left strict instructions to be buried in the clothes in which he died and for there to be no post-mortem, it was revealed that he was a woman and may even have had a child as evidence by striae gravidarum (stretch marks) on his abdomen. However, this can happen in males also if they have certain types of hormonal disturbance, e.g. Cushing's disease etc.

Barry's life is still the subject of mystery and rumours of affairs with nobility persist and there are more questions than answers concerning this doctor. However Barry lived life as a male to be able to pursue an ambition to enter medical school, had studied surgery and made a major contribution to health in general and military surgery in particular. Perhaps James Barry could lay claim to being the University of Edinburgh's first female graduate and the first female from Great Britain to become a doctor.

The Sanitary Commission and its impact, 1855

A series of Commissions were established at the end of 1854 and beginning of 1855 to address many issues in need of attention. Two of these Commissions were sent to the Crimea and the Sanitary Commission inspected hospital facilities in Scutari. The members of the Sanitary Commission which arrived in Scutari on 4th March 1855 were:

- Dr John Sutherland (Inspector, Board of Health and graduate from the University of Edinburgh);
- Dr Hector Gavin (Physician to the Post Office, who previously worked on cholera epidemics);
- Mr Robert Rawlinson, (Civil Engineer, Board of Health);
- Mr Newlands (Sanitary Inspector from Liverpool);
- Mr Milson (Sanitary Inspector from Liverpool).

Nightingale worked with the Commission who set about their work immediately and within 96 hours were able to make critical observations and recommendations which were summarised as follows:[51]

Table 10.4 Key initial findings and recommendations by the Sanitary Commission, March 1855.

HOSPITAL	FINDING
Barrack Hospital	• Lack of ventilation in corridors and wards • Poor toilet facilities • Unhygienic area around the area of the hospital
General Hospital	• Very clean except toilets • Kitchens very damp • Unhygienic area around the area of the hospital
Palace Hospital	• In all respects was poor
"Convalescent" ships at Scutari	• Poor ventilation • Overcrowded • Dirty

From Shepherd, J., *The Crimean Doctors. A History of the British Medical Services in the Crimean War.* Liverpool: Liverpool University Press, 1991, Volume 2, p.457.

Changes were implemented very quickly, which included improvements in drainage and ventilation of all hospitals, cleaning of toilet and washing facilities, cleaning of water tanks, avoidance of burials close to the hospitals, a reduction in the number of patients in each hospital and avoiding keeping patients in corridors. This was a major undertaking which needed structural changes made to buildings and engineering works. The Commission turned its attention to the facilities in Balaclava, and made similar recommendations. The members of the Commission had a terrible experience in Balaclava, because Gavin was accidentally shot and killed by his brother and Rawlinson was shot while inspecting near the front line, although he survived and returned to England! Sutherland remained and worked with Nightingale and the two formed a strong and useful working relationship.

Sutherland made the following astute observation:

> ...we have also found the medical authorities thoroughly alive to the nature of the changes required but without the power to carry them out.[52]

By the end of March 1855 the mortality rate began to drop and this was probably due to falling numbers of sick and wounded admitted to hospitals and less overcrowding. The various structural changes could not have been made within such a short period of time although this must have been a pleasing co-incidence for the Commission. However, the improvements that had been made and put into place benefited the sick and wounded for the remainder of the war when hostilities ceased with the Treaty of Paris on 27 April 1856.

THE CHANGING MEDICAL SITUATION IN SPRING 1855 AND ONWARDS

Health improved due to changes in the provision of medical care and a better understanding of prevention of disease. For example, the following all had a significant impact on improving the quality and availability of medical care:

- Fall in disease incidence and mortality underpinned by better general health of soldiers, so less susceptibility to disease;
- Diseases less virulent;
- Less overcrowding of hospitals;
- Extra beds and accommodation available if required;

- Better regimental care (earlier surgery, better care in the regimental hospitals, washing of clothes and bed linen, fresh food and water, improvements in evacuation to Balaclava and onwards to Scutari);
- Better transport ships (hygiene, food, water, drugs, adequate space);
- Better conditions and hygiene in the soldiers' camps, provision of clean drinking water and adequate amounts of food, good periods of rest and relief from duty to allow soldiers to keep in better condition;
- Fresh vegetables and meat and provision of fruit juice (lemon or lime) containing vitamin C to prevent scurvy;
- Construction of railroads between Balaclava and the camps for transport of provisions and men and the sick and wounded could also be transported now in relative comfort.

The monthly admissions to regimental hospitals fell by about 15% after April 1855 and the mortality for these admissions dropped substantially from 15% to only 6%.

Table 10.5 Comparison of numbers of hospital admissions at the beginning and later during 1855.

	January-March 1855	**April-September 1855**
Admissions to regimental hospitals (approximate monthly average)	7,500	6,500
% of admissions who died	15%	6%
Casualties transferred to Scutari hospitals (monthly average)	2,153	1,294

Contributions of civilian surgeons to the care of the sick and wounded

Civilian surgeons contributed to medical care, although there was no formal mechanism for this in place. Many civilian doctors were associated with militias in Great Britain and some went to the Crimea, either to observe, or to volunteer their services. It will be recalled that surgeon Charles Bell could not resist a trip to Brussels after the Battle of Waterloo. Volunteers were employed as assistant surgeons or full surgeons, depending on their experience. There were approximately 30 attached at different times either to Scutari or other locations close by. There were 46 medical students employed as "hospital dressers" who dressed wounds and this often brought them into conflict with nurses who also wished to do this.[53]

The contribution of Mary Seacole to nursing care

Another woman who made a significant contribution to nursing the sick and wounded was a Jamaican Nurse called Mary Seacole. Her father was a Scottish military officer and her mother a black Jamaican. She stated in her autobiography that:

> I am a Creole, and have good Scotch blood coursing in my veins. My father was a soldier, of an old Scotch family.[54]

Her husband, Edwin Horatio Seacole, who was believed to be a relative of Admiral Lord Horatio Nelson, died at any early age. Mary Seacole had extensive experience looking after patients suffering from cholera and yellow fever. She established a boarding house in Jamaica to treat victims of a cholera epidemic with success and had experience as a nurse working alongside doctors. She moved to Panama to stay with her brother and again nursed patients suffering from cholera, although her help had been initially refused because she was black. She understood the contagious nature of the disease and eventually returned to Jamaica via Cuba, treating the sick wherever she went.

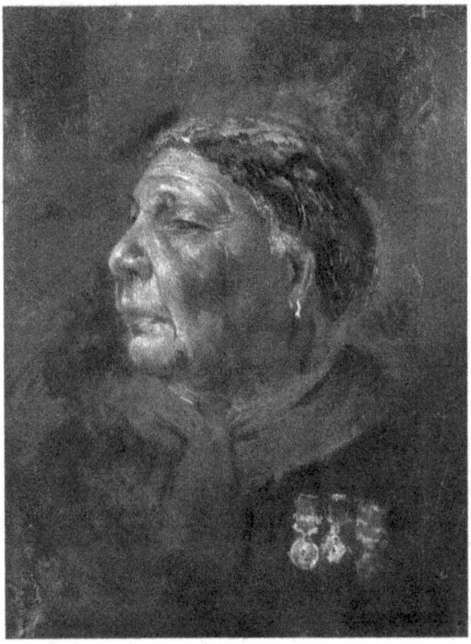

Figure 10.10. Portrait of Mary Jane Seacole by Albert Charles Challen, 1869. (With permission of the National Portrait Gallery, London).

She became involved in the Crimea when Jamaican troops were sent there and reports came back describing the poor conditions. She travelled to Britain and offered her services to the War Office, to the Quartermaster-General's Department and to the Medical Department. She was turned down by them all. She went to Sidney Herbert's house, was interviewed by friends of Nightingale and applied to the Crimea Fund - but they too refused her offer of help. Mary Seacole herself raised the possibility in her autobiography that racial prejudice was the reason for her lack of success.[55]

Undeterred and with help from a friend of her late husband, she bought medicines and supplies and set out at her own expense, where she set up a boarding house called "The British Hotel" just two miles from Balaclava. There was a restaurant on the ground floor and beds for sick and convalescing officers on the upper floor. She even provided care on the battlefields at other times. Nightingale accused her, although not in as many words, of running a brothel which she referred to as a "bad house" and tried to prevent her nurses associating with Seacole.

Despite all her efforts, Seacole was given no official recognition despite being known as the "Black Nightingale" by the soldiers. At the end of the war she was bankrupt. Later, her work was recognised, thanks to officers who knew what she had done and there were public efforts made to support her financially. It has been reported that Nightingale contributed anonymously to this fund. Perhaps she felt guilty. The press acknowledged her contributions with articles appearing in *Punch* and support was given by *The Times* in articles by William Russell. Seacole published her autobiography in 1857, with Russell providing a preface as follows:

> I should have thought that no preface would have been required to introduce Mrs. Seacole to the British public, or to recommend a book which must, from the circumstances in which the subject of it was placed, be unique in literature.
>
> If singleness of heart, true charity, and Christian works; if trials and sufferings, dangers and perils, encountered boldly by a helpless woman on her errand of mercy in the camp and in the battle-field, can excite sympathy or move curiosity, Mary Seacole will have many friends and many readers.
>
> She is no Anna Comnena, who presents us with a verbose history, but a plain truth-speaking woman, who has lived an adventurous life amid scenes which have never yet found a historian among the actors on the stage where they passed.
>
> I have witnessed her devotion and her courage; I have already borne testimony to her services to all who needed them. She is the first who has redeemed the name of "sutler" from the suspicion of worthlessness, mercenary baseness, and plunder; and I trust that England will not forget one who nursed her sick, who sought out her wounded to aid and succour them, and who performed the last offices for some of her illustrious dead. [56]

Eventually the British Government awarded her the Crimea Medal for her work with the sick and wounded. Recognition took a long time but her contributions are now fully acknowledged and the Nursing and Midwifery Council of the UK allocates Mary Seacole Leadership and Development Awards annually in open competition to nurses and midwives. Seacole was voted Greatest Black Briton in an online BBC poll in February 2004. Her portrait hangs in the National Portrait Gallery.

NIGHTINGALE AFTER THE WAR

After the war, Nightingale returned to England, and was hailed a national heroine. Her concern for the care of wounded soldiers remained and to push this agenda she visited Queen Victoria in Scotland at Balmoral Castle in October 1856. She gave evidence to the Sanitary Commission in 1858 (her friend Sidney Herbert being instrumental in this), which certainly valued the evidence that she gave. The work of the Sanitary Commission, along with other important changes, will be discussed fully in Chapter 11. Nightingale remained active and authored two books in 1859 (*Notes on Hospitals* and *Notes on Nursing*) to support her case for the need for reforms. A fund was set up in 1855 to improve nursing care and through her influential connections, and the support of *The Times* she was able to raise almost £60,000, with £44,000 coming from the British Army. This money was crucial to her being able to start the Nightingale School and Home for Nurses.

Even with this help she still faced opposition from the medical profession. The senior surgeon at St Thomas' Hospital, Mr J.F. South (where it was planned for the school to be located), expressed his opinion:

> The very small number of medical men whose names appear in the enormous list of subscribers to the fund cannot have passed unnoticed. Only three physicians and one surgeon from one (London) hospital and one physician from a second, are found among the supporters.[57]

In June 1860, the Nightingale School for Nurses opened and began training nurses but unfortunately her influential personal friend, Sidney Herbert died the following year and this reduced her influence with the War Office, so she focused her attention on sanitary reforms.[58]

Many people questioned why she became so influential and powerful. Her success in the Crimea was attributed to her friendships with ministers and to her association with the Royal Court, both of which allowed her to exert influence when and where it was needed. There is no doubt that she achieved many reforms and was able to cut through red tape and sweep aside administrative delays. However, it is now recognised that many of the reforms attributed to her were done so incorrectly while others had been proposed or even started earlier. For example the establishment of the Army Medical Staff Corps was first proposed by Smith, as was the establishment of a medical statistical branch.[59]

Some surgeons acknowledged Nightingale's contribution, but it is worth noting that if the medical profession had been given access to the resources she had and had enjoyed a similar independence of action, then many lives could have been saved before her arrival.[60] She had her supporters and her detractors including many in the army, as evidence by the report after the war into medical services, which did not mention her once.[61]

Nightingale remained very active in supporting women to attain their chosen careers, unless that career happened to be in the medical profession. She argued that women were better to spend their energies more profitably by becoming nurses. Perhaps, Sir Edward Cook summed up Nightingale very well when he said:

> What was afterwards to characterise her work in a larger field was already observed in Harley Street. It was the combination of masterful powers of organisation with womanly gentleness and sympathy.[62]

When it suited her, she had tact in abundance, diplomatic skills and the ability to make things happen through her contacts! She was also prepared to speak her mind and had numerous difficulties with doctors. She particularly disliked Sir John Hall, and constantly questioned his competence. When he received a KBE (Knight of the British Empire) in 1857, she referred to this as standing for "Knight of the Crimean Burial Grounds". Hall referred to Nightingale as a "petticoat *imperieuse*."

An editorial in the *British Journal* in 1913 concluded that:

> With the fullest admiration of her intellect and energizing power, we think most people will agree that unless she had been the personal friend of the Minister in whose hands were the destinies of the British army at that time, she might never have been allowed to undertake her mission of mercy; or, indeed, she would have had, like so many other spirits burning with the ardour of reform, to retire baffled and heartbroken from a contest with official inertia and ineptitude.[63]

Unfortunately she suffered ill health after the war, perhaps because of it, and she became an invalid requiring full time care, becoming blind before her death in 1910 at the age of 90 years.

COMMON DISEASES OCCURRING AND NECESSITATING HOSPITAL ADMISSION

The state of medical knowledge during the Crimean War was little better than during the Peninsular War. Causes of infectious diseases were not understood. Chapter 13 will deal with the discovery of bacteria and the germ theory of disease.

Diarrhoea

The three commonest diseases to affect the men were diarrhoea (from a variety of causes), dysentery and cholera. The numbers affected who were admitted to hospital are shown in Table 10.6. Different types of diarrhoea were recognised and were categorised as shown below.[64, 65]

Table 10.6 Numbers affected with the common diseases.

DISEASE	NUMBER ADMITTED TO HOSPITAL	NUMBER WHO DIED
Diarrhoea	44,164	3,651
Dysentery	7,882	2,543
Cholera	7,575	4,513

From Cantlie, N., *A History of the Army Medical Department.* Edinburgh and London: Churchill Livingstone, 1974, Volume 2, p.185.

Table 10.7 Recognised types of diarrhoea and their treatment.

TYPE OF DIARRHOEA	TREATMENT
Occurring with cholera	Astringents, mineral oils, creosote, opium
Endemic, summer	Laxatives, mercury, ipecacuahna, silver nitrate enemas
Congestive	Rest, mercurials, anodynes
Atonic	Mineral acids, quinine, cod liver oil, nutritious diets
Scorbutic	1-3 ounces of lime juice given up to three times per day and opium to control diarrhoea if necessary

From Cantlie, N., *A History of the Army Medical Department.* Edinburgh and London: Churchill Livingstone, 1974, Volume 2, p.186.

Dysentery

Two peaks of dysentery (which was differentiated from other causes of diarrhoea by the presence of blood and mucus in the bowel motions) occurred between November 1984 and January 1855 and between July and September 1855. The mortality was greater than 30% (shown in Table 10.6) and various treatments were given including rest and warmth, a good diet, ipecacuahana, mineral acids, charcoal, quinine and opium.

Cholera

Cholera was a major problem during the Crimean War and carried a mortality of 60%. The symptoms, signs and clinical course are summarised in Appendix II. Treatment of the day was based on infusions of arsenic, mercury, opiates and bleeding which did nothing but accelerate death in these sick patients.

Table 10.8 Admissions and deaths from the different types of fever.

TYPE OF FEVERS	ADMISSIONS TO HOSPITAL (DEATHS)
Intermittent fever	2,406 (60)
Common continued fever	25,013 (2,790)
Remittent fever	2,957 (311)
Typhus fever	828 (285)

From Cantlie, N., *A History of the Army Medical Department.* Edinburgh and London: Churchill Livingstone, 1974, Volume 2, p. 187.

Fevers (including typhus)

Fevers of various types accounted for large numbers admitted to the hospitals and the different types of fever which were recognised together with the number of admissions and deaths are shown in Table 10.8.[66]

Treatments tried included quinine, liquor arsenicalis, grey powder and ipecacuanha. Prevention was the key and there was a tenfold reduction in deaths from fevers between the first and second winters of the war after the measures discussed were put in place.

Scurvy

Scurvy was observed approximately three months after the men left for the Crimea and was associated with a diet deficient in fresh fruit and vegetables. Scurvy is associated with bleeding from the gums, loosening of the teeth, bleeding into the skin, muscles and the bowel and progressive weakness and pallor. We now know that the physiological basis for this is a deficiency of vitamin C (ascorbic acid), which is normally present in fresh fruit and vegetables, with a little in meat and milk. It is not synthesised by the body. Vitamin C is important in the formation of collagen which is a key structural part of a variety of body tissues known as connective tissues. A British naval officer called James Lind discovered in 1847 that fresh oranges would cure and prevent scurvy, although he didn't know why. During the initial part of the war, up until April 1855, the number of cases of scurvy was approximately 640 per month, with a mortality of 1 in 12.[67] However, prevention was quite simple and comprised of taking by mouth up to 3 ounces of lime juice given 3 times per day.[68]

SPECIFIC WOUNDS AND THEIR MANAGEMENT

USE OF CHLOROFORM AS ANAESTHESIA FOR THE SURGICAL TREATMENT OF WOUNDS

This is discussed in more detail elsewhere in the book (Chapter 9) but an interesting insight into its use from a surgeon's point of view was published by surgeon Lt. Col. Wrench of the Sherwood Foresters, who was an assistant surgeon with the 34th Foot. He described how the use of chloroform was forbidden because of the fear of using it and causing death. This prohibition for all but the most severe of wounds was issued by the Director-General. Hall declared:

> The cries of the patient undergoing an operation were satisfactory to the surgeon, as an indication that there was no fear of syncope and that pain was a stimulant that aided recovery.[69]

However, the majority of surgeons continued to use chloroform despite Hall's directive.

CAUSATION OF WOUNDS

Wounds were caused by a variety of agents which were often different in the three major battles that occurred. The Battle of the Alma was characterised by wounds caused by the round musket ball; at Balaclava it was the sword and lance; at Inkerman it was the bayonet and musket ball. Wounds were caused by other agents including grape shot, explosives, fragments of shell casing or canister and flying bits of masonry dislodged by exploding shells. Burns were commonly associated with wounds caused by high explosives. It was recognised that when the shape of the musket ball changed from being round to a more conical shape, there were more extensive wounds with greater associated tissue damage.

WOUNDS OF THE LIMBS, IN PARTICULAR, THE THIGH

George James Guthrie served in the Peninsular War and was a most distinguished surgeon who made major contributions to war surgery. He was President of the Royal College of Surgeons in 1854, having been President on two previous occasions, in 1833 and 1841. Although he did not go to the Crimea himself due to his age, he used the experiences of the surgeons in the Crimea to add to his text book and so produced an up to date text of military surgery.[70,71] Forty years before the Crimea he considered that his objective was to save the limb, but if this was not possible and amputation was the only treatment option, then this should be carried out within 24 hours. He specified that there should be an initial period of 3 to 4 hours delay whilst "the first shock had subsided".

Wounds of the thigh were either flesh (muscle) wounds alone, or were associated with damage to major nerves, arteries and fractures of the thigh bone (femur), or damage to the knee joint, or less commonly to the hip joint. There was often a combination of damage to various structures.

A general principle of treatment of wounds to the thigh (and to all wounds of all the limbs) was to explore the wound, enlarge it if necessary and probe it using either specially made instruments or better still the surgeon's finger, considered to be the best instrument of all! By doing this the surgeon gained some understanding of the severity of the wound and was able to remove foreign material, such as clothing, bullets and pieces of debris or metal.

Loose bone fragments could also be removed if the bone had been shattered. If bone fragments were not attached to the surrounding tissues, then they were removed but the significance of retaining a blood supply to the bone was not fully appreciated. Wound exploration by increasing its size surgically or by making other incisions to allow better access was called "dilatation" of the wound. This was an important step to clean out contamination but was only part of what was actually needed for the appropriate management of these wounds.

In modern surgery, the wound would be opened widely to allow direct inspection of damaged and dead tissues before completely excising them. "Dilatation" by its very name implies a limited and therefore inadequate exposure to perform an adequate surgical procedure.

Infection was not understood and surgeons did not realise that retained dead tissue, especially dead muscle, predisposed to bacterial growth and to infection and abscess formation later. This usually occurred from a few days up to 14 days after the wound had been sustained, when pus either burst through the wound or required a surgical incision to allow it to drain. This was accepted as part of the normal course of events after wounding.

Following exploration, the wounded tissues were allowed to fall back into place and if necessary sutures were used to achieve this. Nowadays such primary wound closure would generally not be performed. Delayed primary closure after a few days would be employed, allowing a second look to ensure that all dead tissue had been removed before closing the wound. A piece of wet lint was put over the wound and bandages were applied. The lint was kept moist and the bandage was left in position for up to 72 hours, although some surgeons applied a further dressing over the lint e.g. calamine or gutta percha.[72] It is interesting to note that tetanus seemed to have been relatively uncommon in the Crimean War, if the available figures are an accurate reflection on its incidence. Only 21 cases were recorded between April 1855 and September 1856, and only one patient survived.[73] McGrigor documented 51 deaths from tetanus in two and a half years during the Peninsular War. Treatment of tetanus during the Crimean War was limited and usually involved administration of morphine and chloroform in the hope of relieving the muscle spasms which occur with the disease.

Wounds involving the top part of the thigh were frequently associated with compound fractures of the upper end of the femur and if there was major damage to the femoral artery then an amputation was carried out. Guthrie indicated that if the damage was confined to the top end of the femur (called the femoral head and neck) and if the rest of the limb looked viable and salvable, then a possible alternative to amputation was to excise only the head and neck of the femur where the bony damage had occurred. This was put into practice in the Crimea and several patients were treated in this way, but they all died. Surgeons knew that fractures of the upper femur carried the highest mortality.[74,75] Fractures of the femur below this level but still involving the upper half of the femur were treated by amputation.

Fractures of the lower half of the femur had a better prognosis, provided they did not involve the knee joint. The recommended treatment was to try to preserve the limb if at all possible provided there was no severe damage to major vessels and nerves. The limb was put into various splints to try to keep the fracture in reasonable alignment, with the knee bent, whilst healing occurred. Unfortunately there were no adequate splints to maintain the position, and these fractures were very difficult to manage just as they had been during the Peninsular War. Effective splinting for these fractures would not become available until the Great War.

Infection was almost inevitable and Guthrie explained to readers of his text how this should be dealt with as often there was residual dead and infected bone:

> When the abscess breaks externally, the probe will now pass through the hole in the new bone and rest on the rough, dead, and now perhaps moveable splinter, the extraction of which can alone afford permanent relief. The earlier this is done the softer the ossific matter will be; at an early period, it will cut like Parmesan cheese intermixed with lime.[76]

Mortality rates for this wound were high and there was a school of thought that limb preservation was a mistake and that all compound femoral fractures should be treated by primary amputation. The bones commonly didn't heal or form new bone (fracture callus) and it was felt that general health, especially when patients were suffering from scurvy, was a factor in this respect, although the commonest cause for failure to heal was an infected non-union, where the fracture site became infected and healing thus prevented. Early amputation might have saved many of the wounded from a long course of painful complications resulting in prolonged morbidity, late amputation and death,[77] and many surgeons expressed the view that it was:

> .... better to live with three limbs than die with four.[78]

Mortality for amputations through the thigh at different levels is shown in Table 10.9.[79]

Table 10.9 Mortality following amputation of the limb at different levels.

LEVEL OF AMPUTATION	MORTALITY RATE (%)
Upper third of thigh	87%
Middle third of thigh	60%
Lower third of thigh	57%
Through the knee joint	56%

From MacLeod, G.H.B., *Notes on the surgery of the war in the Crimea, with remarks on the treatment of gunshot wounds*. London: John Churchill, 1862, pp.290-1.

Only 3 soldiers with a compound fracture of the upper one-third of the thigh survived without having an amputation. More survived without amputation if their fractures involved the middle and lower third of the femur but it was considered that the mortality was higher than it would have been had primary amputation been performed. Nevertheless attempts were more commonly made to save the limb at this level.[80] It was universally accepted that if the fracture involved the knee joint then amputation was necessary, because in the unlikely event of surviving this wound without amputation, functional outcome was abysmal. British surgeons expressed their disdain for their French colleagues and surgeon MacLeod stated:

> The French surgeons in the East fully acknowledged the hopelessness of these cases; but the fatality of amputation was, with them, little behind that of preservation.[81]

Whilst the British might have questioned the technical expertise of the French surgeons in carrying out amputations the French philosophy of early amputation was clear:

> ... operate early, and feed your patients, if you wish to save life; operate late, and starve them, if you wish for suppuration, unhealed stumps, pyaemia, dysentery or death.[82]

It was also noted that the different shapes of musket ball produced different effects. Depending on the distance from which it was fired, the round ball might not penetrate the bone if fired from far away, while if very close it might go straight through the bone without splitting it. When fired from middle distances it might shatter the bone. In contrast, the new conical ball used by the Russians would usually shatter the bone, regardless of the range and even if the surgeon only saw a relatively small skin puncture wound, the femur could be split along its whole length.[83] Furthermore, the damage and destruction to the muscles was greater and the risk of complications resulting in death from overwhelming infection significantly higher with this conical ball.

Surgeons began to improve their management of compound fractures when they recognised the importance of removing all the foreign material, e.g. metal, clothing and all the devitalised pieces of bone that had been shattered. They recommended that the exit wound should be enlarged to allow a free flow of pus from the wound, and to keep the "aperture open", and not allow pus to accumulate before making an incision to allow its release.[84] They debated whether or not small pieces of bone which were still attached to periosteum should be retained and recognised that such pieces of bone perhaps helped to generate new bone but also realised that to leave them increased the risk of suppuration. Many survivors had wounds that chronically discharged pus (including bits of dead bone) for many years and had shortening and deformity secondary to loss of bone and mal-alignment of the ends of the fractured bone.

WOUNDS TO THE ABDOMEN

Wounds to the abdomen were recognised as being some of the most serious and were categorised broadly into "blunt" non-penetrating wounds and penetrating wounds. Wounds to the abdominal wall could occur without damage to the contents of the abdomen and these were dealt with by surgical exploration and removal of foreign bodies to facilitate healing. At the most severe end of the spectrum, such wounds might result in destruction of the abdominal wall, with exposure of the abdominal contents, which remained essentially intact at the time the wound was sustained. This was a very serious situation and one which usually resulted in death.

There was a clear understanding that severe blunt trauma could result in major damage to the abdominal contents and could result in death without any apparent injury to the abdominal wall itself. When rupture of the intestines occurred, surgeons knew that the patients would inevitably die.

Often surgeons could not decide whether a projectile (ball or bullet) had entered the abdominal cavity or not on the basis of examining the entry and exit wounds. The situation here was described as follows:

> It is neither allowable nor desirable that we should make such a search as will determine the question; for if the ball be not easily found, we never "amuse ourselves by seeking for it.[85]

The standard treatment was therefore not to try to find the ball or bullet but to follow the treatment regime below:[86]

- The wound was lightly covered with a wet lint compress, if the edges of the wound were widely apart then stitched together;
- The patient was positioned to reduce tension on the abdominal wall;
- Pain relief was provided with opium;
- Food was totally forbidden;
- Enemas (but not purgatives by mouth) were administered;
- If "inflammation" of the peritoneum occurred then the application of leeches to the abdominal wall and/or bloodletting was instituted.

Penetrating wounds of the abdomen commonly resulted in death but surgeons knew that the point of wounding might influence the outcome. They used the patient's symptoms to try to determine which organ within the abdomen had been damaged. For example, vomiting, vomiting blood, passage of blood in the urine or stools, or the appearance of bile stained fluid through the abdominal wound itself helped to localise where the wounded structure was. Whilst surgeons knew that haemorrhage from organs with a rich blood supply occurred, there was a mistaken belief that the blood would subsequently decompose, set up "inflammation" and cause death.[87] If casualties survived and this did occur from time to time, then the wound was re-opened in the hope that any such fluid would escape. Similarly, if there were faeces, urine or blood seen to be coming through a narrow wound then the surgeons would enlarge the wound with the aim of allowing the free escape of these contents.

Some did survive wounds of the liver, kidneys and spleen, when haemorrhage from these organs spontaneously stopped. The fatal consequences of wounds involving the small and large bowel were well recognised, even though in previous wars a handful of survivors had been reported.[88] It was realised that penetrating objects could pass through the abdominal cavity without causing any injury to the contents or significant bleeding and then survival could occur. If the intestine protruded through the abdominal wall it was positioned back into the abdominal cavity but no further surgery within the abdomen was carried out. If there was a hole in the bowel then this was usually left and was in effect a colostomy or ileostomy where the contents of the bowel emerge onto the abdominal wall. The bowel was generally not sutured and when this was tried in a few cases, the outcome was fatal.[89] There were no further developments in abdominal surgery.

WOUNDS OF THE CHEST

There was no effective treatment for chest wounds. Soldiers lived or died depending on what structures within the chest were damaged, and whether or not major infection set in.

Table 10.10 Chest wounds in the 12,094 total wounds in all sites occurring during the Crimea.

	Number	%
Chest wounds compared with all wounds sustained	474	3.90
Actual lung wounds compared with all wounds sustained	164	1.35
Mortality of chest wounds compared with all wounds sustained	135	1.11
Mortality of actual lung wounds compared with all wounds sustained	130	1.07

From Fraser, P., *A treatise upon gunshot wounds of the chest.* London: John Churchill, 1859.

A total of 474 of the 12,094 wounds recorded in the Crimean War were chest wounds (3.9%) but of these chest wounds 80% resulted in death.[90] The late sequelae of blunt, non-penetrating wounds of the chest were recognised with haemorrhage into the lung, contusions and pneumonia.

Penetrating wounds of the chest were usually caused by ball or bullet. The projectile might have passed straight through the chest with an entry and exit wound or it might have become lodged within the chest cavity or elsewhere in the body for that matter. The overall mortality was about 80% for these wounds, but it was thought to be less if the projectile passed through the chest.[91] Even if the casualty survived the initial wounding and did not bleed to death due to injury to major blood vessels within the chest, or to direct damage to the heart, or to the effects of blood accumulating around the heart in sufficient quantities to compress it and to stop it pumping effectively (cardiac tamponade), there was a high probability that infection would occur, with formation of abscesses, within the lung or in the pleural cavity, ensuring a fatal outcome. Autopsy (post-mortem) examinations were carried out, which led to a better understanding of these complications but it was not possible to prevent them.

Management of chest wounds did not involve surgery but did follow the principle to prevent "ingress of air and obviate inflammatory action".[92] Surgeons explored the wound very carefully using their fingers but the only intervention was to carefully remove any foreign bodies, fragments of metal, bits of bone from fractured ribs, if it was easily done. Larrey had done the very same during the Napoleonic Wars. If there was bleeding from an intercostal artery (superficial and next to the rib) then it was stopped using a strong curved needle and a ligature was put around the blood vessel. Wounds were covered using a dressing material but the skin was not sutured. The aim of dressing the wound was to prevent air from entering the chest, but this was almost impossible to achieve.

Although many of the patients who were lucky enough to survive the initial wound had lost blood, surgeons followed the principle that further venesection to remove blood was required since they thought this was the only way to keep blood out of the chest cavity and pressing on the lung.[93] The amount of blood removed was decided upon by the surgeon who relied on his clinical judgement and experience; some surgeons suggested that it should be enough to remain consistent with life-but perhaps only just! These casualties usually died, possibly helped on their way by inappropriate intervention. The only other indication for intervention was if the casualty survived and developed an accumulation of blood in the chest (called a haemo-thorax) which was removed, either by opening the original wound or placing a needle between the ribs to let the blood out of the chest. This may have been beneficial on occasions.

Some patients survived and were carefully guided back to health:

> The strictest regimen should be maintained for ten days or a fortnight after the infliction of a gunshot wound of the lung. Any irregularity in diet, or indulgence in ardent spirits during convalescence, is most apt to cause dangerous if not fatal relapses. Not a few were lost in the East from such carelessness.[94]

WOUNDS TO THE HEAD

Wounds to the head were most commonly caused by musket balls, bullets, grape, shells and sword. The damage caused was variable, ranging from sword wounds where a fragment of the skull might be cleaved off, to wounds from blunt swords which caused extensive splintering and depression of bone. Shell wounds often had a large amount of bone which was driven into the underlying brain causing extensive destruction of brain tissue.

Severe wounds were usually fatal and one of the commonly used classifications and the mortality associated with these wounds in shown in Table 10.11.

Table10.11 Classification and mortality of head wounds.

CATEGORISATION OF HEAD WOUND	MORTALITY RATE (%)
Simple flesh wound	0%
Severe flesh wounds	3.4%
Cranial fracture without depression of bone	36%
Depressed fracture of the skull with contusion	72%

The standard treatment was non-surgical and included many of the following:

- Dressing wounds (e.g. with wet linen);
- Purging and enemas;
- Keeping quiet (described as "utmost quiet");
- Shaving the hair off the head and applying cold either through ice or water;
- Applying leeches to the scalp;
- Minimal diet.

Operative intervention was variable and a subject for extensive debate, but the general view was not to operate unless there were either symptoms of "compression" of the brain, although these symptoms were not clearly defined, or there was a depressed compound fracture of the skull. Surgeon John Bell summed matters up when he stated:

> No injury requires operation except compression of the brain, which may arise from extravasated blood, or from depressed bone, or matter generated from within the skull.[95]

Bell's recommendations would form a reasonable basis today for surgical intervention in a patient with a head wound, although neurosurgeons today have a much more refined and clearer understanding of pathology of wounds of the brain, and are able to employ sophisticated technology such as CT scans and magnetic resonance imaging scans to indicate exactly what the pathology is and where it is to be found.

Some surgeons in the Crimea were more aggressive in their surgical management of head wounds and attempted extensive operations in some instances to remove bullets and balls which may have travelled to the opposite side of the brain. Although some successes are recorded the majority of casualties died, with MacLeod perhaps offering some words or advice and caution when he said:

> "... perhaps the best line of conduct is to let the man die in peace".[96]

The management of simple flesh wounds involved the use of dressings and all patients recovered. Patients with more complex wounds generally experienced a poor result. Those with skull fractures where the skull bones lay in their correct position (i.e. the bone was not "depressed" into the brain) were treated in a variety of ways including use of antimony, purgatives, venesection and the application of leeches. If the patient's condition deteriorated, presumably due to bleeding around the brain with a rise in intra-cranial pressure, then sometimes a surgical operation was carried out to remove any fragments of bone – but the patients always died.

When the bone was depressed into the underlying brain, 72% of patients died. In some cases, surgeons attempted to operate and remove the depressed bone (which was technically relatively straightforward to do) but this was still associated with a very high mortality as a result of complications such as meningitis and brain abscess formation. Nevertheless, some patients did survive although many experienced distressing long term effects such as paralysis, and incapacitating changes in their cognition and mental functions. The most severe wound to be encountered was the penetrating wounds of the brain which carried 100% mortality.

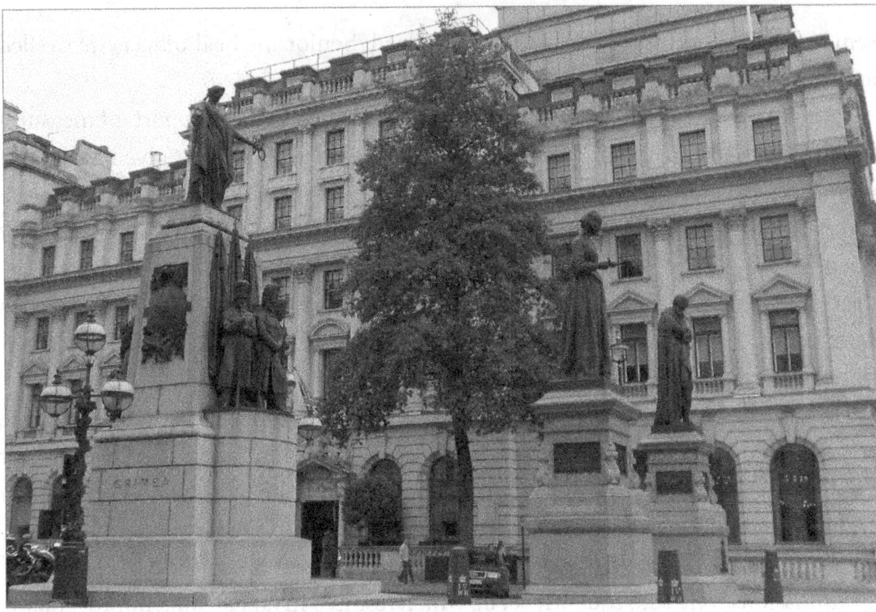

Figure 10.11. The Crimean War Memorial in London, unveiled in 1861, and designed by John Bell. The figures were cast in bronze from Russian cannon captured after the siege of Sevastopol. It was dedicated specifically to the 2,152 members of the Brigade of Guards lost in the Crimean War. It was modified in 1918 to accommodate two more statues of Florence Nightingale and Sidney Herbert. (Authors' photograph).

SUMMARY

By the end of the Peninsular War in 1814, James McGrigor had improved the health of Wellington's forces by many important measures which he had introduced after becoming Wellington's Chief Medical Officer in the Peninsula. He clearly appreciated that hospitals should be clean and well ventilated and that overcrowding should be avoided at all costs since overcrowding in squalid conditions predisposed to various fevers which carried a high mortality. McGrigor was highly regarded by the senior Peninsular surgeon George James Guthrie, who attributed much of the surgical success in the Peninsula to McGrigor's organisational skills. Wellington had complete faith in his senior medical officer and McGrigor made a very significant contribution to the success of the war.

In contrast, the situation in the Crimea was quite the opposite. Senior medical officers were held in very low esteem both by politicians and by senior military service personnel. As a result, communication between military authority and senior medical personnel was very poor indeed. Senior medical officers quarrelled amongst themselves and were simply not up to the job.

All the good work done by McGrigor was forgotten and the important measures he introduced to maintain the health of troops were either never given a thought or were completely disregarded, with the result that hospitals in the Crimea were filthy, overcrowded and without any air circulation because the windows would not open. This was a recipe for disaster which duly occurred when there were so many deaths from disease. McGrigor ensured that over the winter of 1812/13 that troops were well fed to improve their health. The nutrition of soldiers in the Crimea was so bad that men died of scurvy.

It was the first war when reporters informed the public in Britain about the conditions under which soldiers were living, fighting and dying and as a result the Crimean War was rightly regarded as a scandal. Soldiers should never have to endure the appalling conditions that men put up with in the Crimea.

There is no doubt that major lessons were learned from the Crimean War. Commissions were subsequently set up which resulted in far reaching improvements in conditions during the second half of the nineteenth century. Problems of overcrowding and poor hospital sanitation, responsible for so many deaths during the Crimean War were tackled and the education and training of doctors was improved by the establishment of an Army Medical School. Never again would the medical profession be so badly prepared for war as it was between 1854 and 1856.

ENDNOTES

1. Lawrenson, R., "Sir James Mouat, VC KCB FRCS (1815-1899): winner of the first medical Victoria Cross", *Journal of Medical Biography* 2004; 12(4): pp.196-201.
2. Gill, C.J., G.C.Gill, "Nightingale in Scutari: her legacy re-examined", *Clinical Infectious Diseases* 2005; 40: pp.1799-1805.
3. *Medical and Surgical History of the British Army in the War against Russia 1854-1856*. London: Harrison, 1858, Volume I.
4. Cantlie, N., *A History of the Army Medical Department*. Edinburgh and London: Churchill Livingstone, 1974, Volume 2.
5. Evatt, G.V.H., *Army Medical Organisation*. Allahabad: Pioneer Press, 1977, p.3-1.
6. Guthrie, G., *Commentaries on the surgery of the war in Portugal, Spain, France and the Netherlands.* Philadelphia: J.B. Lippincott, 1862.

7. Ballingall, J., *Outline of Military Surgery*. Edinburgh: Adam and Black, 1833.
8. Watson, W.B., "An Edinburgh surgeon of the Crimean War. Patrick Heron Watson (1832-1907)". *Medical History* 1966; 10(2): pp.166-176.
9. *Ibid.*
10. Cantlie, *op. cit.*
11. *Ibid.*
12. *Ibid.*
13. Shepherd, J., *The Crimean Doctors. A History of the British Medical Services in the Crimean War.* Liverpool: Liverpool University Press, 1991, Volume 2.
14. Cantlie, *op. cit.*
15. *Ibid.*
16. *Ibid.*
17. Mitra, S.M., *The Life and Letters of Sir John Hall.* New York, Bombay and Calcutta: Longmans, Green and Co., 1911.
18. *Ibid.*
19. *Medical and Surgical History of the British Army in the War against Russia 1854-1856.* London: Harrison, 1858, Volume I.
20. Cantlie, *op. cit.*
21. *Ibid.*
22. Wrench, E.M., "Midland Branch: The Lessons of the Crimean War". *British Medical Journal* 1899; 2: pp.205-208.
23. *Ibid.*
24. *Ibid.*
25. Duberly, F., *Journal kept during the Russian war: from the departure of the army in England in April 1854, to the fall of Sebastopol.* London: Longman, 1856.
26. Hill B. "Treatment of the sick and wounded in war", *British Medical Journal* 1870; 2 (510): p.375-5.
27. *Ibid.*
28. Wrench, *op. cit.*
29. Osborne, S.G., *Scutari and its hospitals.* London: Dickinson Brothers, 1855.
30. *Ibid.*
31. Bloy, M., *Florence Nightingale (1820-1910).* 2012; available at: http://www.victorianweb.org/history/crimea/florrie.html. Accessed 01/29, 2012.

32. Hibbert, C., *The condition of the British Army in the Crimea.* 2002; available at: http://www.victorianweb.org/history/crimea/condition.html. Accessed 01/29, 2012.
33. Goldie, S., *Florence Nightingale: Letters from the Crimea 1854-1856.* Manchester: Mandolin, 2007, p.23.
34. *Ibid.*
35. Bloy, *op. cit.*
36. *Florence Nightingale.* 2008; available at: http://www.robinsonlibrary.com/medicine/nursing/history/nightingale.htm. Accessed 29/12, 2012.
37. *Florence Nightingale Biography.* 2011; available at: http://www.biography.com/people/florence-nightingale-9423539?page=4. Accessed 01/30, 2012.
38. Cook, E., *The life of Florence Nightingale, 1862-1910.* London: Macmillan and Co, 1913, Volume II.
39. Anonymous. "Florence Nightingale". *British Medical Journal* 1913, pp.1436-3.
40. Dalrymple, T., "The truth about Nightingale". *British Medical Journal* 2012 (overseas and retired doctors' edition). 344: p.35.
41. Cantlie, N., *A History of the Army Medical Department.* Edinburgh and London: Churchill Livingstone, 1974, Volume 2, p.91.
42. Shepherd, J., *The Crimean Doctors. A History of the British Medical Services in the Crimean War.* Liverpool: Liverpool University Press, 1991, Volume 2, p.356.
43. Baylen, J.O., "The Florence Nightingale/Mary Stanley controversy: some unpublished letters". *Medical History* 1974; 18(2) pp.186-193.
44. Woodham-Smith, C., *Florence Nightingale, 1820-1910.* London: Constable, 1950, p.194.
45. Baylen, *op. cit.*, pp.186-193.
46. Dalrymple, *op. cit.*, p.35.
47. Gill, C.J., G.C.Gill, *op. cit.*, pp.1799-1805.
48. Shepherd, J., *The Crimean Doctors. A History of the British Medical Services in the Crimean War.* Liverpool: Liverpool University Press, 1991, Volume 2, p.457.
49. *Alexis Bénoist Soyer.* Available at: http://www.soyer.co.uk/. Accessed 03/12.
50. Scarlett, E.P., "Officer and Gentleman", *Canadian Medical Association Journal* 1967; p.1415.
51. *Shepherd, op. cit., p.457.*
52. *Ibid*, p.474.
53. *Ibid.*

54. Seacole, M., *Wonderful adventures of Mrs Seacole in many lands*. London: James Blackwood, 1857.
55. *Ibid.*
56. *Ibid.*
57. Anonymous. "Florence Nightingale". *British Medical Journal* 1913; pp.1436-3.
58. Williams, K., Reappraising Florence Nightingale. *British Medical Journal* 2008; 337: 2889, pp.1461-2.
59. *Ibid.*
60. Wrench, *op. cit.*, pp.205-208.
61. *Medical and surgical history of the British Army which served in Turkey and the Crimea during the war against Russia during the years 1854-1856.* London: Harrison, 1858.
62. Anonymous. "Florence Nightingale". *British Medical Journal* 1913; pp.1436-3.
63. *Ibid.*
64. Rawlinson, R., "An address on hygiene of armies in the field", *British Medical Journal* 1883;.1(1174): pp.1276-1.
65. Cantlie, *op. cit.*, p.185.
66. *Ibid*, p.187.
67. *Ibid*, p.189.
68. *Ibid*, p.187.
69. Wrench, *op. cit.*, pp.205-208.
70. Shepherd, *op. cit.*, p.474.
71. Guthrie. G., *Commentaries on the surgery of the war in Portugal, Spain, France and the Netherlands.* Philadelphia: J.B. Lippincott, 1862.
72. Shepherd, *op. cit.*, p.474.
73. *Ibid*
74. Guthrie, G., *op. cit.*, p.564.
75. *Ibid*, p.569.
76. *Ibid*, p.152.
77. MacLeod, G.H.B., Notes *on the surgery of the war in the Crimea, with remarks on the treatment of gunshot wounds.* London: John Churchill, 1862, p.251.
78. Guthrie, G., *op. cit.*, pp.140-1.
79. MacLeod, *op. cit.*, pp.290-1.
80. *Ibid*, p.263.
81. *Ibid*, p.267.

82. Guthrie, G., *op. cit.* pp.140-1.
83. MacLeod, *op. cit.*, pp.290-1.
84. *Ibid.*
85. *Ibid.*
86. *Ibid*, p.235.
87. *Ibid*, p.283.
88. *Ibid*, p.230.
89. Shepherd, *op. cit.*, pp.478-481.
90. Fraser, P., *A treatise upon gunshot wounds of the chest*. London: John Churchill, 1859.
91. Shepherd, *op. cit.*, pp.478-481.
92. Fraser, *op. cit.*, p.109.
93. MacLeod, *op. cit.*, p.214.
94. *Ibid*, p.221.
95. *Ibid*, p.171.
96. *Ibid*, p.186

11

Medical Reforms after the Crimean War

Serious medical shortcomings were identified during the Crimean War which became the catalyst for change over the following years. Florence Nightingale was actively involved in many of the reforms, as was her friend, Sidney Herbert, who had been Secretary of State for War during the Crimean War. It was Herbert who sent Nightingale to the Crimea and who became her great ally. Herbert worked tirelessly to improve the health of the army after the war. He was the first Minister to set himself the task of improving the health of the ordinary soldier. The strain proved too much for him and after being compelled to resign through ill health he died on 2 August 1861.

When Florence Nightingale returned from the Crimea, she was quite determined to make changes in the organisation of the Medical Department. She made a direct appeal to Queen Victoria and to the Secretary of State for War, Lord Panmure. This meant that she effectively bypassed the Director General of Army Medical Services, Sir Andrew Smith, whom she regarded with disdain.

As a result of her irregular, but nevertheless effective approach, the Royal Sanitary Commission was set up in 1857, presided over by Sidney Herbert and with Dr Graham Balfour as secretary. Balfour was a statistician, whose previous role has been discussed earlier in this book (Chapter 7). He took over from Henry Marshall when the latter retired after completing his work, the *"Statistical report on the sickness, mortality and invaliding among the troops in the West Indies"*. Florence Nightingale was a most enthusiastic statistician and thoroughly approved of Balfour's appointment.

As well as the Sanitary Commission, other commissions were established and these will be outlined before studying the work of the Sanitary Commission in some detail.

Sidney Herbert was chairman of the Indian Army Sanitary Commission which sat in 1859. Florence Nightingale had vociferously supported the establishment of this Commission when it became clear that soldiers' barracks and hospitals in India were frequently situated in the unhealthiest locations. This of course resulted in soldiers being put at significant risk of catching "fevers", sometimes with fatal consequences. Improvements in hospitals were required, with better ventilation, a safer and purer water supply and improved drainage all being essential to promote a healthy environment for the soldiers and the staff. As a result of the measures introduced the mortality in the Indian Army fell from an average of 68 per 1,000 (between the years 1817 and 1856) to 18.69 per 1,000 by 1871.[1]

The Commission for Soldiers' Day Room and Institutes was established to tackle the problems associated with excessive consumption of spirits by soldiers. It was proposed to build appropriate facilities for troops so that they would spend more time engaged in healthy recreation and exercise and with the hope of spending less time going to public houses and getting drunk. It was recognised that "intemperance" was one of the main factors which predisposed to disease. Furthermore, chronic liver disease secondary to alcohol abuse can impair the body's immune response thus making individuals more susceptible to disease, delaying wound healing and increasing the risk of wound infection. Excessive alcohol consumption by soldiers was endemic and in 1834 Henry Marshall had urged vigorously that consumption of liquor should be abolished and that this would lead to an improvement in the health of garrisons who were overseas.[2]

The Purveyors' Branch, whose role was to make supplies available, had been greatly criticised during the Crimean War both for incompetence and corruption. As a result of experiences in the Crimea, purveyors were now authorised to issue clothing to soldiers admitted to hospital. Previously, soldiers were required to provide clothes for themselves on admission. This system completely failed during the Crimean War and many casualties arrived home from the Crimea dressed in filthy rags.

THE WORK OF THE SANITARY COMMISSION OF 1857

Four sub commissions were set up to deal with various issues, all aimed at improving the health of soldiers. They were established to deal with the following subjects:

- The reorganisation of the Medical Department;
- The creation of an Army Medical School;
- The establishment of a Department of Medical Statistics;
- A barrack and hospital improvement scheme.

The reorganisation of the medical department

Medical officers had grievances about pay and conditions of service including their own promotion prospects. Their pay was not on an equal footing with that of other officers and they were discriminated against. Over the course of many years, there would be various attempts made to rectify this inequality, but unfortunately these would meet with little success.

Without doubt, the principal grievance, which was not resolved by a Commons Select Committee of Enquiry in 1856, was the lack of authority conferred upon medical officers during the discharge of their duties. One of the conclusions of the committee was that the relative position of medical and combatant officers should remain unchanged and medical officers should not be made a military body with the authority that doing so would have conferred upon medical officers.[3]

As part of the overhaul of medical services, educational standards were made more stringent, and doctors, as well as having the diploma in surgery from the Royal College of Surgeons, would now also be required to hold the Licentiate from the Royal College of Physicians.

With regard to the "relative ranks" of medical officers, a staff or regimental assistant surgeon was equivalent to a lieutenant; a staff or regimental surgeon was equivalent to a major; a surgeon-major was equivalent to a lieutenant colonel; a deputy inspector general to a colonel; and an inspector general to a brigadier-general.[4]

This was not a real equivalence in all respects and these were not military ranks. Doctors were regarded as little better than "camp followers". There was a widespread prejudice against them and no matter how long a medical officer served he was always subordinate to the most junior military subaltern.[5]

At first, the Royal Warrant of 1858 was acclaimed by medical officers as important and a step forwards in view of the better pay and conditions it provided for them. It even offered medical officers who sat on courts martial precedence according to relative rank which was a gesture which was welcomed by medical personnel. Any positive feeling, however, was short-lived and the warrant became the subject of much discontent as a result of subsequent actions taken by regular army officers.[6]

Such was the concern amongst regular army officers from Horse Guards (the official home of the British Army) that medical officers would rise above their station, that a further Royal Warrant was issued in 1858. This warrant ensured that medical officers were permanently junior to all regular officers of the same relative rank. This meant that a medical officer, who might have had 30 years of experience, could well be junior to a subaltern who had just joined the army. The number of medical recruits dramatically declined and a total of 70 new entrants a year was required to replace natural wastage of doctors, let alone fuel an expansion in the service. However, there were only 24 who joined in 1861, 51 in 1862 and 54 in 1863.[7]

So great was the disillusionment caused by loss of hard fought for privileges that Florence Nightingale urged that the terms of the original Royal Warrant should be restored otherwise the army would simply not be able to recruit the required number of medical staff. She was quick to point out that medical staff needed proper military status and "gentlemanly treatment".[8]

Apart from inequality of rank, there were recurring issues of poor pay and conditions. By contrast, the Colonial Medical Services offered better pay and conditions and not surprisingly attracted the best candidates. Indeed, some of the candidates for the Army Medical School were regarded as being quite unfit to be doctors. Between 1860 and 1865, there were only six candidates of first class standard, 144 of second class and 180 of third class.[9] The Royal Colleges believed that the poor quality of applicants reflected the poor conditions in the army and that the best candidates looked elsewhere for employment.

Pay and conditions were improved by another Royal Warrant enacted in 1867, but many years would pass before medical officers would be regarded as equals by their other non-medical officer colleagues. The unresolved question of rank would become a festering sore of discontent. Even when the Royal Army Medical Corps came into being in 1898, medical authority over health matters of the troops would take some considerable time.

It would not be until 1906, when Richard Haldane was appointed Secretary of State for War, with a remit to modernise the British Army in preparation for a European war, that doctors would exert real influence in matters that were appropriate for them to do so.[10] Haldane's contribution will be discussed later in this chapter.

The creation of an Army Medical School

The Army Medical School was opened at Fort Pitt in 1860 and was transferred to Netley two years later. Once again, Florence Nightingale played a major role in its formation by exerting pressure on its founding members. It had been the wish of Sir James McGrigor to create a Military School of Medicine,[11] but the cost incurred by the treasury to fund the Napoleonic Wars ensured that it never happened in his lifetime. Edinburgh University created a Chair of Military Surgery in 1806 and led the way in the instruction of medical students in military surgery throughout much of the nineteenth century.[12]

Now, in the wake of the Crimean disaster public opinion finally loosened the purse strings of the Treasury. There were four chairs created in the new Military School of Medicine to push forwards the frontiers of research and ensure that the best care would be given to soldiers. The four chairs were in Medicine, Surgery, Hygiene and Pathology, with all being filled by able and experienced men.

Thomas Longmore, a Deputy Inspector of Hospitals, was appointed to the Chair of Surgery. His remit included field medical organisation and transportation and equipment. He had a long and distinguished career with the Medical School. Longmore published a book in 1877 which covered every aspect of gunshot wounds.[13] He included chapters on all types of projectile, both large and small, along with details of the weapons that fired these projectiles, their range and killing power. The effects of missiles on different types of human tissues and the treatment and complications of wounds, including hospital gangrene which was prevalent throughout the nineteenth century, were discussed in full. He dealt with the regional incidence of wounds and their outcomes and provided statistical analysis of wounds, including the number of expected major and minor wounds sustained in any given engagement.

Longmore's responsibilities included the provision of a strategy for transportation of the wounded and in 1876 a committee was formed to modernise the evacuation pathway for casualties. It was chaired by the then Director General of Army Medical Services, Sir William Muir, and Longmore was on the committee. A complete evacuation pathway was introduced, with stretcher bearer companies, movable field hospitals, stationary hospitals, general hospitals, sanitary detachments and often hospital ships in those campaigns with a maritime base.[14]

The first line of medical care consisted of a regimental medical officer with sixteen stretcher bearers. The bearer company then assumed responsibility to transport the wounded to a field hospital in ambulance wagons. Field hospitals were mobile units, which dealt with soldiers with minor wounds, while more seriously wounded men were transferred to stationary hospitals on the lines of communication. Each field hospital was supplied with 200 beds, and was divided into three or four sections, capable of independent activity. Field hospitals were equipped with bell tents.

Stationary hospitals had marquees since they were larger. There were 13 stationary hospitals of 200 beds each for every army corps. General hospitals were located at the base, each with approximately 500 beds. A hospital ship often functioned as an additional base hospital. Swift steamers attached to hospital ships transported the most serious saveable cases back to Great Britain.

A Commissariat Transport Corps allocated vehicles for the various forms of transport needed by the medical units. There was one very serious problem with this otherwise praiseworthy organisation. To enable it to run smoothly, the Principal Medical Officers invariably asked for transport to be put under medical administrative control. However, this was invariably turned down on the grounds that medical officers, without executive rank, could under no circumstances be allowed to give orders to a Transport Officer of the regular army. As a result, there were frequent and frustrating delays.

Dr E.F. Parkes became Professor of Hygiene and he gave the school an international reputation in the science of field sanitation. His laboratory research included investigation into the purification of water using potassium permanganate and the disinfection of sewage by means of filters. He became a world authority in preventive medicine and was the author of a book entitled "*The Manual of Practical Hygiene.*"[15] Parkes laid great emphasis on regulations which were published in 1859. For the first time a regimental medical officer could officially advise his commanding officer on all matters relating to the health of troops.[16] Needless to say, this was a potentially very important milestone in medical responsibility. However, just because a medical officer became entitled to advise his commanding officer, did not necessarily mean his advice was listened to or followed.

Parkes' Manual of Practical Hygiene covered every aspect of military hygiene. It gave advice on the supply, storage and purification of water, and on the disinfection and deodorisation of sewage. It discussed prevention of diseases and focussed on the well being of soldiers in their barracks, detailing the minimum desirable space for every soldier. The provision of adequate ventilation and nutrition, with close attention to proper diet for maintaining good health was clearly laid out.

Parkes made a study of various diseases which were a great source of morbidity and mortality. Whilst the causes of these diseases were not known in many cases, he nevertheless recommended effective measures which could be adopted to help in their control. One of the most lethal diseases was cholera and Parkes wrote:

> External Cause—as in the case of yellow fever, we have no certain clue to the origin of cholera, and in some respects the propagation of the disease is very enigmatical. The way, for example, in which the disease has spread over vast regions, and has then entirely disappeared and the mode in which it seems to develop and decline in a locality, in a sort of regular order and at certain seasons, are facts which we can only imperfectly explain. But as far as

> preventive measures are concerned, the researches of late years seem to have given us indications on which we are bound to act, though they are based only on a partial knowledge of the laws of spread of this poison.[17]

Parkes went on to say:

> The portability of the disease, i.e., the carriage of cholera from one place to another by persons ill with the disease, both in the earliest stage (the so-called premonitory diarrhoea), the latter period, and in convalescence; the carriage by healthy persons coming from infected districts is not so certain; but there is some evidence. It is clear this last point is a most important one, in which it is desirable to have more complete evidence. The occasional carriage by soiled clothes, though not on the whole common, has also evidence in its favour. All these points were affirmed by the Vienna Conference of 1874. Even Pettenkofer admitted that man is the carrier of the disease germ, although the locality may be the means of rendering it potent. On the other hand, Dr. J.M. Cuningham makes a "tabula rasa" of everything, denies the transportability of the disease either by persons or by water, and says there is a mysterious factor still to be sought for. His evidence, however, cannot be considered as conclusive.
>
> Whatever may be the final opinion on all these points, we are bound to act as if they were perfectly ascertained. It is usually impossible to have rigid quarantines; for nothing short of absolute non-communication would be useful, and this is impossible except in exceptional cases. For persons very slightly ill, or who have the disease in them but are not yet apparently ill, or possibly who are not and will not be ill at all, can give the disease, and therefore a selection of dangerous persons cannot be made.[18]

This is a perceptive account, because clearly Parkes recognised that cholera could be transmitted by patients with only minor symptoms. Furthermore, he also was aware that it could be transmitted by some who were asymptomatic but were still capable of carrying the disease. He did not understand why the disease sometimes appeared and then spread over vast areas, only to subsequently regress and disappear.

We now understand that the disease did not disappear, but rather continued in a low grade and unobtrusive fashion in India, within a population with partial immunity only to re-emerge with a vengeance when conditions were right. Parkes was witnessing the cholera pandemics which swept around the globe, often assisted by the movement of British troops.

Parkes was quite clear that cholera was a water-borne infection, as his following account confirms:

> The introduction of the disease into any place by persons is considered by most observers to be connected with the choleric discharges, either when newly passed, or according to some, when decomposing. The reasons for this are briefly these: the portability being certain, the thing carried is more likely to be in the discharges from the stomach and bowels than from the skin or breath (the urine is out of the question), and for these reasons : Water can communicate the disease, and this could only be by contamination with the discharges ; water contaminated by discharges has actually given the disease, as in Dr. McNamara's cases ; in some cases a singularly local origin is proved, and this is nearly always a latrine, sewer, or receptacle of discharges, or a soil impregnated with choleraic evacuations ; soiled linen has sometimes given it, and this is far more likely to be from discharges than from the perspiration.[19]

Unfortunately Parkes died of pulmonary tuberculosis in 1876 at the relatively young age of 56. Dr William Aitken was appointed to the position of Professor of Pathology. He wrote a text *The Science and Practice of Medicine*, a work which was in great demand and which maintained the high profile of the Medical School.[20]

Dr Morehead became the first Professor of Medicine, holding the chair for one year only before being succeeded by Dr Alexander Maclean. Maclean had previously taught at the Medical School at Hyderabad, and had particular experience in yellow fever. In 1864 there was an outbreak of yellow fever in Bermuda, which killed 14 (18.9%) officers and 173 (14.9%) men. Amongst the officers who died were 4 medical officers. According to Professor Maclean, this epidemic could have been avoided, since medical officers had given warning that it was imminent but their advice had been ignored.[21]

When Sir William Aitken retired from the Chair of Pathology in 1892, his place was taken by Almroth Wright. Wright was a strong advocate of placing medicine on a scientific footing. Netley (to where the Army Medical School moved in 1863 instead of Chatham) gave him ample opportunity for research and he most certainly put his time to good use, performing research into diabetes and acidosis. But it was his work on typhoid fever that really made his reputation.

Typhoid fever is spread by contaminated food and water and was common in India and South Africa. Wright developed a vaccine effective against typhoid. He demonstrated that organisms that had been killed (and therefore likely to be safe) could stimulate immunity against the live organism if an individual was subsequently exposed to it. He first used his vaccine in 1896 and demonstrated the formation of antibodies in "volunteer" subjects who were at Netley! Despite no harm befalling his "volunteers", the War Office would not sanction compulsory vaccination, fearing that the vaccine might not be as harmless as Wright claimed.

It was left up to the individual soldier to decide whether or not to be vaccinated. As a result, in the South African War in 1899-1902 only 14,626 men were vaccinated. There were 1,417 cases of typhoid and 163 deaths in this group. This meant that 313,618 men had not been vaccinated. There were 48,754 cases of typhoid and 6,991 deaths in this group. The mortality per 1,000 amongst the inoculated group was 10 and amongst the un-inoculated group it was 32. Despite these convincing statistics the War Office suspended voluntary inoculation, stating that the case for vaccination had not been made! Wright was furious and resigned from his Professorship! [22]

In 1902, London became the centre of activities, and Netley went in to decline. It finally closed as a military hospital and school in 1905, and in May 1907 the Royal Army Medical College formally opened at Millbank in London.

The establishment of a Department of Medical Statistics

The report of the Committee on the preparation of Army Medical Statistics was published in 1861 and in the same year the first annual report of the Army Medical Department was published.

Florence Nightingale was a passionate statistician and once again she played a prominent role in influencing the setting up of this department. She had a gift for mathematics which she had exhibited from an early age. She was particularly interested in statistics, a field in which her father was an expert. Nightingale made extensive use of statistical analysis in the compilation, analysis and presentation of information relating to medical care and public health.

It was partly as a result of her influence and effort that Dr Graham Balfour (Chapter 7) was appointed to lead the department. He was well qualified having worked previously with Alexander Tulloch. Tulloch and Balfour produced statistical analyses from various parts of the Empire, after Tulloch's initial ground breaking work on diseases in the West Indies carried out in collaboration with the pioneering statistician, Henry Marshall.

All through the first half of the nineteenth century, the nomenclature of disease was based on Cullen's Nosology which was published in 1780. A nosology is a systematic classification of disease.

William Cullen (1710-1790) was a Scottish physician, and a leading academic at the University of Edinburgh Medical School. He was a leading figure in the Scottish enlightenment and was Adam Smith's personal physician. The hallmarks of Scottish medicine were close clinical observation, hands-on diagnosis and a systematic approach.[23] Cullen, in his day, revolutionised the practice of medicine and produced many important publications. This perhaps explains why his text was still being used nearly one hundred years after its publication. Alternatively, it might also reveal how little medical science had progressed during that time.

Now a new and improved nomenclature of disease was introduced to replace Cullen's Nosology as a symbol of modernisation and enlightenment of military medicine in the second half of the nineteenth century. In 1870 the classification of diseases was changed by the Royal College of Physicians. Disease caused by miasma, or march vapours, was finally laid to rest and medicine was on a new and more scientific footing.

The publication of the first practical statistical analysis quickly established Balfour as the leading statistician amongst Europe's armies.

Table 11.1 shows the mortality at various locations around the world with the figures in column 2 for the years 1817-21. They have been taken from a paper in *Proceedings from the Royal Society of Medicine* in 1916. The years 1817-21 were chosen because the British Empire was at peace during those years. This means that the figures therefore represent deaths caused exclusively by disease and thus not affected by the result of enemy action.[24]

Because these are mean figures they tend to "flatten out" peaks and troughs. For example, in the cholera outbreak in Lahore in 1861, the mortality reached two-thirds with 837 deaths out of 1,303 admissions in Bengal, and 425 out of 643 cases in Punjab, giving mortalities per 1,000 of 642 and 660 respectively.[25]

A barrack and hospital improvement scheme

The final sub-commission of the Royal Sanitary Commission was put in place to improve the observed sanitary deficiencies which had been made all too obvious by the Crimean War. Often barracks and hospitals were constructed in the unhealthiest of places, with those building them having no knowledge of basic sanitary and other health requirements. The committee drew up a code of practice for sanitary requirements for all future constructions. They proposed major changes

Table 11.1 Mean annual mortalities for 1860-1898 and for 1817-1820. All columns are mortalities per 1,000.

LOCATION	MEAN ANNUAL MORTALITY	MEAN ANNUAL MORTALITY PER 1.000 FOR EACH DECADE			
	1817-21	1860-69	1870-79	1880-89	1890-98
U.K.	17	9.95	12.67	6.40	9.03
W. Indies	185	5.58	10.99	14.94	9.56
S.Africa	12	13.16	39.12	37.96	7.38
Ceylon	111	13.03	14.90	14.34	9.66
China		52.04	14.14	9.82	11.03
India	85	25.46	19.25	16.36	16.42
Egypt				26.72	13.22
W.Africa	362				45.13

Data column 2: From Chaplin A., "The rate of mortality in the British Army 100 years ago". *Proceedings of the. Royal Society of Medicine.* 1916; 9 (section History of Medicine); pp.89-99. Remainder of data from: Rosenbaum S., "More than a century of Army medical statistics." *Journal of the Royal Society of Medicine.* 1990; 83: pp.456-463.

to every aspect of any building to militate against any possible adverse impacts on the general health and well being of the soldiers.

FURTHER ADMINISTRATIVE CHANGES: THE CARDWELL REFORMS OF 1870-1873

Further changes for medical officers came about in 1870 at the time of a widespread reorganisation of the army. Separate regiments were replaced by two linked battalions which constituted a regiment. One battalion was always abroad in some part of the Empire, whilst the other was at home. The overseas battalion was kept up to full strength, and the home based unit provided drafts for the overseas battalion to make good any losses. Therefore, the home-based battalion always tended to be under strength. Much of the impetus for medical change was as a result of observations made on the performance of the Prussian Medical Services during the Franco-Prussian War, when it became clear what could be achieved with scientifically trained personnel and an organised system of medical care. [26] Medical officers were removed from the regiment, and put under the control of the Principal Medical Officer (PMO), and were detailed by him to go where directed.

In 1873, the regimental hospital system which had existed for 200 years was abolished, in what became defined as "unification" (see below). Many senior military commanders were resistant to change and the eviction of medical officers who had perhaps been with a regiment for many years caused great consternation. Some medical officers who perhaps thought that they were safe at home now found themselves at risk of an overseas posting with all its attendant diseases and dangers, let alone wars and decided to leave the service.[27]

A new Royal Warrant in 1873 provided better pay and conditions for doctors but a career in the army medical services failed to keep pace with the many opportunities which were available in civilian practice and consequently recruitment continued to slide. Although the relative ranks of officers were re-defined again, these were changes in name only and nothing had fundamentally altered for the medical officer. With the coming of the Royal Warrant of 1873 control of military hospitals was handed to the Medical Department, with the exception of hospital ships and the General Hospital for Invalids at Netley. As well as having control over supplies and the administration of medical affairs, they also became responsible for cooking, repairs and general maintenance. This brought with it some "power" and new responsibilities; although many of them did not particularly appreciate this and felt that some of their new responsibilities had nothing to do with medical matters.

The medical officer became the official advisor to his commanding officer on sanitary arrangements. In theory at least, the commanding officer could no longer ignore the recommendations of his medical officer and this was potentially one of the most important changes ever introduced.

THE REORGANISATION OF THE HOSPITAL SERVICE - UNIFICATION

The regimental hospital system was abandoned for what became known as "unification" because the small hospitals could not provide separate wards for different groups of patients. The regimental system made it more difficult for medical officers to keep up to date with advances in medical practice because they worked in isolation and were denied the opportunity to consult with and learn from others. There was a duplication of a range of items including instruments and dressings, which was an unnecessary expense. During the Crimean War, some regimental hospitals worked excessively hard, whilst others didn't have enough to do. Some maintained that the regimental system provided better continuity of care because the medical officer knew his own soldiers better, but others refuted this argument.

The new organisation had stationary and garrison hospitals and resources were pooled, resulting in a better available expertise to deliver more efficient treatment. Female nurses were employed for the first time in peacetime in 1870 and they went overseas to Egypt in 1882. However, too much change which occurs to quickly may not promote the best morale and this has been cited as one of the reasons why the number of recruits declined. Between 1871 and 1876 there were four occasions when no examinations for entry of doctors into the medical services were held because there were no candidates who put themselves forwards to be considered.

The field reorganisation was brought into effect in 1876. This has been discussed under the responsibilities of the Professor of Military Surgery at Netley, in a previous section of this chapter.

In 1884, the medical relative military ranks were abolished completely, as though by abolishing them the problem might go away. This move did nothing to improve the feeling between the medical profession and the War Office. Since medical officers had no rank at all, they were effectively excluded from all decision-making and were simply not recognised as an integral branch of the service.

There was an entrenched prejudice on the part of Horse Guards, where the notion was harboured that a medical officer of higher rank than a service office might want to assume military control of a fighting unit. This of course was what would have happened. Doctors, however, had more than enough to do looking after the health and fitness of soldiers. This stance displayed a staggering and irrational fear on the part of regular army officers.

Most medical schools refused to supply candidates for the army, and there was a great deal of lobbying by the British Medical Association (BMA) to bring about change. The Medical Royal Colleges, whilst not supportive of army careers for doctors, did emphasise that army doctors *must* have equivalent military rank to non-medical officers to enable them to carry out their medical duties with appropriate authority.

Resistance persisted, both from the War Office and other military personnel. There were no new entries to the School in the two years after 1877. Yet another committee sat in 1889 and reached the same negative outcome. There was very little hope of improvement when General Wolseley, the most senior army commander of his day expressed the desire to close the Army Medical School. Wolseley also felt there was no need for a sanitary officer to be in the field:

> As long as this fad continues my recommendation is to leave him (the sanitary officer) at the base, where he may find some useful occupation as a member of the sanitary board.[28]

It was because of this attitude displayed by senior officers that twice as many soldiers died from disease in the Boer War as were killed in action or died of wounds.

A parliamentary committee reported on Doctors' Injustices in 1890, while the campaign for equality for medical officers continued, with persistent lobbying by the BMA and Royal College of Physicians of London. The President of the College of Physicians of London, Sir Andrew Clark, protested in the strongest possible terms to the Secretary of State for War, enumerating in a letter the many causes of discontent amongst medical officers. He even cited the disgraceful example of Surgeon Major Home, winner of the Victoria Cross at Lucknow, who was the only officer not to be invited to the palace to be presented to the Queen. Home had felt so slighted by this that for many years he refused to wear his decoration. The number of honours granted to the medical department was disproportionately few in number compared with those received by other units in the army. It is noteworthy that when these issues were finally addressed and medical officers were viewed on equal terms, that two of the three double Victoria Cross winners in the history of the award were medical officers, who demonstrated on multiple occasions outstanding acts of bravery and heroism for which there were rightly awarded this highest of all honours.

In 1898, the most powerful deputation of Britain's most senior doctors ever assembled met the Secretary of State for War, Lord Lansdowne. Sir Thomas Granger Stewart, President elect of the British Medical Association led the deputation. He was accompanied by Surgeon General Mouat VC, and by Professor Sir Alexander Ogston of the University of Aberdeen. It was pointed out, that under the prevailing conditions the army would never get good doctors and that no one would consider applying for a commission in the army unless medical officers were treated equally.[29]

The British Medical Association was particularly active in finally bringing about a solution. Professor Ogston worked tirelessly for many years to reform army medical services. He had attended as an observer during the Sudan Campaign in 1885 and during the Second Boer War (1899-1902). He was called to give evidence to numerous committees.

Ogston was also an outstanding clinician and his enquiring mind led him to investigate the principal cause of wound infections, which were such a major

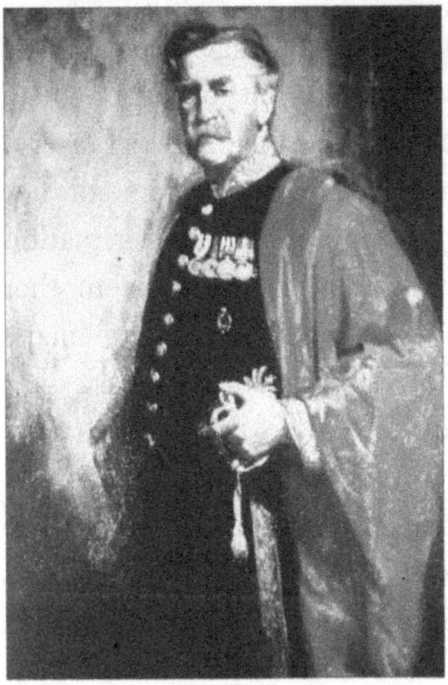

Figure 11.1. Sir Alexander Ogston, Professor of Surgery, University of Aberdeen, was a surgical pioneer who discovered the staphylococcus, and who championed the cause of army doctors leading to the establishment of the Royal Army Medical Corps. (Courtesy of Aberdeen Medico-Chirurgical Society).

complication of surgical and war wounds throughout the nineteenth century. He successfully isolated a micro-organism from patients with wound infections, which appeared in grape-like clusters. This organism differed morphologically from streptococci which were aligned in a chain when they grew and were observed under the microscope. Ogston named his new discovery the staphylococcus.

On 1 July 1898, officers and other ranks providing medical care became the Royal Army Medical Corps (RAMC). It emerged after nearly half a century of strife. "In Arduis Fidelis" (Steadfast in Adversity) is its motto which is a most appropriate one for this Corps.

In spite of the creation of the RAMC, inequality persisted and doctors still did not see joining the army as an attractive career option. Not only were there no new doctors joining but there continued to be a boycott by many medical schools for a variety of reason including the uncertainty about the structure of careers within the army. Army doctors had to retire after 10 years service and moreover they did not have the same conditions governing leave as other officers.[30]

During the Boer War, mortality from infectious disease, especially typhoid fever, significantly exceeded deaths sustained during fighting. Medical officers still had little influence in managing health issues, whilst the higher command had concerns which they regarded as of a higher priority and paid little heed to medical matters.

A key figure in the development of the RAMC and in bringing about a radical change in the medical officer's standing was Sir Alfred Keogh who joined the Army Medical Services in 1880. Keogh was a doctor of exceptional ability, gaining the highest marks during his time at the Army Medical College. As his career developed, he distinguished himself in the Boer War and rose rapidly through the ranks becoming Director-General Army Medical Services in 1904.

Medical officers often experienced difficulties with other officers during the Boer War, who showed lack of respect for their commitment and professional

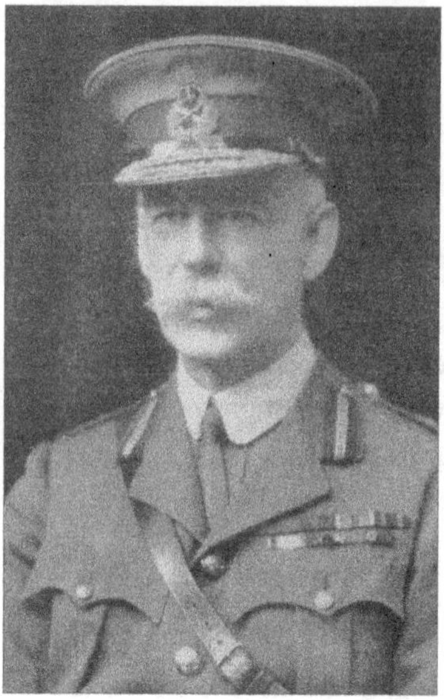

Figure 11.2. Sir Alexander Keogh. (Courtesy BMJ Publishing Group Ltd).

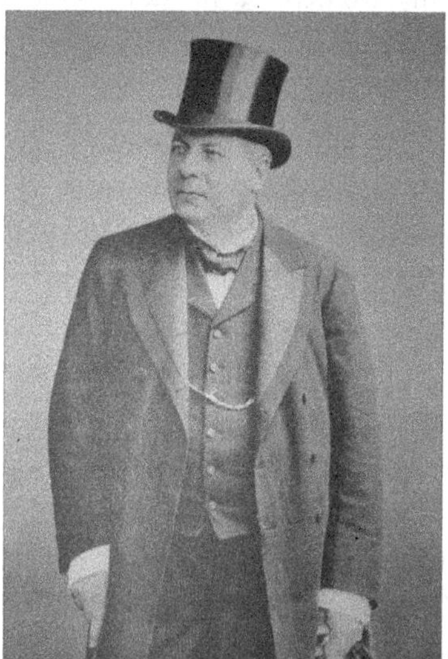

Figure 11.3. Richard Haldane (1856-1928) Secretary of State for War 1906-1912, the minister responsible for army reforms. (Private collection).

skills. There was even a suggestion that the Victoria Cross should not be awarded to doctors (no matter what their acts of bravery) and their terms and conditions were still not equivalent and appropriate. This situation could not be allowed to continue and another Royal Commission was set up to make recommendations to bring about the necessary changes to put an end to this longstanding inequality.

Keogh made important contributions in the RAMC to improvements in hygiene and to the reorganisation of the service during his tenure of this post until his initial retirement from the army in 1910.[31,32] Poor hygiene and communicable diseases was a cause of substantial morbidity and mortality during the Boer War. The Army School of Hygiene was established by Lt-Col Richard Firth. As Professor of Hygiene, he particularly addressed such issues as good sanitation, clean water supplies (use of chlorination), effective typhoid vaccination and the education of soldiers in all matters pertaining to their health and well being. Keogh ensured that different hospitals in existence were reorganised to create larger, fit for purpose military hospitals where appropriate expertise and facilities for treating the wounded were to be found.[33,34]

In 1906, Richard Haldane was appointed Secretary of State for War, with a remit to modernise the British Army in preparation for a European war. He was arguably the most capable Secretary of State for War that Great Britain has known. Haldane was very aware of financial restraints and he knew that the army had lost too many men to various preventable diseases in previous campaigns.

It was very much in his interest to ensure that the soldiers received the best possible medical care, minimising losses from disease, and maximising the fighting capability of the troops. In Keogh, Haldane found a very supportive ally, and at long last, medical officers were to play a significant role in health matters, with due attention being given to proper sanitation and appropriate education of medical personnel. Haldane created the British Expeditionary Force for overseas service, and formed the Territorial Force from Volunteers and Yeomanry, to protect the United Kingdom while the BEF was overseas. He created Special Reserves from Militias, and to encourage plenty of officer recruits, he created the Officer Training Corps (the OTC). This ensured a great interest amongst medical students and a plentiful supply of young doctors, willing and able to serve when the time came, which it would with the outbreak of the Great War in 1914.

ENDNOTES

1. Cantlie, N., *A History of the Army Medical Department.* Edinburgh: Churchill Livingston, 1974, Volume 2, p.207.
2. Blanco, R.L., "Henry Marshall (1775-1851) and the health of the British Army". *Medical History,* 1970. July; 14(3). p.266.
3. Cantlie, *op. cit.*, Volume 2, p.199.
4. Royal Warrant, 1st October 1858.
5. Whitehead, I.R. *Doctors in the Great War.* Barnsley: Leo Cooper, 1999, p.7.
6. Cantlie, *op. cit.*, Volume 2, pp.267-268.
7. *Ibid,* p.270.
8. *Ibid,* p.268.
9. *Ibid,* p.270.
10. Maurice, F., *Haldane 1956-1915. The Life of Viscount Haldane of Clone.* London: Faber and Faber Limited, 1937.
11. Cantlie, N., *A History of the Army Medical Department.* Edinburgh: Churchill Livingston, 1974, Volume 1, p.439.
12. Kaufman, M.H., *The Regius Chair of Military Surgery in the University of Edinburgh* 1806-55. Amsterdam and New York: Wellcome Trust Rodopi BV, 2003.
13. Longmore, T., *Gunshot Injuries. Their History, Characteristic Features, Complications and General Treatment.* London: Longmans Green and Co, 1877.
14. *Ibid,* pp.426-488.

15. Parkes, E.A., *A Manual of Practical Hygiene*. London: John Churchill and Sons, 1864.
16. Cantlie, *op. cit.*, Volume 2, p.395.
17. Parkes, *op. cit.* p.134.
18. *Ibid*, p.135.
19. *Ibid.*
20. Aitkin, W. *The Science and Practice of Medicine*. Philadelphia: Lindsay and Blakiston, 1866.
21. Cantlie, *op. cit.*, Volume 2, p.366.
22. *Ibid*, p.230.
23. Herman, A., *The Scottish Enlightenment. The Scots' Invention of the Modern World*. London: Harper Perennial, 2006, pp.310-312.
24. Chaplin, A., "The rate of mortality in the British Army 100 years ago". *Proceedings of the Royal Society of Medicine*.1916; 9 (section History of Medicine); pp.89-99.
25. Rosenbaum, S., "More than a century of Army medical statistics". *Journal of the Royal Society of Medicine* 1990; 83: pp.456-463.
26. Whitehead, I.R., *Doctors in the Great War*. Barnsley: Leo Cooper, 1999, p.10.
27. *Ibid.*
28. Cantlie, *op. cit.*, Volume 2, p.286.
29. *Ibid*, p.359.
30. Blair, J.G.S., "Sir Alfred Keogh – the early years". *Journal of the Royal Army Medical Corps* 2008; 154: pp.268-269.
31. *Ibid*, pp.268-269.
32. Murray, J., "Sir Alfred Keogh: Doctor and General". *Irish Medical Journal* 1987; 80: pp.427-432.
33. Blair, *op. cit.*, pp.273-274.
34. Obituary: Sir Alfred Keogh. *British Medical Journal* 1936: 2: pp.317-318.

12

American Civil War

In 1860 Abraham Lincoln was elected President of the United States of America. He was a Republican who was opposed to slavery. Seven Southern States which endorsed slavery and whose economy depended upon them withdrew from the Union to form the Confederate States of America. A further four States joined the Confederacy after the first shots of the Civil War were fired. Twenty five states supported the Federal Government, or the "Union".

The first shots of the American Civil War were fired on 12 April 1861 when Confederate forces fired on a US military installation at Fort Sumter in South Carolina. Lincoln responded by calling for a volunteer army from each state to seize federal property and this was enough to persuade four of the remaining slave States to join the Confederacy. Both sides raised armies as the Union seized control of the Border States.

In the context of the American Civil War, Border States were those states which did not declare their secession from the United States before April 1861. Four states, Delaware, Kentucky, Maryland and Missouri never did declare secession, while Virginia, Arkansas, North Carolina and Tennessee declared their secession after the 1861 battle at Fort Sumter. Four years of bitter fighting followed, marked by historic battles in now famous locations such as Bull Run, Antietam, Chancellorsville, Gettysburg and Vicksburg. By the time the war ended in 1865 when the Confederate Army surrendered, the Civil War had proved to be the costliest war ever fought on American soil in terms of the numbers of men killed and wounded.

WEAPONRY

The Civil War introduced a great variety of new weaponry which greatly increased the efficiency of inflicting wounds. The American Civil war may be regarded as the first war which saw casualties on a massive scale. An example of the new weaponry was the Spencer repeating rifle, which was a manually operated lever-action rifle fed with cartridges from a tube magazine. The Spencer was very reliable and with its magazine was capable of firing in excess of 20 rounds per minute. Compared to standard muzzle-loaders, with a rate of fire of 2-3 rounds per minute, this represented a significant tactical advantage for those who possessed it. The Spencer carbine was a shorter and lighter version of the repeating rifle and was used mainly by the cavalry.

The Spencer did not replace the standard issue muzzle-loading rifled musket in use at the time which was the Springfield rifle. This was a single shot, muzzle-loading weapon which used a percussion cap firing mechanism. It had a long rifled barrel and using a .58 calibre ball, it was possible to hit a man-sized target as far away as 500 yards (460 m). To reflect this longer range, the Springfield was fitted with two flip up sights, one set for 300 yards and the other for 500. Along with a revised 1863 model it was the last muzzle-loading weapon ever adopted by the US Army.

In the late 1860s, the Spencer Company was sold to the Fogerty Rifle Company and ultimately to Winchester. With almost 200,000 rifles and carbines made, it marked the first use of a removable magazine-fed infantry rifle by any country. Many Spencer carbines were later sold as surplus to France where they were used during the Franco-Prussian War in 1870.

There were crude hand grenades used during the Civil War which were equipped with a plunger that would detonate upon impact. The Union relied on the experimental Ketchum grenade, which was patented on 20 August 1861 by William F. Ketchum. It was fitted with a tail to ensure that the nose would strike the target first and start the fuse. The Confederacy used spherical hand grenades that weighed about six pounds and were sometimes fitted with a paper fuse.

The Civil War marked the first occasion when a machine gun was used. The Gatling Gun was a hand-crank-operated weapon with 6 barrels revolving around a central shaft. The cartridges were fed to the gun by gravity through a hopper mounted on the top of the gun. The gun was capable of firing 600 rounds a minute, each barrel firing 100 rounds per minute. There were various teething problems with this new weapon and so it was not used widely. Nevertheless, it was the first stage in the development and application of what was to become a most feared weapon in subsequent conflicts.

Land mines were invented and were first used by Confederate Americans. Brigadier-General Gabriel J. Rains of the Confederate Army first experimented with booby traps in 1862 when he ordered his men to prepare artillery shells so that they could be detonated by concealed trip wires when unsuspecting enemy soldiers walked over them. This led to the development of a primer which exploded on the slightest pressure and by 1863 his mines were being used widely.

During the Civil War there were many types of artillery pieces, both field guns and siege artillery. Field artillery was lighter and travelled with the armies whereas in contrast siege and garrison artillery pieces were heavy and were used either to attack or defend fortified positions. Seacoast batteries were the largest of all and were designed for use in permanent coastal fortifications against attacking warships.

All these developments resulted in the ability to inflict wounds on a scale not previously encountered. As a footnote it is of interest to point out that the very first use of a "wire obstacle" as an aid to defence may be attributable to General Ambrose Burnside during the American Civil War Battle of Fort Sanders in November 1863, when telegraph wire was strung between tree stumps 30 to 80 yards in front of one part of the Union line. Barbed wire was invented in America after the Civil War and became a very important defensive aid in future conflicts.

CASUALTY FIGURES

At least 618,000 Americans died in the Civil War and some experts say the toll reached 700,000. This exceeded the nation's loss from the combined total of all other conflicts including the Revolutionary War, the Great War, the Second World War, Vietnam and Afghanistan.[1] The Union armies had between 2,500,000 and 2,750,000 men and the losses they sustained are difficult to determine exactly but the best estimates are summarised in Table 12.1.

Table 12.1 Deaths in the Union Army in the American Civil War.

Deaths	Number	Percentage of deaths
Battle Deaths	110,070	31%
Disease Deaths	250,152	69%
Total Deaths	360,222	

From: Davis, B., *The Civil War - Strange and fascinating Facts.* New York: Wings Books, 1994,

Assuming a total manpower of 2,500,000, deaths in the Union Army amounted to approximately 14.4% of the total force.[2]

The Confederate strength is known less accurately because of missing records but it was thought to be in the region of between 750,000 and 1,250,000. Its estimated losses are summarised in Table 12.2.

Table 12.2 Deaths in the Confederate Army in the American Civil War.

Deaths	Number	Percentage of deaths
Battle Deaths	94,000	36%
Disease Deaths	164,000	64%
Total	258,000	

From: Davis B., *The Civil War - Strange and fascinating Facts.* New York: Wings Books, 1994.

Assuming a manpower of 1,000,000, then 258,000 deaths amounted to 26% of the total force. This difference in percentage has not been fully clarified but it is possible that it reflects the inferior medical services which were available to the Southern forces.

MEDICAL DEVELOPMENTS

There were significant medical developments, which must be viewed against the background of huge numbers of casualties dealt with during the American Civil War compared with previous conflicts. In the Crimean War, for example, the total number of British deaths from all causes was 21, 827.

Bitterly acquired experience during the American Civil War contributed to the knowledge base for the further development of military surgery. Britain sent observers to the Civil War, no doubt partly out of curiosity, but also partly to see if lessons could be learned. The important medical developments made during the Civil War may be summarised as follows.[3]

Data collection

The collecting of adequate records and detailed reports for the first time in North America permitted a complete military medical history for every wounded soldier to be kept. This led to the publication of the *Medical and Surgical History of the War of the Rebellion*, which was identified by European authorities as the first major academic accomplishment by US military medicine.

The *Medical and Surgical History of the War of Rebellion* (MSHWR) was a six volume work published between 1870 and 1888 by the U.S. Government Printing Office, under the direction of J.K. Barnes, Surgeon General US Army. It statistically analysed wounds and diseases, in both Union and Confederate Armies and formed an important source of medical information and data on the War. It also provided important information on medical histories of individual soldiers and detailed tens of thousands of medical and surgical cases which occurred during the conflict.

The development of a system of managing mass casualties

This included aid stations, field hospitals and general hospitals. This system set the American pattern for management of the wounded in the Great War, World War II and the Korean War.

Aid Stations and field hospitals

Aid stations close to the front permitted the first dressing to be applied to a wounded soldier, who could then return to the front if his wound was very minor, or go back to a field hospital if further treatment was required. The Union Army used tents for field hospitals for the first time at the Battle of Shiloh on 6 and 7 April 1862. Dr B.J. Irwin, Medical Inspector of the 4th Division, made use of the abandoned tents of an infantry division by making them into a field hospital, which included an operating theatre and dispensary for 300 patients. [4] It was quickly appreciated that the use of large field hospitals using tents was much more efficient than trying to establish medical facilities in church halls or other such buildings.

A Field Ambulance System

An efficient Field Ambulance system was introduced by Dr Jonathan Letterman, Medical Director of the Union Army of the Potomac, as part of the strategy to deal with the large numbers of casualties. Upon taking up his appointment on 1 July 1862, he immediately set about improving the inadequate means at his disposal for evacuation of the sick and wounded:

> The subject of the ambulances became, after the health of the troops, a matter of importance. No system had anywhere been devised for their management. They could not be depended upon for efficient service in time of action or upon a march as if they had been made for the convenience of commanding officers. The system I devised was based upon the idea that they should not be under the immediate control of medical officers, whose duties, especially on the day of battle, would prevent any proper supervision; but that other officers, appointed for that special purpose, should have direct charge of the horses, ambulances, etc, and yet under such regulations as would enable Medical officers at all times to procure them with facility when needed for their legitimate purpose.[5]

Letterman devised the following system. No doubt he studied the ambulance of Larrey (see Chapter 4) before developing his own method of evacuation.

Ambulance Corps personnel had a command structure with a captain as commandant who was responsible for ensuring ambulance availability for an entire army corps. To help him, he had first lieutenants each of whom was responsible for a division; there was a second lieutenant for each brigade, and one sergeant for each regiment. Transport for the wounded was carefully organised and distributed. Every regiment was allocated one transport cart, one four-horse and two two-horse ambulance vehicles. Each battery of artillery received one two-horse ambulance wagon. In addition, the headquarters of each army corps was allocated two two-horse ambulances.

Each ambulance vehicle was provided with two stretchers. The vehicles of the Ambulance Corps were driven by private soldiers, with two men and one driver allocated to each ambulance wagon and one driver to each transport cart. The captain was commander of all the ambulance and transport vehicles in the army corps and he was answerable to the Medical Director. The captain's responsibility was to ensure that the sick and wounded were treated with gentleness and care and were removed from the field as quickly as possible to reach their destination:

> It will be perceived that the ambulance system, with that of supplies and of field hospitals, were ordered as essential parts of that new organisation from which, I earnestly hoped, the wounded and sick would receive more careful attendance and more skillful treatment.[6]

Letterman's system was first employed at the Battle of Fredericksburg in 1862, but it was at Gettysburg 1-3 July 1863 when it was tested to the limit:

> At the Battle of Gettysburg, the ambulance vehicles, medicine wagons and ammunition wagons were placed in forward positions, while the hospital wagons and battle supply wagons (carrying all the important equipment) were sent to the rear, around twenty five miles from the front.The exposure of the whole battle front to enemy fire meant that it was impossible to place field hospitals to the rear of their divisions. When wounded were taken to the rear, there was therefore nowhere near at hand for them to go. There was a regrettably severe shortage of tents and cooking apparatus, since all the vital equipment and supplies had been sent further back. As a result, it meant that the wounded had to lie out in the open, with what little shelter could be found, and they were cold and wet. Without proper means, the Medical department can no more take care of the wounded than the army can fight without ammunition.[7]

In one of the corps, the order to move most supplies to the rear had not been carried out and the Medical Director of that corps wrote:

> It is with extreme satisfaction that I can assure you that it enabled me to remove the wounded from the field, shelter, feed them, and dress their wounds within six hours after the battle, and to have every capital operation performed within twenty four hours after the wound was received.[8]

After the battle was over, Letterman reflected:

> The Ambulance Corps performed its duty well. Before daylight on the morning of the 4th July, all wounded within our lines (numbering on those two days about twelve thousand) were removed to the hospitals.[9]

The importance of immediate, definitive treatment of wounds and fractures

It was clearly demonstrated that major operative procedures, such as amputation, were optimally carried out within 24 hours of being wounded. These operations were performed at the field hospitals. This corroborated the findings of others in earlier conflicts and was not a new observation. Amputations carried out early were shown to be the best way to treat such wounds by George James Guthrie in 1815.

Pavilion-style general hospitals

There had been an awareness for a long time that hospitals should have adequate space and be well ventilated. Sir James McGrigor demonstrated this during the Peninsular War in 1812 and John Bell recognised that hospitals were often dangerous places to be when he described the clinical features of hospital gangrene during this period (see Chapter 4).

The devastating number of British deaths from disease during the Crimean War prompted improvements in sanitation and hospital design. Florence Nightingale provided better hospital accommodation with the "Nightingale ward" following the Crimean War. This was a long ward, well ventilated by windows on both sides and at one end, with plenty of room between patients' beds which were lined up against the walls facing inwards.

During the American Civil War, general hospital pavilions were designed to offer the benefits of a tent but with the protection of a solid structure. They were warmer and better ventilated than a tent and were approximately 150 feet long, 25 feet wide, with a ceiling approximately 12 to 14 feet high. Each pavilion ceiling had a series of adjustable shutters on the ridge of the roof that allowed ample ventilation yet gave protection from inclement weather. They were often connected by a common passageway that allowed quick access by hospital staff to any pavilion ward. The design of military pavilion hospitals was copied by large civilian hospitals over the next 75 years.

The Sanitary Commission

Just as disease caused more deaths than wounds during the Crimean War, the same was true for the American Civil War. The American Sanitary Commission was set up in response to this. What made the American system unique was that it was organised and run by civilians. It had its origins in the Women's Central Relief

Association of New York, a charitable organization inspired by the British Sanitary Commission of the Crimean War.

An effort to create an effective system of collection and distribution was begun by the ladies of New York in 1861 and subsequently they held a conference to coordinate all the individual efforts of relief societies throughout the United States. Doctors, clergymen, lawyers and other interested parties who recognized a need for better coordination of relief efforts, attended the conference. As a result they developed an organisation which would become the Sanitary Commission on 9 June 1861.

The first President of the Commission was Rev. Henry W. Bellows, D.D. of New York and the General Secretary of the Commission was a noted landscape architect Fredrick Law Olmstead. Volunteers raised money and collected donations. They worked as nurses, ran kitchens and looked after soldiers' homes. They generally worked in a charitable way. Amongst the volunteers was Louisa May Alcott, author of *Little Women*.

American Red Cross

Clara Barton (1821-1912) was also involved in voluntary work. She trained as a teacher and at the start of the war she established the concept of soldier aid and formed an organisation to help locate men listed as missing in action. She interviewed Union soldiers returning from Southern prisons and was successful on several occasions in being able to notify families about the fate of their loved ones.

After the Civil War, she went to Europe in 1869, ostensibly for a restful vacation. While there, she became involved in the work of the fledgling International Red Cross during the Franco-Prussian War (1870-71) and brought the ideas and principles of the organisation home with her to America. It was generally thought that the US would never again find itself exposed to the terrible hardships experienced and imposed by the Civil War, but Barton finally succeeded in bringing about the creation of the American Red Cross during the administration of President Chester A Arthur, on the basis that the new American Red Cross organization could also be available to respond to other types of crisis and not just war.

Female nurses introduced to hospital care

Although Florence Nightingale had firmly established the role of nurses in the Crimea, this was the first occasion when female nurses were used in America.

Professor SD Gross, of the Jefferson Medical College in Philadelphia, made some observations on the attributes he thought a nurse should possess. One can only hope that others were perhaps more liberally minded and less patronising, otherwise it is a wonder they attracted any nurses at all:

> It is not my purpose here to point out the qualities which constitute a good female nurse. It will suffice to say that she should be keenly alive to her duties, and perform them, however menial or distasteful, with promptness and alacrity. She must be tidy in her appearance, with a cheerful countenance, light in her step, noiseless, tender and thoughtful in her manners, perfect mistress of her feelings, healthy, able to bear fatigue, and at least twenty-two years of age. Neither the crinoline nor the silk dress must enter into her wardrobe; the former is too cumbrous, while the latter by its rustling is sure to fret the patient and disturb his sleep.
>
> In regard to the cleanliness of a sick-room, it is advisable to use a mop occasionally for the removal of flue from under the bed; when, however, the patient is in too critical a situation for dampness, a few tea-leaves scattered over the apartment will absorb the dust, and can be quietly taken up with a hand-brush.[10]

Improved experience and training of doctors

Doctors were introduced to new ideas and standards of care. These included familiarity with prevention and treatment of infectious diseases, experience with anaesthetic agents (chloroform and ether) and with surgical principles. All of this led rapidly to an advance in the overall quality of American medical practice. It is often stated that the only good thing ever to come out of war is the advance of surgery and the American Civil War was no exception.

TREATMENT OF WOUNDS

S.D. Gross was Professor of Surgery at Jefferson College in Philadelphia. He published a book in 1861 at the outset of the American Civil War which gave considerable insight into how wounds had been managed up to that point in time. In *A Manual of Military Surgery; or Hints on the Emergencies of Field, Camp and Hospital Practice*, Gross described how wounds should be dealt with:

> This (cleansing of the wound) should be done at once and effectually; with sponge and water, pressed upon the parts, with finger, or finger and forceps. Not a particle of matter, not a hair, or the smallest clot of blood must be left behind, otherwise it will be sure to provoke and keep up irritation. As soon as the bleeding has been checked and the extraneous matter cleared away, the edges of the wound are gently and evenly approximated and permanently retained by suture and adhesive plaster, aided, if necessary, by the bandage.[11]

At the time of the outbreak of the American Civil War, existing knowledge came from previous European conflicts, since the United States had not fought in any significant war since the Mexican-American War of 1846-1848. Consequently Gross made frequent references to the work of Percy, Larrey, Hennen and Guthrie, as well as to work done in the Crimean War. It is clear that military surgery had made little significant progress by the outbreak of the Civil War, although Gross provided us with a useful window to view surgical thinking at the time.

For example, Gross reviewed all the military cases of hip disarticulation to that point in time. As already discussed,the operation of hip disarticulation was a "hot topic" during the Peninsular War and Guthrie made frequent reference to it in his book *A Treatise on Gunshot Wounds: on Inflammation, Erysipelas and Mortification, on Injuries of Nerves* published in 1827. Gross reviewed 44 cases of hip disarticulation; 30 were primary, and all ended fatally; 11 were early secondary or intemediate in timing, and 3 recovered; 3 were late cases, and one recovered. Thus 4 patients survived out of 44, giving a mortality of 90.9% for this particular procedure. Some of the primary procedures died on the table and all the rest, except two, before the tenth post operative day.

Clearly hip disarticulation was not a procedure to be undertaken early, unlike other limb amputations which did much better when carried out soon after the wound had been sustained. Hip disarticulation was a procedure of such great magnitude, that the challenge to the body of operative trauma super-imposed upon an already major wound was too much to withstand. Some of the cases operated on late after the wound had occurred survived because after initial severe blood loss, there had been haemodilution and stabilisation of the casualty's cardiovascular system which can occur using the body's mechanisms if the wound is not severe enough to be quickly fatal. This might have allowed the patient to withstand the trauma of the surgery better.

Fractures

Of fractures Gross wrote:

> Most of the cases of fractures occurring on the field of battle are the result of gunshot injury, and are frequently, if not generally, attended by such an amount of injury to the soft parts and also to the bone as to demand amputation. The bone is often dreadfully comminuted, and consequently utterly unfit for preservation. The more simple fractures, on the contrary, readily admit of the retention of the limb, without risk to life. If the fracture be attended with splintering of the bone, all loose or detached pieces should at once be extracted; a proceeding which always wonderfully simplifies the case, in as much as it prevents, in great measure, the frightful irritation and suppuration which are sure to follow their retention.[12]

Wounds of joints

Wounds of the knee joint carried a poor prognosis throughout the history of warfare. Gross's views were no different:

> Gunshot wounds of the knee-joint are among the most dangerous of accidents, and no attempt should be made to save the limb when the injury is at all extensive, especially if it involves fracture of the head of the tibia or condyles of the femur. Even extensive laceration of the ligament of the patella should, I think, as a general rule, be regarded as a sufficient cause of amputation.[13]

Gross had definite views about anaesthesia, which had yet to gain acceptance:

> Anaesthetics should be given only in the event of thorough reaction; so long as the vital powers are depressed and the mind is bewildered by shock, or loss of blood, their administration will hardly be safe, unless the greatest vigilance be employed, and this is not always possible on the field of battle, or even in the hospital. Moreover, it is astonishing what little suffering the patient generally experiences, when in this condition, even from a severe wound or operation.[14]

The reasons why anaesthesia was unsafe have been discussed in detail elsewhere in this book.

Abdominal wounds and chest wounds

Soldiers who had sustained wounds of the abdominal or chest cavities generally died and surgical intervention did not occur.

Wounds of the skull and brain

Understanding of the pathology of head injuries had certainly improved:

> Compression of the brain arises, surgically speaking, from two causes only: effusion of blood and depressed bone. In the former case, the characteristic symptoms —insensibility and coma, dilated and fixed pupil, stertorous breathing, and paralysis — frequently do not come until some time after the receipt of the injury. The first symptoms will probably be those of concussion, or exhaustion. By-and-by, the patient regains his senses and his strength, gets up, talks or walks and then suddenly drops down, as if he had been shot, in a state of utter unconsciousness. The effusion of blood, kept in abeyance during the collapse, has had full play, filling empty places, and causing unmistakable effects. Such an occurrence will be most apt to happen when there has been extensive separation of the dura mater, or rupture of the middle meningeal artery. If, on the other hand, the compression is due to depression of the skull, the symptoms are nearly always immediate.[15]

Despite this better understanding of pathology, surgical management made little progress. Brain compression by a developing haematoma was treated by the ineffective use of purgatives and bleeding. As for surgery, there was thought to be little role for this to be carried out with this type of wound:

> The trephine is not thought of unless the unconsciousness obstinately persists, and there is reason to believe, from the nature of the phenomena, especially the existence of a wound or contusion on the head, that the blood may be reached by the instrument.[16]

Neurosurgeons now know that under the circumstances just described, immediate surgery is required to remove the expanding intracranial clot, which will result in ever deepening unconsciousness leading to death from respiratory and cardiac arrest. One of the problems encountered before accurate imaging of the brain was available (such as is now available with CT or MRI scanning) was that very often surgeons were unsure as to where to drill a hole through the skull and be able to find such a blood clot and remove it.

In contrast, when a bullet had caused a compressed fracture of the skull, there was a perceived clear case for immediate surgery, and this was probably partly because a depressed skull fracture is clinically obvious and it seemed logical to operate to remove splinters of broken bone from the surface of the brain as this would also lead to death:

> When, on the contrary, the bone is badly fractured, comminuted, or forced greatly beyond the natural level, the proper plan is to trephine, whether there be any external wound or evidences of compression or not. If the operation be neglected, loss of life from inflammation will be sure to arise within the first six or ten days after the receipt of the injury. In the punctured fracture, as it is named, the trephine is invariably employed at the earliest moment, however flattering, apparently, the head symptoms may be. If the instrument be withheld, fatal cerebritis or arachnitis will be no less certain than when the bone is shattered and driven down upon the brain.[17]

Massive blood loss

Acute major blood loss was the main cause of early death in severely wounded soldiers. In wounds of the limb, blood loss is obvious and readily seen and it was relatively easy for surgeons of that time to control the bleeding by the use of tourniquets as a temporary measure before ligating bleeding blood vessels. Blood loss deep within the chest or abdomen is not at all obvious and no clear solution was available to surgeons at the time of the American Civil War any more than it was to Guthrie and Hennen during the Peninsular War 50 years before.

The general supportive measures available at the time would clearly have been of no value, and it is little wonder that those with abdominal or chest wounds usually died:

> Internal haemorrhage is more dangerous than external, because it is generally inaccessible. The chief remedies are copious venesection, elevated position, opium and acetate of lead, cool air, and cool drinks.[18]

Gross was of the opinion that the aim of treatment of the wounded should be to prevent shock, to arrest haemorrhage, to remove foreign matter, to approximate the edges of the wound and to limit resulting inflammation, in that order of importance. He pointed out that haemorrhage may be arterial, venous or both and that when severe it may prove fatal within a few minutes. Furthermore, hundreds of men may die on the battlefield from acute blood loss which may or may not have been prevented with appropriate immediate medical care in some of the wounded:

> They perish simply from their ignorance, because the regimental surgeon has failed to give the proper instruction. It is not necessary that the common soldier should carry a Petit's tourniquet, but every one may put into his pocket a stick of wood, six inches long, and a handkerchief or piece of roller, with a thick compress, and be advised how, where, and when they arc to be used. By casting the handkerchief round the limb, and placing the compress over its main artery, he can, by means of the stick, produce such an amount of compression as to put at once an effectual stop to the haemorrhage. This simple contrivance, which has been instrumental in saving thousands of lives, constitutes what is called the field tourniquet. A fife, drum-stick, knife, or ramrod may be used, if no special piece of wood is at hand.[19]

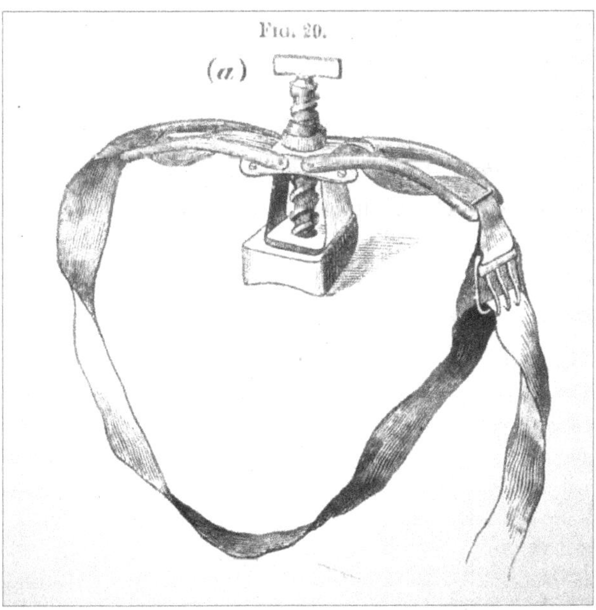

Figure 12.1. Petit's Tourniquet.

In modern civilian trauma, experts talk about the "golden hour", during which it is possible to influence whether a patient lives or dies following serious trauma depending on what actions are taken. Nowadays, in "modern" warfare, there is the so-called "platinum ten minutes", where a very brief opportunity exists to arrest catastrophic haemorrhage by applying a field tourniquet and soldiers are currently being taught how to do this. This was, of course, advocated 150 years previously in the American Civil War!

ENDNOTES

1. Davis, B., *The Civil War - Strange and Fascinating Facts.* New York: Wings Books, 1994.
2. *Ibid.*
3. Blaisdell, F.W., "Medical advances during the Civil War". *Archives of Surgery,* 1988 Sept; 123 (9); pp.1045-1050.
4. Laffan, J., *Surgeons in the Field.* London: J.M. Dent and Sons Limited, 1970, p.162.
5. Letterman, J., *Medical Recollections of the Army of the Potomac.* New York: D. Appleton and Company, 1866, pp.22-23.
6. *Ibid,* p.64.
7. *Ibid,* p.156.
8. *Ibid,* p.157.
9. *Ibid,* p.158.
10. Gross, S.D., *A Manual of Military Surgery; or Hints on the Emergencies of Field, Camp and Hospital Practice.* Philadelphia: J.B. Lippincott and Co, 1861, pp.40-41.
11. *Ibid,* p.57.
12. *Ibid,* pp.46-47.
13. *Ibid,* p.67.
14. *Ibid,* p.81.
15. *Ibid,* p.99.
16. *Ibid,* p.100.
17. *Ibid,* p.10.
18. *Ibid,* p.56.
19. *Ibid,* pp.53-54.

13

The Franco Prussian War (1870–1871)

In 1870, Emperor Napoleon III of France based his foreign policy on two assumptions. The first was that France was the greatest European power and the second was that France's supremacy must never be challenged by a unified Germany. Prussian Chancellor Otto von Bismarck's pre-occupation was precisely what the French Emperor was determined to prevent, namely the unification of the German nation which was composed of many individual German states, including Prussia.

Prussia had already been victorious in a war against Austria in 1866 and as a result of this Austria no longer played a dominant role over the German states. There was, however, a North German Federation which had been formed between Prussia and the north German states. By showing itself superior to Austria, Prussia now challenged France as the dominant force in Europe. Napoleon III was not prepared to permit any further expansion by Prussia, which he now perceived as a serious threat. Bismarck, however, wanted more than this; he wanted to unite all German states but with Prussia occupying the dominant position. His mission was to find a way to achieve this political ambition.

The opportunity to unite Germany came not from any scheming on Bismarck's part, but as a result of the throne of Spain happening to become vacant following the deposition of Queen Isabella II in 1868. The Spanish Government searched for a new monarch and this resulted in the Spanish crown being offered to a distant cousin of King William I of Prussia. Neither Spain nor Prussia shared this information with France. When France finally did become aware of the developing situation in July 1870, perhaps not surprisingly there was an outcry. A member of the House of Hohenzollern (Prussian Royal Family) on the Spanish throne would have the potential to upset the balance of power in Europe; a prospect which Napoleon found intolerable.

Napoleon insisted that William I should renounce any claim that the Hohenzollerns might have to the Spanish throne and furthermore that William should also give an undertaking never to aspire again to such a position. William refused to give any such assurance and all the remaining independent states in Germany rallied behind Prussia. They considered that Napoleon had greatly overstepped the mark by demanding assurances from William that he would never again seek to expand his sphere of influence towards Spain.

France declared war on 19 July 1870 and what followed became known as the Franco-Prussian War. Although Prussia undoubtedly played the leading role, it was aided by the North German Federation of which it was a member and the South German states of Baden Württemberg and Bavaria. It would be more accurate to describe this war as the Franco-German War. However the Prussians were so dominant that on occasions the word "Prussian" will be used, whilst on other occasions the word "German" is more appropriate. France was convinced that because she was the most powerful military nation in Europe, the Prussians would be soundly defeated. However, this was not the case and the Prussian commander, General von Moltke, immediately planned an invasion of France with a coalition force of some 400,000 troops. He did this with remarkable speed thanks to the very efficient rail network in Germany which allowed the rapid movement of troops.

After a series of quick defeats in the East, Napoleon surrendered on 1 September 1870, with his army of 104,000 at Sedan, with a most humiliating defeat. Bismarck was of the opinion that the war should then be stopped and that negotiations with France should follow. However, von Moltke wanted Germany to have security in case there might be future conflicts between the two nations. He wanted to establish a buffer zone between France and Germany; which would be Alsace and Lorraine. To achieve this goal he continued to advance on Paris, laying siege to the city, during which von Moltke made his headquarters at the Palace of Versailles. Paris capitulated on 28 January 1871 and an armistice was signed.

Bismarck's goal was a unified Germany and a new German Empire, with the King of Prussia as Emperor of Germany. The Princes of all the independent German states agreed and so Bismarck achieved his unified Germany with Emperor William of Prussia becoming Kaiser William I of Germany.

Von Moltke was successful in achieving a buffer zone because when Alsace and Lorraine were stripped away from France as war indemnity, they then became part of Germany. This left France filled with rage and thirsting for revenge. However, the indisputable fact was that the balance of power had indeed shifted and Europe now had a ticking time bomb; a key factor in the build-up to the start of the Great War in 1914.

THE SCALE OF CONFLICT IN THE FRANCO-PRUSSIAN WAR (1870-1871)

The Franco-Prussian War was a European conflict associated with massive numbers of casualties. The French used a new breech-loading rifle (the Chassepot), which had twice the range of the Prussian needle rifle, so named because a long needle inside the bolt functioned as the striker. The French also had the Mitrailleuse, a machine gun with twenty five barrels which could fire 125 rounds per minute. It was a war of great mobility, associated with large numbers of troops moving rapidly by rail to engage the enemy. These troops were capable of delivering devastating blows using artillery and high velocity bullets to cause many casualties. It was a conflict during which the fledgling Red Cross played a significant role. It was also the first European war where a very efficient evacuation pathway involving hospital trains played a part in influencing outcomes of the surgical treatment of wounded soldiers.

The total German and French losses for the conflict, which began on 19 July 1870 and ended on 10 May 1871 are summarised in Table 13.1.[1]

Table 13.1 Total German and French losses Franco-Prussian War (1870-1871).

Nationality	Killed /died of wounds	Wounded, not fatally	Missing/ Prisoner of War	Total
German losses	28,400	88,000	13,000	130,000
French losses	60,000	140,000	370,000	580,000

From: Bodart, G., *Losses of Life in Modern Wars.* Oxford: Clarendon Press, 1916, pp.148-149.

All causes of death amongst German forces are given in Table 13.2.[2]

Table 13.2 All causes of death amongst German troops.

German Losses Killed	Officers	Men	Total
Killed in Battle	1,046	16,539	17,585
Died of wounds	671	10,050	10,721
Died from Accident	9	281	290
Committed Suicide	3	26	29
Died from Disease	207	11,940	12,147
Missing, presumed dead	3	4,006	4,009
Total	1,939	42,842	44,781

From: Bodart G., *Losses of Life in Modern Wars.* Oxford: Clarendon Press, 1916, pp.148-149.

DEATHS FROM WOUNDS AND DEATHS FROM DISEASES

Of the total German deaths, 12,147 or 27.1% were caused by disease. The diseases causing greatest losses in German ranks were typhus fever and dysentery, the former causing 7,000 deaths and the latter 2,000. While this is a high percentage of total deaths, it nevertheless represents a significant reduction in the percentage of deaths from disease compared with previous conflicts such as the Peninsular and Crimean Wars. Indeed, the Franco-Prussian War was the first conflict where German deaths resulting from enemy action exceeded those caused by disease. Perhaps this was partly due to the mobile nature of the warfare coupled with its short duration.

During times of siege, disease played a more significant role because besieged large populations crowded together in unhygienic conditions are at much greater risk of communicable diseases. The siege of Metz in Eastern France began when German forces invaded France on 19 August 1870 and lasted till 27 October 1870. Approximately 35,000 French people died from disease, mostly louse-borne typhus fever. The average strength of the German armies was 887,000 men and this figure may be used as a basis for the percentage calculation of total German losses, as demonstrated in Table 13.3.[3]

Table 13.3 Total German Battle Casualty Losses.

Total German Losses	Officers	Men	Percentage of effective strength (887,000)
Killed	1,939	42,842	5.0%
Wounded	3,725	86,007	10.1%
Missing/Prisoners	103	10,026	1.4%
Totals	5,767	138,875	16.24%

From: Bodart, G., *Losses of Life in Modern Wars*. Oxford: Clarendon Press, 1916, pp.148-149.

The exact number of French battle casualty losses is not known, but many sources place them at a figure at least double that of German losses.[4]

GERMAN EVACUATION PATHWAY

The Germans used a very efficient evacuation pathway using hand-wheeled litters to evacuate the wounded. This method of evacuation had been developed during the brief Prussian conflict with Denmark in 1864. There were 124 litter bearers for every corps, each of which comprised 30,000 men. There were collecting posts just behind the front line and dressing stations yet further behind the collecting posts. Each corps had twelve 200-bed field hospitals which followed the army as it advanced, whilst at the same time kept as close to rail heads as possible. Hospital trains transported the wounded back to hospitals in Germany.

Having learned from their past experiences of recent wars against the Danes and Austrians, the Prussian dominated combined force had 3,853 medical officers, increasing to 5,548 as the war progressed. There were 5,858 attendants, 2,921 nurses and 468 apothecaries. In contrast, the French had only 1,020 military surgeons, despite their experiences in the Crimea when they had the same number of medical staff; they were ill-prepared for this war.[5]

Both French and German armies had voluntary assistance provided by non-combatant nations, making this a landmark occasion in humanitarian efforts to minimise human suffering in warfare.

THE RED CROSS

The flag of the Red Cross flew over battlefields for the first time during the Franco-Prussian War. The international movement was founded in 1863 by Henry Dunant "to protect human life and health, to ensure respect for all human beings, and to prevent and alleviate human suffering, without any discrimination based on nationality, race, sex, religious beliefs, class or political opinions".

Dunant, a Swiss businessman, had been an observer at the Battle of Solferino on 24 June 1859. Fought between an Austrian army of 175,000 men and an allied force of 150,000 French, Piedmontese and Sardinians, the battle took place a few miles to the south of Lake Garda in Italy. Austria lost this battle. Allied losses were 14,415 killed and wounded, with 2,776 missing. Austrian losses were 13,317 killed and wounded with 9,220 missing. Solferino was a catastrophe of medical mismanagement. Men died unattended and in appalling conditions. Dunant personally intervened to help when he could and from his experience at Solferino he nurtured the hope and belief that the treatment of wounded soldiers could, and should, be significantly improved. His firm conviction that this would be so became the starting point for the International Red Cross and he used some of his personal fortune to help.

The concept of the Red Cross was built on the foundations of the Geneva Convention, which dated from 1864. This was first applied during the Prussian war against Denmark in 1864, and then the Austro-Prussian War in 1866. The Convention guaranteed neutrality to medical staff and to wounded soldiers[6] and it also specified neutrality of ambulances (field hospitals). However, during the Franco-Prussian War, the French employed buildings near to the field hospitals as defensive positions and the ambulances became strongholds to be destroyed by the advancing Prussians.[7]

The British effort was stimulated by the outbreak of hostilities and on 4 August 1870, after a public meeting, the 'British National Society for Aid to the Sick and Wounded in War' (the precursor of the British Red Cross) was established seven years after the formation of the international movement in Switzerland. By coincidence this was on the same day that Prussian forces marched into Alsace. One of the main figures involved setting this up was John Furley, who had already been instrumental in setting up the St John's Ambulance Brigade. At the inaugural meeting, with the Queen as Patron, Colonel Loyd-Lindsay (Lord Wantage), VC, MP, was its chairman. The project was supported by Florence Nightingale, who "if not sick she would have gone out as a nurse." She gave welcome advice on the nursing services, the administration of field ambulances and equipment.[8]

Later, in 1905 the organisation was renamed the British Red Cross Society and received its first Royal Charter in 1908.

In France, the Societé de Secours began canvassing for money in July 1870, but the general public could not understand why there was any need for such an organisation. As far as they were concerned, there was an apparently perfectly adequate military medical service in place, and there was no need for civilian volunteer ambulances. Needless to say, after early heavy defeats at the hands of the Prussians, this point of view quickly changed and donations of money started to dramatically rise.[9]

As the various precursors of the Red Cross blossomed throughout Europe, different countries became involved and rendered aid. Sometimes there was a hidden agenda concealed beneath a philanthropic exterior. For example, an Irish ambulance was put into service during the Franco-Prussian War, but it took sides and even became involved when the 300 Irishmen forming this unit started fighting Prussians troops. It says much for the general goals of the Red Cross that it survived such a blatant example of abuse.[10]

Other nations took the opportunity during this war to gather medical intelligence. The Russians were particularly interested in the wounds caused by small calibre high-velocity bullets, whilst the Italians looked at the uses and advantages of hospital trains. Of course, all nations including the British, Dutch, Austrian and Belgian sent ambulances to both help the wounded and observe the effects of modern warfare.[11]

Men who had played their part during the American Civil War also made important contributions. The Anglo-American ambulance had experienced men such as James Marion Sims and Charles C. Mayo, who had served during that bloody conflict. Mayo's unit served with the Prussians, while Sims served with the French, until the surrender at Sedan.

British Red Cross Contribution to the War

Initially, the Committee of the British National Society sent ten surgeons and five nurses and by the end of September 1870 the number had risen to sixty two surgeons and sixteen nurses. They served in equal distribution between the French and German forces.

Those who served with the Germans were very impressed by German medical services, which were well-organised thanks to Prussian experience. Each soldier carried a field dressing and had a card around his neck so that if wounded, medical officers could record the wound for the guidance of ambulance wagon personnel who would be caring for that soldier. Evacuation was rapid and trains left every hour and a half to two hours for towns and cities in Germany.

Dr William MacCormac served with the French and noted that they did not generally employ anti-septic surgery. During the Battle of Sedan, there were 12,500 wounded and wounded and dead lay side by side. MacCormac was critical of the very inefficient and cumbrous French system which often arrived too late to be of any use.[12]

ANTISEPTIC SURGERY

Between 1864 and the outbreak of the Franco Prussian War there were two very important scientific developments which changed the face of surgery for ever. The first was the discovery of bacteria by Louis Pasteur and their implication in the causation of disease. The second came about as the direct result of Pasteur's discovery and was the use of antiseptics in surgery by Joseph Lister. Inspired by

Pasteur's groundbreaking work, Joseph Lister, who was Professor of Surgery in Glasgow, first used antiseptics (specifically carbolic acid spray) to kill bacteria in wounds in 1865. Lister's techniques using anti-septic surgery were enthusiastically employed by the Prussians.[13]

Louis Pasteur and the Germ Theory of Disease

Louis Pasteur was a research chemist who in 1854, at the age of 32, became Dean of the Faculty of Science at the University of Lille. At the time, Lille was the centre of alcohol manufacture in France. Pasteur's early work was focussed on trying to understand why beer turned sour. Using a microscope he identified thousands of micro-organisms in sour beer and was convinced they were the cause of, and not the result of, souring of the beer. He did further work on milk and wine and drew the same conclusions. He also discovered that the organisms could be destroyed by heat, a process which became known as pasteurisation. This process is well known in the sterilisation of milk and used to this day.

In 1865, he was asked to investigate his first disease called "pébrine" which was affecting the silk worm industry. Larvae of the silkworm affected by this disease are unable to spin thread. If affected, adult moths transmit the disease to their larvae then the larvae die. Pasteur established a bacterial cause for the disease and became convinced that bacteria were also responsible for diseases in humans as well. Pasteur was strongly motivated to pursue his research into micro-organisms and disease because two of his own daughters had died after contracting typhoid fever.

Despite suffering a stroke in 1868, he persevered with his work. Pasteur was not medically qualified and had no detailed medical knowledge. Therefore, he enlisted the help of two brilliant young doctors, Emile Roux and Charles Chamberland. In 1880 when working with chicken cholera, Pasteur accidentally discovered an effective vaccine. He inoculated chickens which had been previously exposed to a mild infection of the disease and by so doing he successfully rendered them immune from attack by a more potent strain. Pasteur believed that their bodies had somehow been able to make use of the weaker strain of germ to form a defence mechanism against the more powerful germs in the fresher culture.

Subsequently and following the principles he had discovered, he went on to develop an effective vaccine against anthrax in 1882 and then against rabies three years later. For the latter he used a vaccine, previously untried on humans, on a young boy who had been bitten by a rabid dog. Rabies is caused by a virus and not a bacterium but a vaccine may be prepared in the same way with the same underlying principles. Pasteur employed the technique of collecting infected material from dead rabbits inoculated with the disease and weakening the strain of the causative organism by allowing it to dry for 5 to 10 days. The boy survived, but without the vaccine he would almost certainly have died.

Joseph Lister and Antisepsis

In August 1865, Professor Joseph Lister applied a piece of lint which had been soaked in carbolic acid, to the injured leg of an eleven year old boy who had been admitted to Glasgow Royal Infirmary. His young patient had sustained a compound fracture of his tibia and fibula as a result of an accident where his leg had been run over by the wheel of a cart. Until then, such an injury would almost certainly have resulted in a major infection. After four days, he renewed the pad and discovered to his delight that the wound looked clean. After five weeks he was amazed to discover that the boy's fractured bones had united. This had occurred without the usual complication of infection which almost invariably previously occurred. Lister published his findings in the *Lancet* in a series of articles, and in the *British Medical Journal* on 21 September 1867.[14]

Lister's inspiration was unquestionably derived from the work of Louis Pasteur and his following statement is surely a landmark moment in the history of surgery. The era of anti-septic surgery had begun:

> When it had been shown by the researches of Pasteur that the septic property of the atmosphere depended not on the oxygen or any gaseous constituent, but on minute organisms suspended in it, which owed their energy to their vitality, it occurred to me that decomposition in the injured part might be avoided without excluding the air, by applying as a dressing some material capable of destroying the life of the floating particles.[15]

Lister used carbolic acid, derived from creosote, which had been discovered by Friedlieb Runge, who was a prominent German analytical chemist. Creosote was used by Runge to protect wood from rotting and to treat railway sleepers from decomposition. Runge did not understand that it was bacterial action which brought about the decomposition and disintegration of the wood. Lister tested the results of spraying instruments, surgical incisions and dressings with a solution of carbolic acid. He found that carbolic acid solution swabbed on wounds remarkably reduced the incidence of hospital gangrene. This was an advance which would revolutionise surgery.

Lister left Glasgow in 1869, and returned to Edinburgh to succeed James Syme as Professor of Surgery at the University of Edinburgh. He continued to develop and to improve his methods of antisepsis. His fame had spread by then and he regularly addressed large audiences on the use of antiseptics in surgery.

One surgeon who was convinced of the benefits of Lister's work was Alexander Ogston, who is credited with bringing antiseptic surgery to Aberdeen, Scotland. Ogston later went on to discover the staphylococcus, as already mentioned in Chapter 11, which was, and still is, the most important organism causing wound infections in surgical patients.

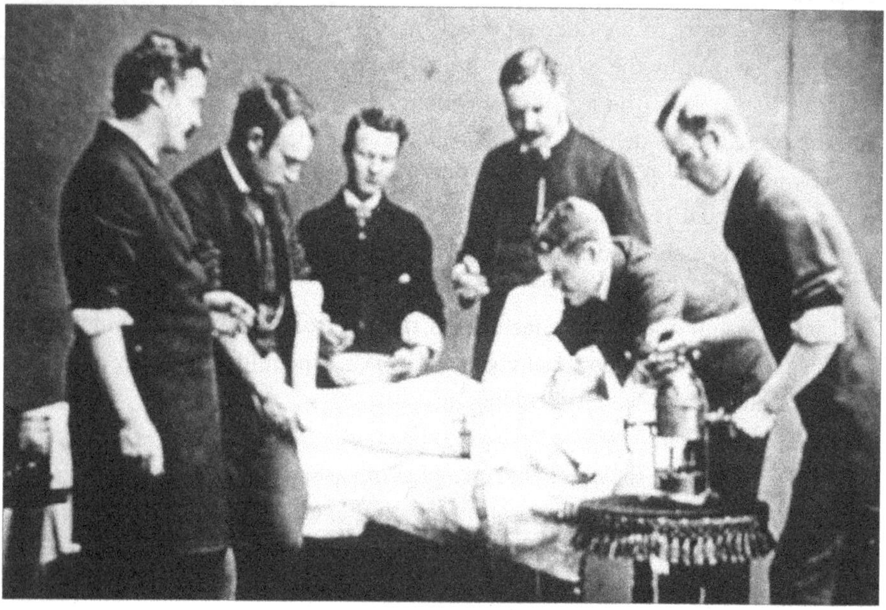

Figure 13.1. This photograph shows an operation being performed in Aberdeen by Alexander Ogston using antiseptic spray. Ogston was one of the first surgeons to adopt Joseph Lister's method. Ogston is at the extreme left of the photograph. (Courtesy of Aberdeen Medico-Chirurgical Society).

The development of aseptic surgery

As the germ theory of disease became more widely accepted, it was realised that infection could be better avoided by preventing bacteria from getting into wounds in the first place. While Lister and his contemporaries used antiseptics to destroy bacteria within wounds, they were still operating wearing coats and tails and moving freely from one patient to the next wearing their blood-caked garments.

If surgeons wore gowns which had been sterilised and if the surgical instruments were likewise sterilised, then bacteria would have had much less chance of gaining access to the wound. Prevention of wound infection during surgery made further progress when methods for sterilising gowns and instruments became available.

Ernst von Bergmann made a major breakthrough in aseptic surgery when he successfully sterilized surgical instruments by steam in 1885. Born in Latvia in 1836, Bergmann was Professor of Surgery at the Universities of Berlin and Würzburg. He is also credited with using a similar method to sterilize wound dressings and other medical equipment used during surgical operations. Bergmann's method used steam under pressure and is the basis for modern sterilization procedures using autoclaves.

Bergmann worked as a surgeon in the Austro-Prussian War (1866) and also in the Franco-Prussian War, where he gained experience treating cranial trauma and neurological disorders. Bergmann published several surgical works, including a classic treatise on cranial surgery entitled *Die Chirurgische Behandlung der Hirnkrankheiten.*[16]

The Prussians made some use of Lister's methods of antisepsis, whilst the hard-pressed French did not and they used non-sterile lint to pack the wounds of their men.[17] McCallum documented a higher incidence of gas gangrene amongst French troops and most likely due to their not using anti-sepsis.[18]

Lister evolved a famous bandage, which consisted of a rather complex eight fold thick bandage of gauze treated with carbolic. There was a strip of mackintosh at the outer end to act as a waterproof layer and impermeable silk against the skin to protect the skin from the corrosive effects of the carbolic acid. It was only during the siege of Paris that both sides were provided with the necessary materials to put Lister's antiseptic method into practice.[19]

Further developments in microbiology by Robert Koch

Robert Koch was born in 1843 in Clausthal in the Harz Mountains and was the son of a mining engineer. He graduated in medicine from the University of Göttingen and trained in Berlin and Hamburg. Whilst Pasteur was convinced that microbes were associated with disease, he never managed to link a specific organism with a specific disease. Robert Koch's work would change all that. Koch's work took place during the years after the Franco-Prussian War and while it may seem that he followed very much in the footsteps of Louis Pasteur, the two men were bitter rivals. This rivalry was partly on a personal level, since they did not like one another but also on a nationalistic basis after France's defeat in the Franco-

Prussian War. Their bitterness towards each other was particularly vehement when they clashed over their work on anthrax.

The Pasteur-Koch controversy reflected, at least in part, the contemporary political antagonism which prevailed between France and Germany, while on a scientific level, the Pasteur and Koch schools of microbiology adhered to different methods and philosophies. Pasteur was deeply interested in questions of immunity and in developing specific ways to protect humans against specific infectious diseases. In contrast, Koch favoured public health measures for controlling infectious diseases. Pasteur's method was to vaccinate individuals, whereas Koch's approach was to rely on sanitary methods to protect populations.[20] The fact of the matter, however, is that both men made outstanding contributions to the advance of evidence-based medicine, and their bitter rivalry and nationalistic tendencies should not obscure their major contributions to medicine.

In 1872, Koch became district medical officer for a rural area near Berlin. He started to experiment with microbes in a small laboratory he had built for himself in his surgery. He investigated anthrax in animals and identified the anthrax bacillus in 1877. He discovered that the anthrax bacillus produced spores which were capable of surviving for a long time in a dormant state, but were still capable of growing under suitable conditions into the anthrax bacillus and causing clinical infection with the disease.

In 1880 he was appointed to a post at the Imperial Health Office in Berlin where he perfected the technique of growing pure cultures of germs using a mix of potatoes and gelatine. This was a firm basis to allow and support the germs to be studied in more detail.

In 1881 he began to work on one of the worst killer diseases of the nineteenth century and indeed of the first half of the twentieth century. This was tuberculosis (TB). He successfully cultured the causative bacterium, mycobacterium tuberculosis, in 1882.

In 1883, he isolated vibrio cholerae, the organism responsible for cholera and which had ravaged armies throughout the nineteenth century.

Koch's pupils went on to discover the organisms responsible for diphtheria, typhoid, pneumonia, gonorrhoea, cerebrospinal meningitis, leprosy, bubonic plague, tetanus, and syphilis by using his methods. Microbiology had truly arrived on the medical scene and never again would there be talk of "miasma" in the causation of disease.

A MAJOR DISADVANTAGE OF RAPID MOVEMENT OF TROOPS: SMALLPOX EPIDEMIC OF 1870

During the Franco-Prussian War there was a European pandemic of smallpox. There is evidence for its presence in Paris as early as New Year's Day in 1870. By the time war was declared on 17 July 1870 there was a frightening level of this disease in the capital. The work of Edward Jenner in 1796 had led to the development of a successful vaccine against smallpox. However, it required its proper implementation in the population for it to be effective in preventing disease. Unfortunately it had not been generally employed by the French, and subsequent events serve to illustrate how troop movements in time of war may bring them into contact with civilian populations with devastating consequences.

The smallpox epidemic of the war of 1870-71 is well documented and may be used to illustrate other epidemiological disasters throughout history. As with conflicts in other historical periods, troop mobilization resulted in the mixing of both military and civilian populations. This resulted therefore in an increased likelihood of disease transmission.

Large numbers of French prisoners of war were rapidly removed to Prussia by train and were sent to internment camps. The close contact of the prisoners with each other led to a marked spread of the disease within the French soldier population and from there to the surrounding civilian population.

In effect, this represents a reversal of the usual pattern of disease in society. Normally if an individual is ill, that individual usually separates himself from others, or is isolated from the population and stays at home until the illness has resolved or is fatal. This naturally benefits the general population, since by staying at home he will not transmit the disease to others. In contrast, during conditions of war, the concentration of sick people together in overwhelming numbers facilitates the transmission of disease.

There was a vigorous vaccination and re-vaccination programme in the German forces, whilst the French were less fastidious in their approach. A programme of compulsory vaccination of all new French recruits had been introduced in 1859. However, the reputedly high failure rate of the army's re-vaccination schedule in the years immediately preceding the war with Prussia, coupled with the outbreak of hostilities, ensured that a large sector of the French army was susceptible to smallpox. Civilian populations in Germany and France were not vaccinated.[21]

Table 13.4 provides a very clear demonstration of what happened.

Table 13.4 Deaths from smallpox in military and civilian populations in France and Germany 1870-1871.

Country	**Smallpox deaths**
France	Soldiers - 25,077 Civilians - 89,954
Germany	Soldiers - 297 Civilians - 176,977

From: Smallman-Raynor, M., A.D. Cliff. "The Geographical Transmission of Smallpox in the Franco-Prussian War: Prisoner of War Camps and Their Impact upon Epidemic Diffusion Processes in the Civil Settlement System of Prussia, 1870-71". *Medical History*, 2002, 46: pp.241-264.

SUMMARY

There were two significant medical advances made between the end of the American Civil War and the start of the Franco-Prussian War which were the discovery of bacteria and the introduction of antiseptic surgery. These developments required a combination of genius in scientific research, a certain amount of luck and hard work. The face of medicine had changed forever. The discovery of bacteria established micro-biology as an essential medical specialty and greatly added to the understanding both of disease and wound infection, while antiseptic surgery led to aseptic surgery, which is the basis of modern surgery as practiced today.

Unfortunately, counter-balancing the beneficial effects of these medical advances was the arrival of ever more powerful weapons. These were capable of inflicting more terrible wounds, employed by ever increasing numbers of troops who were able to move very quickly from one location to another by ever improving transport systems. The result was a massive number of casualties, as exemplified by Dunant's experience at Solferino, which in turn of course led to the birth of the International Red Cross. The ability to rapidly evacuate the wounded soldiers was beneficial, but also carried the potential risk of assisting in the transmission of disease, as illustrated by the smallpox pandemic of 1870.

The methods employed during the American Civil War and the Franco-Prussian War to evacuate and treat huge numbers of wounded during these conflicts were duly noted and meant that an effective evacuation pathway with adequate numbers of doctors could be put into place for subsequent conflicts as exemplified by the Great War in 1914.

ENDNOTES

1. Bodart, G. *Losses of Life in Modern Wars* Oxford: Clarenden Press, 1916, pp.148-149.
2. *Ibid.*
3. *Ibid.*
4. *Ibid.*
5. McCallum, J.E., *Military Medicine from ancient times to the 21st Century.* Santa Barbara, California: ABC-CLIO, 2008, pp.124-127.
6. 6 Cooter, R., M. Harrison, S. Sturdy. *War, Medicine and Modernity.* Stroud, Gloucestershire: Sutton Publishing Limited, 1998, p.25.
7. *Ibid*, p.27.
8. Swain, V.A.J., "Franco Prussian War 1870-1871 Voluntary Aid for the wounded and sick", *British Medical Journal* 1970; 3: pp.514-517.
9. Cooter, *op. cit.*, p.30.
10. Laffin, J., *Surgeons in the Field.* London: J.M. Dent and Sons Limited, 1970, p.170.
11. Cooter, *op. cit.*, p, 30.
12. Swain, *op. cit.*, pp.511-514.
13. Laffin, *op. cit.*, p.169.
14. Lister, J., "On the antiseptic principle in the practice of surgery." *British Medical Journal*, 1867; 2 (351): pp.246-248.
15. *Ibid.*
16. Bergmann, E., *Die Chirurgische Behandlung der Hirnkrankheiten*, Berlin, 1899: A Hirschwald.
17. Laffin, *op. cit.*, p.168.
18. McCallum, *op. cit.*, pp.124-127.
19. Laffin, *op. cit.*, p.169.
20. Ullman, A. Pasteur-Koch: "Distinctive ways of thinking about infectious diseases". *Microbe*, Volume 2, Number 8, 2007; pp.383-387.
21. Smallman-Raynor, M., A.D. Cliff. "The Geographical Transmission of Smallpox in the Franco-Prussian War: Prisoner of War Camps and their Impact upon Epidemic Diffusion Processes in the Civil Settlement System of Prussia, 1870-71". *Medical History*, 2002, 46: pp.241-264.

14

More Minor Wars

Following the Crimean War, many shortcomings were identified in medical services in the British Army which resulted in the major policy changes discussed in Chapter 11. The recommendations of the Sanitary Commission were published in the Royal Warrant of 1858 and the Cardwell Reforms of 1870-1873 resulted in the abolition of the regimental hospital system. Several colonial wars were fought between the conclusion of the Crimean War (1853-1856) and the beginning of the Boer War (1889-1902) against this background of administrative change. These wars reflect how medical services responded to the reforms as they were adopted and implemented.

Many scientific discoveries were made during the nineteenth century and without doubt the most important advance in surgical practice was Joseph Lister's use of antiseptics. This alone resulted in a significant reduction in the incidence of wound infection. Whilst this was a very important development, the health and well-being of troops was helped much more by other changes. These included better sanitation, proper sewage disposal and water purification, better quality of barrack and hospital accommodation and better siting of these facilities in healthier locations.

There were several important medical developments which were introduced during these colonial wars which brought about a significant improvement in the health of troops together with a corresponding reduction in mortality from disease. Some of the conflicts will be discussed in greater detail because they highlight particular issues, while the developments during others are summarised in Table 14.1.

Table 14.1 Important medical developments which were introduced during minor conflicts during the second half of the nineteenth century.

CONFLICT	RELEVANT MEDICAL CHANGES	MORTALITY PER 1,000 FROM DISEASE	COMMENTS
Indian Mutiny (1857-59)	Sanitary Commission recommendations not published till 10 October 1857.	89.42 per 1,000.	High death rate from heat stroke, malaria and dysentery;
Second & Third China Wars (1857-60)	Sanitary officer appointed for first time; Drinking water filtered, which clarified but did not sterilise water supplies; Quinine issued to deal with malaria; Regimental hospital system scrapped as unworkable;	Deaths varied between 22.65 & 65.54 per 1,000; This compares with 178 per 1,000 in First China War; In 10 years from 1870-79, death rate only 14.4 per 1,000;	Two modern hospital ships with full facilities; Big effort made due to high mortality which occurred in First China War; Well organised campaign; Growing dissatisfaction with regimental hospital system;
New Zealand Wars (1860-67)	Regimental hospital system again scrapped as unworkable; Sanitary officer again appointed; Field hospitals well ventilated; hand washing encouraged; New disinfectant (Condy's Solution);	Deaths 23.02 per 1,000 in 1864; 13.94 per 1,000 in 1865; 12.86 per 1,000 in 1866;	Sanitary officer frequently ignored; Persisting problem of lack of proper rank for medical officers; Small field hospitals with 30 beds and base hospitals in Auckland, New Plymouth and Wanganui;
Abyssinian War (1867-68)	Water purification by condensation of sea water and piping it; Sanitary officer again important in controlling disease;	17.2 per 1,000;	Growing awareness of inadequacies of regimental hospital system;
JOSEPH LISTER DOES HIS WORK ON ANTISEPTICS IN SURGERY IN1867. THIS WAS A MILESTONE IN SURGERY.			
Kaffir Wars and First Boer War(1877-1880)	First time stretcher bearer company used;	32.24 per1,000;	Stretcher bearers put a stop to healthy combat troops accompanying the wounded to the rear; L/Cpl. Joseph Farmer became the first Army Hospital Corps man to be awarded the VC;

Zulu War (1879)	Charcoal filters - but ineffective against transmission by flies carrying disease;	26.63 per 1,000;	All medical services under the control of Principal Medical Officer (PMO);
2nd Afghan War (1878-1880)	British troops employed the new reorganised field medical units;	74-128 per1,000, depending on which part of the force;	Cholera in Khyber Pass Extremely hostile terrain and very hot;
Ashanti (1873-74) War	Sanitary officer responsible for major reduction in mortality from disease;	The annual mortality per 1,000 in the First Ashanti War was 668 per 1,000. In the Second Ashanti War (1873-1874) there were only 38 deaths in a country that had once been "the white man's grave".	Better water; better living conditions; better nutrition; "Sanitary success unparalleled in the long history of armies;"
Third Burma War		48.49 per 1,000 in 1888 30.19 in 1889 483 per 1,000 in First Burma War (1824).	Improvements down to better sanitation and better drinking water;
Egypt (1882)	Antisepsis using carbolic acid	13.21 per 1,000	First major war since reforms of 1873; Problems with base hospitals too far away on Cyprus and Gozo;
Sudan (1884 & 1885)	Carbolic acid dressing employed;	14.37 per 1,000;	Antisepsis now being employed more regularly;
Sudan (1898)	Sterilisation of water by Bromine; X-rays were used in this war, having been used first in the Tirah Campaign, an Indian Frontier War (1897-1898).	36.18 per 1,000.	Royal Army Medical Corps in being; They would not have full impact till 1906-07.

From Cantlie, N., *A History of the Army Medical Department*, Edinburgh: Churchill Livingston; 1974, Volumes 1 and 2.

THE INDIAN MUTINY (1857-59)

The Indian Mutiny was a pivotal conflict because it effectively brought an end to the East India Company. Following the Indian Mutiny, the Government of India Act 1858 led to the British Crown assuming direct control of India in the new British Raj. The East India Company was dissolved in 1874 because by then it was effectively powerless and obsolete.

The Mutiny was sparked by rumours that new cartridges to be issued to troops of the East India Company were lubricated with animal fat derived from beef and pork. This caused great concern amongst native troops because to a Hindu the cow is sacred and the Holy Qur'an forbids Muslims to touch the meat of swine. There were other deep rooted causes for the Mutiny, for example, frustration felt by native troops at poor prospects for promotion in comparison with those of their European counterparts and promotion and recruitment of native troops based on caste rather than ability.

The General Service Enlistment Act of 1856 was a potent predisposing factor, since before its introduction, men of the Bengal Army were exempt from overseas service. On the other hand, soldiers of the Madras and Bombay Armies were obliged to serve overseas if required. This arrangement seemed unfair to Governor-General Lord Dalhousie who instigated the General Service Act and which was signed into effect by Governor-General Lord Canning.

New recruits in the Bengal Army then had to accept a commitment for general (i.e. overseas) service. This was much to the chagrin of serving high caste sepoys in the Bengal Army who were fearful that this directive would affect them and would discourage sons from following fathers into an Army with a strong tradition of family service.

There was also a belief that their culture was being interfered with in what they perceived was a plot to "Christianise" the sub-continent.

The Mutiny began on 10 May 1857 and was characterised by fighting under extremely adverse conditions. There were many deaths due to the effects of heat and disease, a point best illustrated by considering the siege of Lucknow at the commencement of the Mutiny. When hostilities began, Sir Henry Lawrence, the British Commissioner in Lucknow, gathered all the British residents together and took them to the Residency for their safety. There were about 1,700 fighting men and 1,300 non-combatants. Lawrence fortified the Residency against rebel forces, who attacked on 4 July 1857. Lawrence was killed soon after by an exploding shell.

On 25 September 1857, a relief force led by General Havelock fought its way into Lucknow and made its way to the Residency. It was a debilitated and weakened force by then, because for every mile marched and fought over, Havelock's force sustained many casualties from heat stroke and it was not strong enough to both overcome the rebels and lift the siege. The survivors were compelled to join the besieged defenders within the Residency. This action became known as the First Relief of Lucknow. In early 1858, a further rescue mission was mounted and led by Sir Colin Campbell, who had led the Highland Brigade in the Crimea and who was in command of the 'Thin Red Line' at the Battle of Balaclava. His rescue mission was successful.

Four Victoria Crosses were won by medical personnel during the "First Relief" as Havelock fought his way through the streets of Lucknow. Some idea of the conditions may be appreciated by reading the citations of the four medical officers who were awarded the Victoria Cross:

Surgeon Jee

> At Lucknow he displayed great courage in tending to the wounded. He escorted them towards the residency on cots and on the backs of his men as many of the doolie bearers had fled. Whilst approaching the Residency, he was besieged by the enemy in the Mote Mahal. He continued to tend the wounded in an open position. On the following day, he managed to bring many of them in to the Residency under heavy crossfire.[1]

Surgeon McMaster

Assistant surgeon McMaster won his VC in a unique way. All the officers of 78th Foot had acquitted themselves with such great bravery that the Regiment was awarded the VC. All the other officers were of the opinion that McMaster should receive the honour:

> At Lucknow, he exposed himself to the heavy fire of the enemy throughout the night, whilst bringing in and attending to the many injured.[2]

Surgeon Home

> At Lucknow, as the British column was forcing its way into the Residency, he was in charge of the wounded men left behind in the streets. Under fierce fire, he and the others were forced to take refuge in a house, which was soon set ablaze. The occupants retreated to a shed, firing at rebels who

had climbed onto the roof. Soon after dawn, when the small party had lost all hope of survival, they were rescued.[3]

Assistant surgeon Bradshaw

For intrepidity and good conduct when ordered by Surgeon Home to remove the wounded men left behind the column that forced its way into the Residency at Lucknow on 26 September 1857. Many wounded were left behind in the streets. Under heavy fire from the enemy, he persuaded many litter bearers to retrieve the wounded and without the aid of any troops led them to the safety of the Residency.[4]

DISEASES AFFECTING BRITISH TROOPS DURING THE INDIAN MUTINY

Admissions and death rates were high during the Indian Mutiny. Overall figures for British military casualties revealed 792 deaths due to heat stroke. The death rate was 89.4 per 1,000 men. The majority of deaths were caused by malaria and dysentery. Individual regiments suffered heavy losses. The 32nd Foot at Lucknow suffered the heaviest casualties of any regiment, losing by death 384 officers and men from a strength of 510.[5]

THE SECOND AND THIRD CHINA WARS (1857-1860).

The First China War, also known as the Opium War, was discussed in Chapter 8 and began when China tried to stop the lucrative trade in opium to the Chinese market by merchants of the East India Company. China subsequently failed to meet its obligations to permit trade and after diplomatic attempts to bring about a solution failed, British, French and Indian troops invaded China to begin the Second China War. When a new treaty granting additional rights to the British was ignored after the conclusion of the Second War, a Third China War began.

Staff Surgeon Rutherford was appointed as the first ever Sanitary Officer and drinking water was filtered. Troops were issued with quinine to treat intermittent fever (malaria) and this was given to soldiers at morning parade under medical supervision.[6]

The sick rate was significantly reduced compared with the First China War. Between May and July 1860 there were 22.6 deaths per 1,000, whilst in contrast, between August and November of the same year, that figure was 65.5 per 1,000. Comparative figures from the First China War revealed 178 deaths per 1,000. China was still a very unhealthy place to be, but matters had improved significantly. In the ten years from 1860-69 there were 43.3 deaths per 1,000 and for the years 1870-79 there were 14.1 per 1,000, providing conclusive evidence that the sanitary measures taken to improve the health of the troops were proving to be effective.[7]

The regimental hospital system was abandoned during the Third China War (since it was perceived to be inefficient) following consultation with the commanding officer in favour of a more flexible system. This new system required that all regimental medical officers (RMOs) were put under the control of the Principal Medical Officer (PMO). Medical officers were deployed as the PMO saw fit. RMOs went into action with panniers on horseback, whilst ambulance barrows were provided to remove casualties to field hospitals in the rear, and from there to general hospitals. This was a campaign noteworthy for its good organisation of medical care now in place.

THE NEW ZEALAND WARS (1860-1867)

War broke out with the Maoris after a dispute over the sale of Maori land to settlers. Deputy Inspector Mouat VC, (awarded the VC for bravery during the Crimean War), the PMO, once again abandoned the regimental hospital system because it was too unwieldy to work well in rough scrubland. RMOs on horseback tended the wounded, whilst ambulance wagons took the wounded back to small field hospitals. Each field hospital was equipped with 34 beds and had excellent ventilation. A strict hand washing policy was introduced to try to improve and ensure good standards of cleanliness.

During this war men were well fed and were fit and well nourished before battle and in a much better condition to withstand wounding and physical traumas should they occur. Wounds were not interfered with unnecessarily and a new disinfectant called Condy's fluid was employed. As a result surgical complications were reduced and erysipelas, hospital gangrene and secondary haemorrhage did not occur. Henry Bollmann Condy was a chemist and industrialist who had an interest in disinfectants. He developed and patented "Condy's fluid" in 1857 which was a solution of potassium permanganate. His work predated Pasteur's germ theory of disease. From the field hospitals the wounded were taken to general hospitals in

Auckland, New Plymouth and Wanganui which were manned by men from the Army Hospital Corps. The statistics showed that this was a relatively disease free campaign, with deaths per 1,000 at 23.0, 13.9, and 12.9 for the years 1864, 1865 and 1866, respectively.[8]

Therefore, in two consecutive wars, the regimental hospital system was discarded in favour of a more practical and manageable system which was flexible and more adaptable to the conditions in which fighting occurred. Once again, there was a sanitary officer, Surgeon Major MacKinnon, but sometimes his suggestions were ignored. MacKinnon recommended that all combatant officers should attend lectures on hygiene, since most of them knew nothing about the subject. Generally, senior combatant officers neither knew, nor cared, about the sanitary measures necessary to maintain the health of the men for whom they were responsible. This mindset continued throughout the remainder of the nineteenth century and it is salutary to remember that during the Second Boer War (1899-1902) twice as many men died from disease as were killed by the enemy or died from their wounds.

There were many other minor wars in the remaining years of the nineteenth century and the pertinent medical matters of importance are highlighted in Table 14.1.The regimental system of medical care was formally abolished in 1873 in favour of the more flexible system of care under the control of the PMO which had been unofficially adopted as already explained. A sanitary officer was attached to every expedition and this made a significant difference although as has been pointed out his advice was not always heeded and the difference made actually could have been greater.

Nevertheless, as a result of the measures introduced and implemented the death rate from disease in the second half of the nineteenth century when compared with the first was significantly reduced as shown in Table14.2. Figure 14.1 presents the same information in graphical format, where the impact of the post-Crimean changes can be very clearly seen.

Table 14.2 Mortality per 1,000 in minor wars of the nineteenth century.

LOCATION	MORTALITY PER 1,000
Jamaica (1817-1836)	121.3
First Burma War (1824)	483
First Ashanti War (1824-26)	668
First Afghan War (1838-42)	147.5
First China War (1839-42)	178
Second Burma War (1852)	236
Indian Mutiny (1856-59)	89.42
Third China War (1857-60)	65.54
New Zealand (1860-67)	23.02
Abyssinia (1867)	17.2
Zulu War (1879)	26.63
1st Boer War (1880)	32.24
2nd Afghan War (1878-80)	128.15
Egypt (1882)	13.21
Sudan (1885)	14.37
3rd Burma (1885-87)	30.19
Sudan (1898)	36.18

From Cantlie, N., *A History of the Army Medical Department*, Edinburgh: Churchill Livingston, 1974, Volumes 1 and 2.

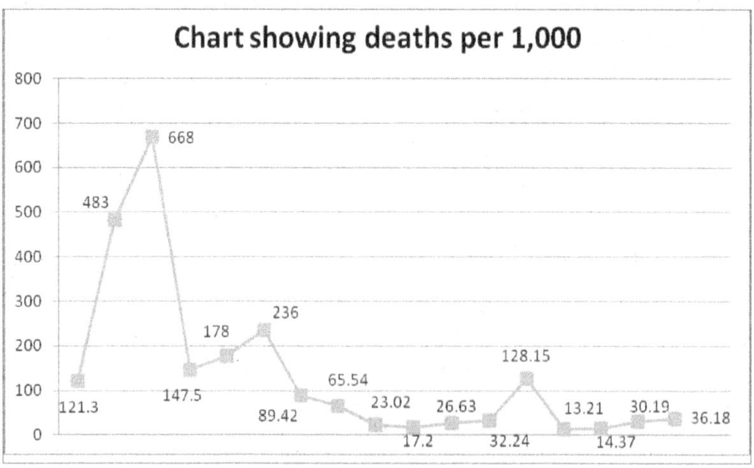

Figure 14.1. Mortality per 1,000 troops in minor wars throughout the nineteenth century. Each point on the graph corresponds chronologically to the data in Table 14.2. (Data compiled from data from Cantlie, N., *A History of the Army Medical Department*, Edinburgh: Churchill Livingston, 1974, Volumes 1 and 2)

SECOND AFGHAN WAR (1878-1880)

This war had its origins in the perceived threat of an invasion of India by Russia through Afghanistan. When a Russian mission was temporarily welcomed to Kabul, the Indian Government became alarmed. When the ruler (Amir Dost Mohammed) in Afghanistan died, his son, Sher Ali succeeded him. When Sher Ali would not admit a British mission to Kabul, Lord Lytton, Viceroy of India declared war on Afghanistan.

The invasion of Afghanistan was carried out by a force of 40,000 men and was split into three military columns which penetrated Afghanistan at different points. Much of the country was occupied and after vague assurances of help against foreign (Russian) aggression, a peace treaty was signed in 1879. British representatives were installed in Kabul and other locations and the British Army withdrew. The mountainous terrain caused particular hardship and returning troops were faced with a journey through the Khyber Pass in extremely hot weather. There was a known outbreak of cholera moving up the Khyber Pass towards them from the south. So began the so called "death march" through the Khyber Pass, in temperatures of 46°C. There were 350 deaths from cholera among British troops during this march, a rate of 74 per 1,000. [9]

Mounting resentment at British presence in Afghanistan led to the declaration of a "holy war". On 3 September 1879 an uprising in Kabul led to the slaughter of Sir Pierre Cavagnari, the chief British administrator, together with his guards and staff. This provoked the next phase of the Second Afghan War.

Major General Sir Frederick Roberts led the Kabul Field Force over the Shutargardan Pass into central Afghanistan and defeated the Afghan Army at Char Asiab on 6 October 1879 before occupying Kabul. An Afghan force of tribesmen attacked a British detachment at the Battle of Maiwand in July 1880 and besieged Kandahar. Roberts led the main British force from Kabul and marched 280 miles with 10,000 men from Kabul to Kandahar in 20 days. This was a formidable undertaking, and when Roberts reached Kandahar he defeated the besieging tribesmen.

Overall death rates amongst British troops in the Afghan War were very high. In 1879 there were more than 1,000 deaths from disease amongst British troops from a strength of 11,000 men. Indian troops suffered a total number of 1,282 deaths, 1,222 from disease and 60 from combat. The main causes of death were cholera, typhoid, dysentery and malaria. During active service on the baking hot plains in soaring temperatures the rate for British soldiers was 138.15 per 1,000.[10]

European troops could not be exposed to hot weather without great sickness and mortality.

No British force which invaded Afghanistan during the nineteenth century performed well under the adverse climatic conditions and the extremely difficult terrain. It proved easy to invade Afghanistan but it was an altogether more difficult proposition to leave it and the cost in lives lost from disease was high.

ANTISEPTIC SURGERY

Lister's work on antiseptic surgery was published in 1867 and involved the use of carbolic acid to destroy bacteria that contaminated wounds. He developed a special bandage which consisted of a rather complex eight fold thick bandage of gauze treated with carbolic. There was a strip of mackintosh at the outer end to act as a waterproof layer and impermeable silk against the skin to protect the skin from the corrosive effects of the carbolic acid. He used a spray of carbolic acid during surgical operative procedures so as to kill micro-organisms that might be in the wound.

His methods were used by the Prussians during the Franco-Prussian War of 1870-1871 but were not quickly embraced by military surgeons in the British Army. In an address delivered in 1880 to mark the twentieth anniversary of the foundation of the school at Netley, Surgeon General Longmore stated that it had never yet been used consistently in the field by British surgeons even although it had been used in civilian surgery for up to fifteen years previously. Although the use of antiseptic treatment in surgical management was on the increase it was by no means universally accepted.[11] Surgeons working in the Russo-Turkish War (1877-1878) used Lister's method and the writings of Volkmann and Esmarch clearly showed that a surgical revolution was taking place in the prevention of infections complicating surgery.

In an address to the Woolwich Military Medical Society, published subsequently in the *British Medical Journal* in 1884, Surgeon-Major Godwin referred to the work of Professor Carl Reyher who was in charge of an ambulance in the Caucasus during that conflict.[12]

Carl Reyher (1846-1890) was a Russian military surgeon, who had also demonstrated the role of debridement in gunshot wounds and fractures.[13] Reyher's work clearly demonstrated the value of antiseptics in military surgery and Godwin summarised Reyher's findings in 81 cases involving the knee joint as follows:

- 18 were treated antiseptically throughout their treatment and three died. 15 recovered with mobile joints;
- 40 cases were operated on without antiseptic surgery before coming under his care. 34 died, six recovered but five of these lost their limbs;
- 23 cases had no "Listerism" at all and one survived.

There was 95% mortality when no antisepsis was employed, 85% mortality when patients were partially treated by the antiseptic method and a much reduced mortality of only 16% when antiseptics were used from the outset.[14]

Lister's antiseptic surgery was used by the British Army in Egypt in 1882 and in the Sudan in 1884, by which time it was a firmly established technique.

WATER PURIFICATION SYSTEMS

Whilst Lister's antiseptic method made great improvements to the outcome of surgery the provision of clean and disease free water was every bit as important. The improved mortality figures in the second part of the nineteenth century were more attributable to the sanitary officer than to the surgeon.

Water was sterilised by one of three methods:

- Filtration (for both clarification and sterilisation);
- Sterilisation by heat;
- Sterilisation by chemicals.

When the Army Medical School was established, the supply of fresh clean water to the troops was studied and over a number of years improvements were made. Table 14.3 summarises the progress made and the methods employed. At first, filtration methods simply clarified the water i.e. made it look clean but did not sterilise it since they did not extract harmful bacteria responsible for typhoid fever and cholera. While the ensuing development improved the rate of filtration (Maignon's Filtre Rapide) it did nothing to address this important issue. Chamberlain's filtration systems both clarified the water and filtered out pathogens using kaolin. They were thus effective but they were too liable to breakages. Heat exchange mechanisms were employed but were cumbersome and had to be centrally located at fixed points which were inconvenient. In 1887 a radical new development using chemical sterilisation was used for the first time to destroy pathogenic organisms. Bromine was the first agent used but was unsatisfactory as

Table 14.3 explains and in the fullness of time chlorine was employed and was used during the Great War.

Table 14.3 Water Purification Systems

War	Water Purification System Employed	Details of System	Observations
Second & Third China Wars (1857-60)	Condensed sea water used before filtration plants set up on shore; Filtration system which only clarified water; Staff Surgeon Rutherford was appointed as the first ever Sanitary Officer; As well as overseeing other sanitary affairs he was responsible for drinking water;	Individual soldiers were given a small flannel bag with charcoal sewn in to the lining, whilst a method employing two barrels (one inside the other and with sand or gravel between the barrels) was used for filtering larger volumes of water; This latter method was a slow and cumbersome procedure.	In 1854, Snow demonstrated that water carried disease; This first significant attempt to purify water used filtration which only clarified the water; It did not destroy pathogenic organisms, which were not recognised at the time.
Abyssinian War (1867)	Condensation of sea water and piping it to combat area;	Later in the conflict porcelain filters were issued to every soldier;	Individual filters were very slow, and porcelain often broke
Zulu War (1879)	Charcoal & sand filters (produced clarification only);		Greatest danger in this campaign was drinking contaminated water. Existing filtration did not prevent typhoid fever.
Ashanti (1873-4)	Filtration (produced clarification only);	Individual porcelain filters to troops; Wooden water bottles issued; Large porcelain filters in hospitals;	Individual filters broke, clogged and were useless;

Sudan (1885)	Maignon's Filtre Rapide; Filtered 1,000 gallons/hour; While it had speeded things up, it did not remove pathogenic organisms;	Water was sucked up by a hand-operated pump, and delivered into copper tanks with a filtering interface of asbestos cloth, charcoal and chalk. It could filter 1,000 gallons an hour;	Individual filters were supplied to the troops once again but they were useless; In 1887 it was realised that water might contain pathogenic bacteria and that existing filtration did not destroy them.
Ashanti (1895-96)	Purifying filters of Pasteur Chamberland type in static installations. These also filtered out organisms.	Individual porcelain filters abandoned. Potassium permanganate and boiling water in forward area	What was once described as "The White Man's Grave" was now safe.
Sudan (1898)	Radical new chemical method of sterilisation employed; Sterilisation using Bromine after experimental work at Netley;	Bromine was unsuccessful because the glass ampoules containing the bromine would not stand up to field conditions; The water tasted awful;	By now it was realised that water might contain bacteria which are harmful if ingested (pathogenic) and this meant that more than simple filtration was required. It was this knowledge that led to the work using bromine.
Subsequent Progress in 20th Century; Sterilisation by filtration ;now there was both clarification and sterilisation;	Bromine replaced by filtration with two sets of filters (1) Sponges to clarify (2) Chamberland porcelain filters containing kaolin	Kaolin in the Chamberlain system prevented the passage of typhoid and cholera bacteria	Porcelain filters cracked on active service allowing pathogenic bacteria top pass through;
Sterilisation by heat exchange;	Sterilisation by heat; Heat exchange mechanism introduced;	With a large enough metallic surface of good conductivity and with sufficient time, a given quantity of liquid will yield all its heat to an equal volume of the same type of liquid;	Too cumbersome; had to be centrally located; not a practical solution

Sterilisation by chemicals	Clarification by sterilisation by chloride of lime; Any taste of chlorine removed by detesting tablets of sodium hyposulphite;	Chemical Clarification by passing water through flannelette wrapped round perforated tin cylinder;	Major General Sir William Horrocks, Professor of Hygiene at Royal Army Medical School made the final development before the Great War.

From Cantlie, N., A History of the Army Medical Department, Edinburgh: Churchill Livingston; 1974, Volumes 1 & 2.

SUMMARY

The British fought many colonial wars in far-flung corners of the Empire throughout the nineteenth century and were usually victorious. They often paid a very high price in lives lost, mostly from disease. The Crimean War was a very important watershed, after which the British Army underwent very important reforms. These were implemented in subsequent smaller wars and resulted in a significant improvement in the general health of soldiers with a corresponding reduction in mortality. Nevertheless, deaths from disease still outnumbered deaths from enemy action and while the appointment of a sanitary officer was without doubt a very important step in the right direction, his advice was often disregarded.

Great Britain was involved in another major war with the outbreak of the Second Boer War in 1899 and as will be seen in Chapter 15, deaths from disease outnumbered deaths from enemy action by 2:1. This was in no small part due to senior combat officers ignoring the advice of sanitary officers. There were important scientific discoveries made during the second half of the nineteenth century including the discovery of bacteria and anti-septic surgery. These were of inestimable importance to the advance of surgery but were of minor importance compared with improvements in hygiene, sanitation, accommodation and education.

ENDNOTES

1. Arthur, M., *Symbol of Courage; The Men Behind the Medal.* London: Pan Macmillan Ltd, 2005.
2. *Ibid.*

3. *Ibid.*
4. *Ibid.*
5. Cantlie, N., *A History of the Army Medical Department.* Edinburgh: Churchill Livingston, 1974, Volume 2, p.249.
6. *Ibid*, Volume 2, pp.250-251.
7. Cantlie, N., *A History of the Army Medical Department.* Edinburgh: Churchill Livingston, 1974, Volume 1, p.478.
8. Cantlie, N., *op. cit.*, Volume 2, p.258.
9. *Ibid,* Volume 2, p.303.
10. *Ibid*, Volume 2, p.306.
11. *Ibid*, Volume 2, p.409.
12. Godwin, C.H., "Antiseptic Surgery in its application to field service". *British Medical Journal* 1884; 1(1208).
13. Wangensteen, O.H., S.D.Wangensteen, "Carl Reyher (1846-1890) - Great Russian military surgeon: his demonstration of the role of debridement in gunshot wounds and fractures". *Surgery* 1973 Nov (5): pp.641-649.
14. Godwin, *op. cit.*, *British Medical Journal* 1884; 1(1208).

15

The Second Boer War

INTRODUCTION

The Second Boer War began on 11 October 1899 and was fought between the British Empire and two independent Boer Republics of Afrikaans-speaking Dutch settlers living in the South African Republic (Transvaal) and the Orange Free State. To understand the origins of the war it is necessary to go back to the beginning of the 19th century to 1805.

In 1805 Cape Colony was in the hands of the French-controlled Netherlands (which was then known as the Batavian Republic) and was protected by a small number of troops from the Netherlands supplemented by local militia men. Both the British Government and Napoleon understood the importance of the Cape with particular respect to sea routes and in the summer of 1805 Napoleon sent troop ships to the Cape to bolster its defence. The British Government countered Napoleon's initiative by sending a fleet of 63 ships commanded by Commodore Sir Home Popham together with some 7,000 British troops.

On 6 and 7 January 1806, under the command of Lt General David Baird, over 5,000 British troops landed and moved towards Cape Town to be met the following day by approximately 2,000 defending troops under the command of Lt General Jan Willem Janssens. The defending Dutch forces were defeated at the Battle of Blaauwberg, following which Baird advanced to Cape Town and reached it the following day. The Commandant of Cape Town surrendered on 10 January 1806 although fighting continued in the surrounding mountains for a few more days. The Articles of Capitulation were published in the Cape Town Gazette and African Advertiser on 25 January 1806. Some key points are summarised below which actually did not appear unfavourable to the defeated troops and the civilians they had been protecting:

- the colony, including all dependencies would be surrendered to the British;
- Batavian troops were to move to Simon's Town. Officers would be allowed to keep their swords and horses, but everything else must be handed over to the British;
- the Batavian troops would not be regarded as prisoners and the British Government would pay for their subsistence until they departed;
- The wounded and sick who could not travel would stay and be cared for by the British before being returned to the Netherlands;
- the rights and privileges allowed to the citizens of Cape Town would also apply to those in the rest of the colony, except that the British could quarter troops in the homes of residents in the country districts;
- Janssens would be allowed to send a despatch to the Netherlands and the British commanders would assist in forwarding.

Immigration of British settlers was encouraged subsequently and this led to increasing tension between the settlers and the Dutch farmers. The word "Boer" is the Dutch and Afrikaans word for farmer and approximately 15,000 Boers moved away, initially towards the east coast and then towards the interior to set up two independent Boer republics called the South African Republic (also called the Transvaal Republic) and the Orange Free State.

The British annexed the Transvaal in 1877 to resolve a border dispute between the Boers and the Zulus. This manoeuvre also saved the Transvaal from financial ruin, as its government had completely run out of money. However it precipitated the very short lived First Boer War which began in December 1880 and finished in March 1881.

In 1867 diamonds were discovered in the Orange Free State and gold was discovered in the Transvaal 21 years later. These discoveries led to large numbers of foreigners, termed "uitlanders", flowing into the areas to exploit the vast resources, with the majority coming from Britain. This massive influx of foreign workers caused tensions to rise even higher and the Jameson raid in January 1896, designed to cause an uprising of "uitlanders" in Johannesburg, failed and made matters worse as the British attempted to bring these two states, with their vast natural wealth, under their control. Furthermore, the Boers realised that if the "uitlanders" were given voting rights then they would lose political control of these territories to the British.

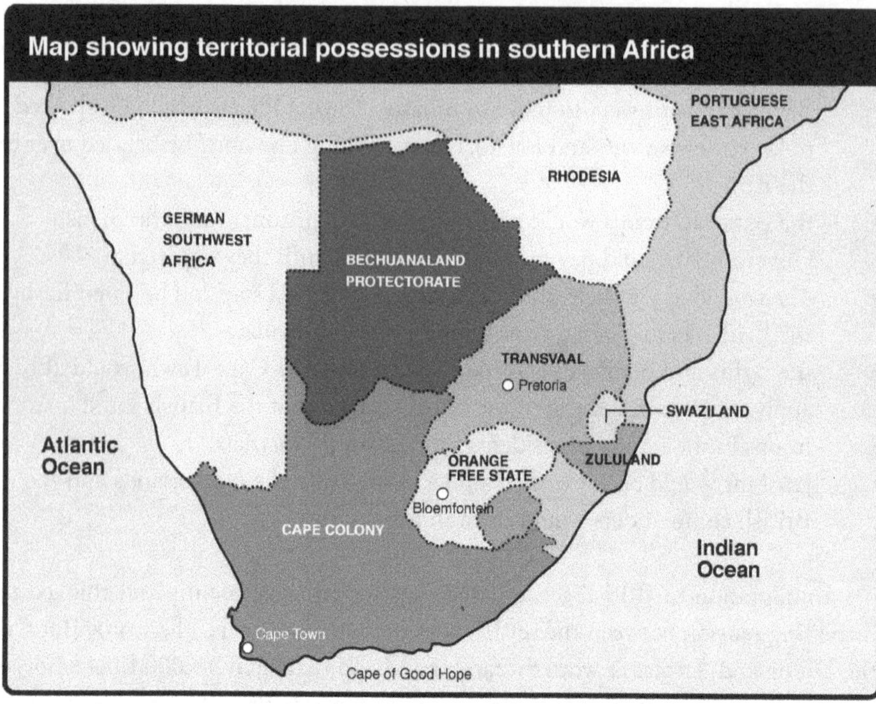

Figure 15.1. Map of South Africa at the time of the Boer War showing the situation in general.

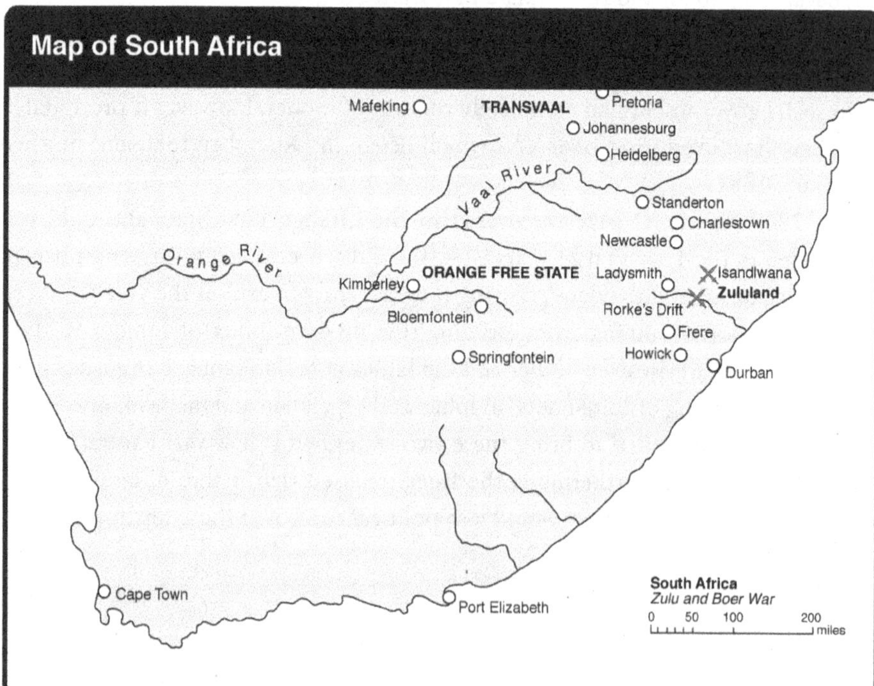

Figure 15.2. Map of South Africa at the time of the Boer War.

In 1899 the British Colonial Secretary, Joseph Chamberlain, demanded that full and proper voting rights be given to "uitlanders" living in the Transvaal. Tensions were clearly rising and the President of the South African Republic, Paul Kruger, responded by issuing an ultimatum to the British on 9 October 1899 giving them 48 hours to withdraw all their troops from the borders of the Transvaal and the Orange Free State. However Kruger's ultimatum was rejected and war was declared on 11 October 1899.

Whilst a detailed description of the military aspects of the campaign is beyond the scope of this book, the key points of the Second Boer War are outlined to provide a background to understanding the surgical and medical response. The war had three distinct phases:

- In the first phase, the Boers attacked British territories in Natal and Cape Colony and laid siege to British garrisons in Ladysmith, Mafeking and Kimberley;
- In the second phase, after strengthening their forces, British troops were sent to relieve the besieged and secured their hold of Natal and Cape Colony. They advanced into the Transvaal and by June 1900 its capital, Pretoria, was in British hands;
- In the third and final phase of the war, commencing in the spring of 1900 and lasting for two years, the Boers began a guerrilla war. They attacked specific targets such as supply depots, telegraph lines and isolated groups of British troops. This was particularly difficult to deal with given the large area in which the guerrillas operated, the isolated nature of events, their sporadic occurrence and the relatively small number of British troops present overall. The British responded by depriving the Boers of supplies and to facilitate this 8,000 block houses which guarded supply lines were built. They were linked by barbed wire, and manned by small numbers of troops (less than 10). The British employed a "scorched earth" policy both against the Boers and Black Africans. This was implemented by expeditionary columns of troops which systematically destroyed crops and farms, maimed animals and left them to die, poisoned wells and spread salt on the fields. Civilian women and children were moved into "concentration camps". To assist the British, Boer auxiliaries who had changed sides were employed to act on their behalf by acting as blockhouse guards, labourers and scouts.

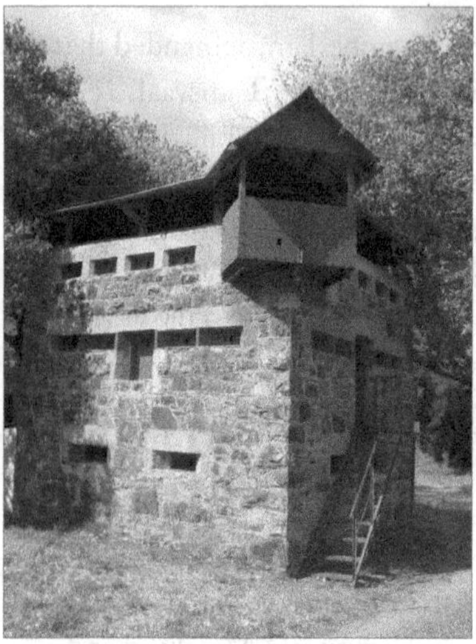

Figure 15.3. Boer Block House. (Kind permission of DanieVDM@flickr.com)

Boer losses continued to rise and the war was costing Great Britain some £2.5 million a month. Very importantly, concern was expressed both nationally and internationally about the treatment the Boers were receiving at the hands of the British. With these pressures on the British continuing to rise, the war came to an end on 31 May 1902 with the signing of the Treaty of Vereeniging. As a result of this the two Boer republics became part of the British Empire. It had been a long and bloody war and the losses sustained during this conflict were greater than those occurring in the Crimea as shown in Table 15.1.

Table 15.1 British casualties occurring during the Second Boer War (1899-1902).

KILLED IN ACTION AND DIED OF WOUNDS	DIED OF DISEASE	TOTAL DEATHS (including accidental)	WOUNDED
7,782	13,139	21,942	19,457

From Mitchell, T.J., G. M. Smith, *History of the Great War: Medical Services Casualties and Medical Statistics*. London: His Majesty`s Stationery Office, 1931, pp. 268-273.

Table 15.2 Numbers admitted to hospital and treated by the medical services (other ranks only).

	WOUNDED	SICK OR INJURED	TOTAL
Admissions	21,292	404,126	425,418
Deaths	1,835	13,682	15,517
Returned to duty	12,523	324,828	337,351
Invalided overseas	6,934	65,617	72,551

From Mitchell, T.J., G.M. Smith, *History of the Great War: Medical Services Casualties and Medical Statistics*. London: His Majesty`s Stationery Office; 1931, pp. 268-273.

CAUSES OF WOUNDS DURING THE BOER WAR

Wounds caused by shellfire were relatively uncommon except during the sieges of Ladysmith and Mafeking. Most wounds were caused by bullets from small-arms fire. Weapons firing small calibre bullets had recently been introduced and the mass produced German Mauser with a magazine holding five bullets was used by many armies on a world-wide basis using a 7mm or 7.6mm bullet. The Boers used the 7mm bullet with a muzzle velocity of 2,400km/hour and with a range of up to 2,000 meters.

Experimental trials in which bullets were fired from this weapon into cadavers and animals suggested that it did have an extensive destructive capacity. The metal casing of the bullet (its jacket) was important as it was this that actually dictated the type of wound. The entry wound was small, as was the exit wound. There was a reduced chance of large amounts of foreign material entering the wound with one exception – the Scottish soldier's kilt which was made from heavy material. This material was carried into the wound, in contrast to the light khaki uniforms worn by other soldiers, and this finding of kilt material in wounds was an important reason in Highland soldiers considering discarding the kilt in favour of a khaki uniform.

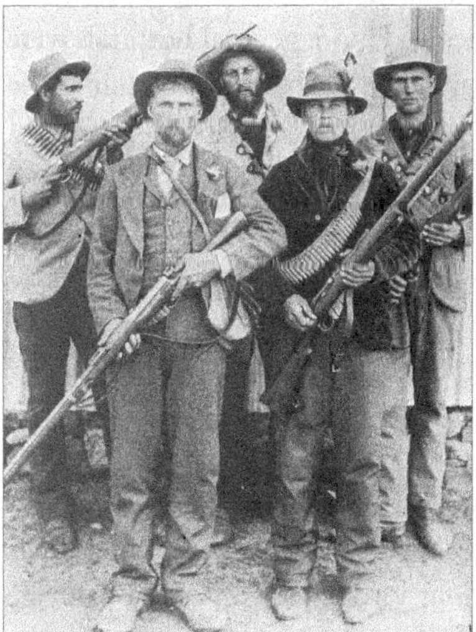

Figure 15.4. Boer guerrillas. (Wikimedia Commons)

Tissue destruction caused by the bullet during its transit appeared to be less than predicted from experimental tests. The range at which men were being shot was much greater, thus reducing the bullet's velocity.[1] In contrast, the rounded ball type projectiles used in previous conflicts and the pointed bullets which would be used in the Great War caused more extensive damage.

Concern was even expressed that this type of bullet did not cause enough damage and Benton summarised discussions which took place regarding the "humanity" of this bullet.[2] Some took the view that war should be made "completely humanitarian" while others were unhappy about the lack of damage caused by this bullet[3] and were of the opinion that the bullets being used were "too merciful".[4] The ratio of soldiers dead to wounded during the Boer War revealed that for every man killed outright, four survived the initial wounding, although 8.7% of them died subsequently.[5] The Boers also used the Martini-Henry rifle which fired a much heavier bullet which caused more extensive tissue damage and they were known on occasion to put poison-impregnated animal fat onto the bullets to increase their killing potential even further.

THE ROYAL ARMY MEDICAL CORPS

The Royal Army Medical Corps (RAMC) was established in 1898 and incorporated the officers and other ranks in the army who had been providing medical care to the soldiers as the Army Medical Staff and the Medical Staff Corps. The Boer War was its first test of how it would respond and function when challenged by a major conflict.

Cape Town was the centre of military operations for the planning and provision of medical care. It was a major port and it had a very efficient railway network leading to the interior. Surgeon General Sir WD Wilson was in charge of the medical war effort and was based in Cape Town. Existing hospitals in Cape Town included two military establishments at the outbreak of the war, but these were not sufficient for the anticipated number of casualties and more general hospitals were opened. By the spring of 1900 some 3,000 hospital beds were operational in Cape Town and Cape Colony.[6]

CHAIN OF MEDICAL CARE DELIVERED TO THE WOUNDED AND THE SICK

First aid on the battlefield

All soldiers carried a field dressing to be applied to any wound that they sustained. This was not a new idea and had originated from the Franco-Prussian War of 1870-1. The field dressing had a pad of gauze and a four yard length of woven bandage which was to hold it in place. A piece of waterproof jaconet was placed over the gauze and bandage and two safety pins held everything together. All the dressing materials were impregnated with a solution of 1 in 1000 mercuric chloride.[7] The waterproof covering was found to be disadvantageous, since wounds dressed in this way and left for a long time were more likely to become infected. Therefore the waterproof component was discontinued and this resulted in the incidence of wound infections reducing.

Casualties were evacuated to the first medical facility which was the regimental aid post. Each battalion had 16 stretcher bearers to perform this duty. The regimental medical officer and a medical NCO then did whatever they could to attend to the wound. Interestingly, they were not protected as "neutrals" by the Geneva Convention and so they themselves were at risk from the enemy. Their most important job was to stop bleeding and save life. There were inventive and ingenious methods which they developed and used to do this when circumstances dictated as illustrated in the following description:

> Shrapnel had exposed a main artery in the forearm and the man came down safely with a tourniquet on his brachial artery comprised of a plug of cake tobacco and the tape of a puttee.[8]

Casualties were taken by stretcher bearers to a casualty collection post and from there to a field hospital by the RAMC Bearer Company. This was often a very long and difficult journey over rugged terrain and could be especially distressing for those who had sustained fractures. The wounded were transported in ox-drawn carts and sometimes they had to be taken in and out of the carts and moved on stretchers when conditions were too difficult. There were specially designated "Maltese Carts" to transport medical equipment but many of these did not reach South Africa in time and medical teams had to purchase whatever carts they could locally in the areas where fighting was occurring.[9]

In addition to RAMC stretcher bearers, others helped to remove the wounded from the battlefield. The Natal Volunteer Ambulance Corps was raised by Colonel Gallway who was the Principal Medical Officer in Natal. It had a complement of 1,000 men from Pietermaritzburg who came from a variety of occupations and backgrounds, e.g. dentists, miners and clerks. The Indian community in Natal also offered to provide a similar corps, which was initially refused. As casualty figures mounted their offer was finally accepted and the Natal Indian Ambulance (Stretcher Bearer) Corps, comprising more than 1,000 Indians (300 free and the remainder employed, indentured labourers) and led by Mahatma Gandhi was formed. At the Battle of Colenso and Spion Kop, men of the Natal Indian Ambulance Corps carried wounded men to the field hospital 20 miles away at Frere. They were known as "the body snatchers" with 12 men taking their stretcher wherever necessary to retrieve the wounded, no matter what the danger to them personally. The excellence and devotion to duty of the Indian stretcher bearers was commented upon in the *British Medical Journal* during the war:

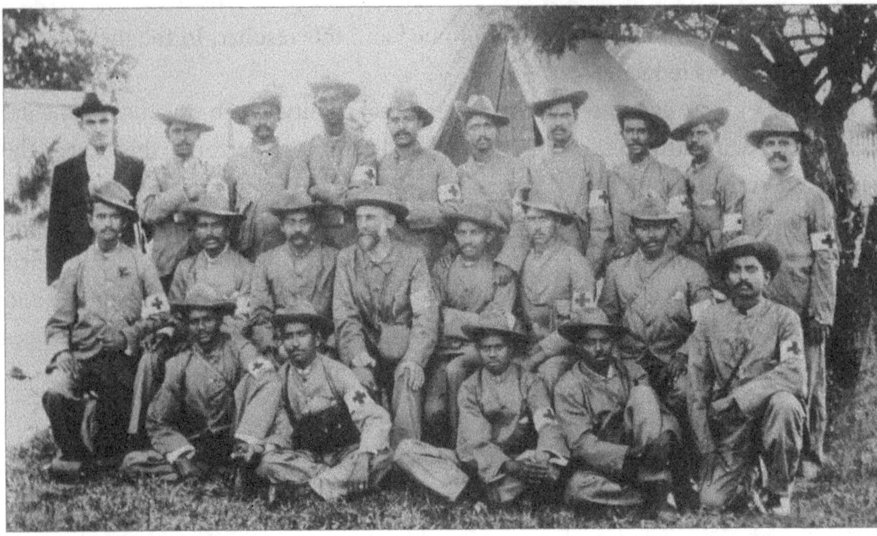

Figure 15.5. Stretcher-bearers of the Indian Ambulance Corps during the Boer War, South Africa. Ghandi is the fifth from the left on the middle row. (Wikimedia Commons)

> Men who were there write to me that the Indian bearers are preferred to their white comrades, having as one phrases it "the hands of a woman" and they exhibit an absolute indifference to the risks of being under fire.[10]

An interesting description of what it was actually like there with these men comes from a very vivid description by Thomas Pakenham:

> At sunset, a wild-looking procession had stumbled into Frere. They were nearly two thousand strong, dressed in tattered khaki tunics, and a strange assortment of hats: helmets, bowlers and tam-o'shanters. They were the 'body-snatchers': uitlander refugees and Gandhi's Indians, recruited as stretcher-bearers. They brought in the last of the wounded: 150 bad cases, covered in brown blankets, with their special belongings, boots, haversack and perhaps a pot of jam and a lump of tinned meat, carried in the hood of the stretchers. Most of the wounded were too shocked, or deeply encased in bandages, to speak. But sometimes a head would peer out of the hood to look at its neighbour. 'Fancy you here, Tom? Thought you were stiff.' Many men were delirious. One shouted that he was going to 'chuck it', and promptly rolled off the stretcher. Another was babbling about the harvest and the great time he was having at home. These were the latest instalment

of the 3,400 casualties the South Natal Field Force had suffered in the last three months".[11]

The Field Hospital

There were four field hospitals per division and the staffing of each hospital usually comprised the following:

- 5 officers;
- 1 warrant officer;
- 34 non-commissioned officers.

Each hospital could treat hundreds of soldiers with minor wounds until they were transported back to stationary and general hospitals further to the rear.[12] The surgeons manning the field hospitals had to deal with the wounded as expeditiously as possible, receiving the wounded one day and working non-stop to ensure that as many as possible were transferred down the line the next day in anticipation and readiness for the next batch coming along.

Field hospitals were tented and as an example, the 4th Field Hospital consisted of a central marquee, which was the operating theatre and a dressing area. It was surrounded by bell tents which provided accommodation for 100 wounded soldiers. Additional tents were erected before and after major battles to cope with the increased numbers of wounded that were expected. For example in preparation for the battle of Spion Kop, 100 additional bell tents were employed to accommodate an additional 500 casualties. All six hundred beds were utilised on that dreadful day.[13] However, the facilities were relatively poor; beds were not provided for the men and casualties had to lie on ground sheets on the floor or wherever there was space for them. There were no nurses because the field hospital was located too close to the front line. Instead, the wounded were cared for by male orderlies.

The operating theatre was relatively well equipped according to surgeons of that time and Frederick Treves, a surgeon of the 4th Field Hospital at Frere, in his book *A Tale of a Field Hospital* provided a detailed description of what actually happened and how life was in such a facility.[14]

He described how the central operating marquee had an operating table in the middle, with panniers all around the sides acting as tables for surgical instruments and dressings with just enough room for the surgeon, his assistant, anaesthetist and orderlies.[15] Water had to be supplied from wherever it could be found and was often brought to the hospital by train. On many occasions there was an insufficient

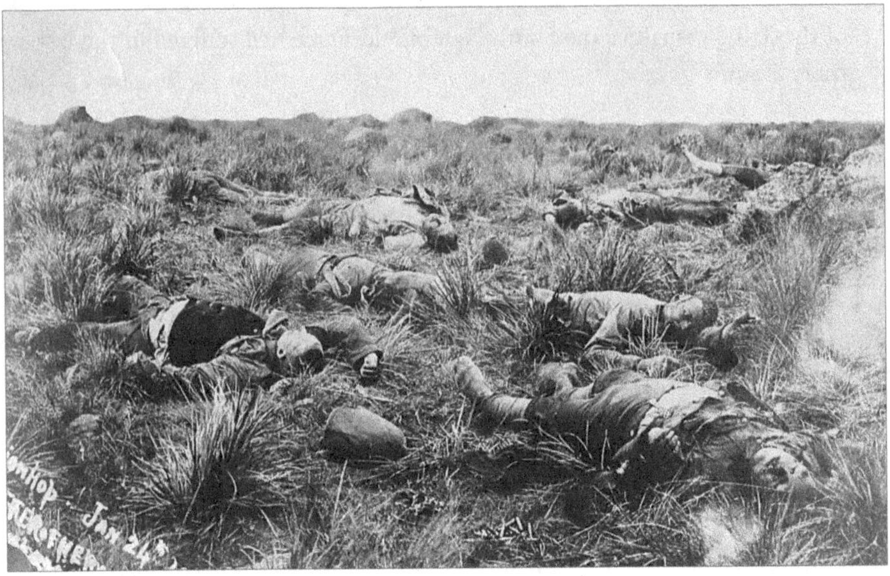

Figure 15.6. British dead shown after the battle at Spion Kop on the 24th January 1900 (Wikimedia Commons)

quantity of good quality water to prepare antiseptic solutions. Surgeons worked for long hours in their shirtsleeves, riding breeches and helmets, assessing the wounded and then operating on them. Sometimes the wounded were examined on the operating table under general anaesthetic (usually chloroform and morphia) if the wound was so severe that this would be the least painful option for the casualty.[16,17]

The wounded usually arrived at the field hospital in ambulance wagons which were pulled by 10 mules and driven by an African. They were either carried as "lying down cases" on stretchers or the less severely wounded were regarded as "sitting up cases".[18] The surgeons would assess them as they were being unloaded from the wagons and placed on the ground; Treves gave some very vivid descriptions of what it was like:

> Here was a man nursing a shattered arm with blood-stained rags of a torn-up sleeve. There was another with his head bandaged up and his face painted with streaks of dried blood, holding a crushed helmet beneath his arm like a collapsible opera hat ... One or two of those who were lying on the ground were vomiting, while near by a poor fellow who had been shot through the lung was coughing up blood.[19]

He went on to say:

> The saddest cases among the wounded were those on the stretchers, and stretchers were lying on the ground everywhere, and on each was a soldier who had been "hard hit" ... One or two were delirious, and had rolled off their stretchers on to the ground; others were strangely silent.[20]

The spirit amongst the wounded was high and they supported each other even in these most adverse of circumstances. What would happen to them? Would they live, or would they die? Would they survive with terrible disability? They constantly encouraged each other even as they were being taken into the operating theatre for surgery:

> Keep your chivey up Joe ... Good luck to yer old cock; you won't feel nothing ...[21]

Treves described a soldier, Private Goodman of the King's Royal Rifle Corps, who had been brought off Spion Kop after being wounded in that battle. He was alive and conscious, but with terrible wounds and had undergone a journey of more than eight hours to finally arrive at the hospital:

> He had been struck in the face by a fragment of shell which carried away his right eye, the right upper jaw, the corresponding part of the cheek and mouth and had left a hideous cavity at the bottom of which his tongue was exposed ... He was unable to speak and as soon as he was settled in a tent he made signs that he wanted to write ... After going through the form of wetting the pencil with what was once a mouth wrote simply "Did we win"? No one had the heart to tell him the truth.[22]

Goodman survived and returned to England, where he managed to establish a life for himself and to return to some sort of "normality".

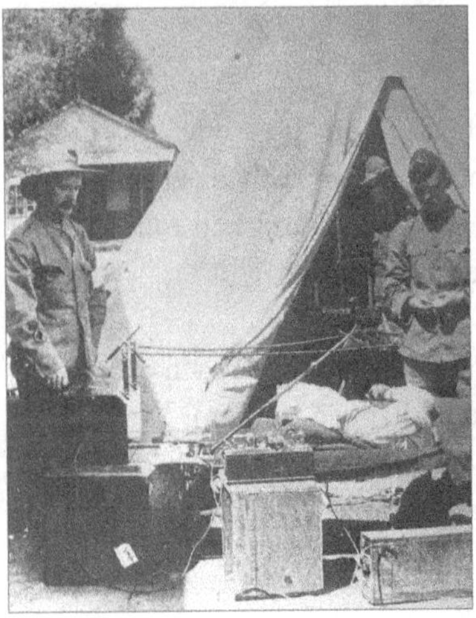

Figure 15.7. Medical tent in use during the Boer War for treating the wounded, 1900. (Wikimedia Commons)

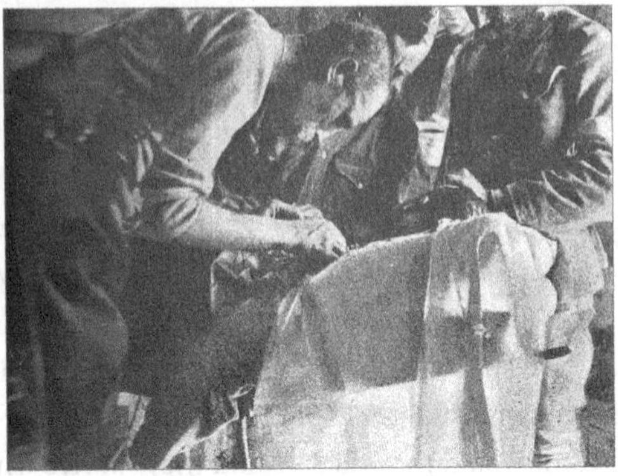

Figure 15.8. Surgeon operating tent during the Boer War. (Wikimedia Commons)

Of course not all the wounded survived and they were buried near the hospital. Teams of six men were assigned to dig graves, led by a corporal, armed only with spades and a sense of humour to make this daily task more bearable. Graves were marked by wooden crosses hand made from any source available, e.g. provision crates and whiskey boxes. Crosses were elaborately carved with pocket knives and can-openers![23] Much thought went into the planning of burials to avoid upsetting survivors. Bodies would be moved quietly to chapels close to the cemetery at 5pm each evening, with the burial ceremony at 8am the following morning.

After the war the bearer company and the field hospital combined to become a single functional unit called a "Field Ambulance" which greatly simplified command and control and utilised available staff more effectively. This concept had been discussed immediately prior to the war in 1899 and was similar to the Indian Field Hospital, but it had been decided not to make any changes at such a crucial time.

An ambulance was defined as: [24]

> a moving hospital which follows its army in its movements, so as to afford the speediest possible succour to the wounded.

Stationary Hospitals

From the field hospital casualties were transferred to stationary or general hospitals by a hospital train. The journey often began with a convoy of carts and horses or oxen. Sometimes patients were transferred as soon as four hours after undergoing an amputation if room had to be made for a new influx of casualties. Stationary hospitals had accommodation for 100 casualties and were usually positioned along railroad links and were an intermediate step between the field hospitals close to the fighting and the general hospitals at the base.[25]

Stationary and general hospitals were equipped with X-Ray facilities, and had operating theatres where more extensive aseptic surgery could be undertaken. Although the X-ray equipment was primitive (it became better developed during the Great War), it was of some help in localising bullets if they could not be found during surgery at the field hospital.[26]

As the war went on, the stationary hospitals increasingly functioned as general hospitals, except they were smaller, having between 100 and 400 fewer beds. There was considerable debate after the war as to what their function should be in future conflicts. During the Great War, the perceived role for stationary hospitals was once again to provide a link between medical facilities in the forward area, and general hospitals on the French coast. They performed the same kind of work as general hospitals, and largely because of this their intermediary role was abandoned and they functioned as general hospitals although with fewer beds.[27]

General Hospitals

General hospitals were located at the main bases, although as the war progressed they were moved closer to the fighting. These were large hospitals with a capacity for 520 or more casualties. They were either tented facilities or were established in existing public buildings and were distributed as follows:

- No. 1: Wynberg Military Camp from existing buildings (520 beds);
- No. 2: Parade ground at Wynberg Military camp and a new tented structure (504 beds);
- No. 3: Rondesboch and made up of buildings and marquees. It was joined by the civilian Portland hospital working together;
- No. 4: Mooi River;
- No. 5: Cape Town (700 beds and took over the existing hospital on Woodstock beach);

- No. 6: Johannesburg;
- No. 7: Pretoria;
- No. 8: Bloemfontein;
- No. 9: Bloemfontein;
- No. 10: Norvals Pont;
- No. 11: Kimberley;
- No. 12: Springfontein;
- No. 13: Johannesburg;
- No. 14: Newcastle;
- No. 15: Howick;
- No. 16: Elandsfontein;
- No. 17: Standerton;
- No. 18: Charlestown.

Lunatic Hospital

Knowledge and understanding of psychological aspects of warfare was rudimentary at best during the Boer War. A small hospital given the name "Lunatic Hospital" confirms a lack of understanding of these important illnesses. It was set up in Pretoria to serve up to 80,000 men at any one time and at the centre of the arrangements the following was provided:

> One or two wards should be reserved for officers, and the name of the lunatic attendants of the corps noted in the P.M.O.'s *(Principal Medical Officer)* office, so that their services can be secured at a moment's notice. [28]

Private Hospitals

In addition to military hospitals a small number of privately funded hospitals were established to support the military ones and these have been discussed in detail elsewhere [29] but some of these are outlined below:

Portland Hospital

This was named after the Duke of Portland. It had 130 beds and was initially situated adjacent to No 3 General Hospital in Rondebosch, before moving to Bloemfontein in April 1902. It was commanded by an RAMC officer and the remainder of the staff, including four surgeons were civilians.

Claremont Sanatorium
By all accounts this was perhaps the best hospital of all, and was located 6 miles from Cape Town. It had European fittings and furniture including electrical lighting and lifts. There were 106 single bedrooms with about half of the hospital being for officers.

Imperial Yeomanry Hospital
This was a small hospital which was located at the Maitland Camp which was then a base camp for the Imperial Yeomanry. It began with 50 beds to serve the camp but due to men coming from other areas the bed complement was increased to 150. In March 1900, its size was increased further due to a typhoid epidemic and its control was taken over by the Government.

NURSING PROVISION DURING THE WAR

An Army Nursing Service was established in 1881 although prior to this 6 nurses were employed at Woolwich in 1861 and six more were subsequently employed at the Royal Victoria Hospital in Netley. In 1882 the military campaign in Egypt needed more nurses and a selected group were trained and sent to Egypt. By 1898 there were many army nurses working in 22 military hospitals.

It was appreciated that in time of war more nurses would be needed. An Army Nursing Service Reserve was formed in 1897 and run by a committee which was led in peacetime by one of Queen Victoria's daughters, Princess Helena (better known by her married name, Princess Christian). This was also called the Princess Christian's Army Nursing Service Reserve. However, in time of war, it was intended to be transferred to be under the command of the War Office.

Just before the outbreak of war there were 88 nurses employed by the British Army. Initially in South Africa this service had a female Superintendent with 18 Superintendent Sisters and 56 Sisters.[30] This was clearly an inadequate number of nurses to undertake what was expected of them and the Army Nursing Service Reserve responded by providing a further 1,500 nurses. Many of these nurses subsequently joined the regular nursing service and served also during the Great War in 1914. One of these nurses was Emma Maud McCarthy who later became the Matron-in-Chief to the British Expeditionary Force, France and Flanders, 1914-19. She had command of more than 6,000 nurses. Nurses also came from the colonies to support the medical services. For example, Australia provided a further 60 nurses.

Nurses worked in general hospitals, stationary hospitals, hospital trains and railheads, as well as in hospital ships and troop ships returning to Britain with the wounded. Treves commented in his book not just on the quality of their work but of the uniqueness and specialness in this situation:

> They brought to many of the wounded and dying that comfort which men are little able to evolve, or are uncouth in bestowing, and belongs especially to the tender, undefined and indefinable ministrations of women.[31]

Some nurses also provided whatever care they could in the concentration camps established by the British as described in this chapter but there were difficulties in providing an adequate service. In 1902 the Queen Alexandra's Imperial Military Nursing Service was formed and replaced the Army Nursing Service with 67 nurses transferring to the new service.

THE NATAL VOLUNTEER MEDICAL CORPS

In 1899 a "Natal Voluntary Medical Corps" was established and consisted of 14 officers, 46 other ranks and 18 nurses. Their main base was Ladysmith, where Captain O.J. Currie, who was from Greenwich and of Scottish parentage, commanded the Volunteer Hospital. The hospital itself was made up of 6 marquees (each with the capacity for 10 patients), an operating room and a nurses' sitting room. However, on one occasion there were more than 340 patients, so the workload could be substantial. This hospital remained in Ladysmith until early November when they were instructed to move to Ndomba's Spruit in Ntombi.

CIVILIAN SURGEONS

Due to heavy demands placed on RAMC personnel, approximately 500 civilian surgeons offered their services and went to South Africa. Many became well known and Anthony Bowlby, Cuthbert Wallace and Watson Cheyne played major roles in the provision of surgical services during the Great War.[32] Also, serving was Dr Arthur Conan Doyle who was subsequently knighted for his contributions to literature being the creator of the fictional character Sherlock Holmes. In addition to civilian doctors a number of other privately supported ventures assisted the newly formed Royal Army Medical Corps including ambulances, ambulance trains, hospitals and ships.

ROLE OF THE BRITISH RED CROSS SOCIETY

The British Red Cross made an invaluable contribution in a number of ways over a 12 month period. It provided hospital trains, one hospital ship and "lucky bags" of supplies for wounded soldiers as they were taken away on hospital trains. It was involved in the running of the hospital ship "The Princess of Wales", and provided supplies (food, medical and practical items) to British prisoners of war in Pretoria. By the end of the war, it had assisted some 200 hospitals, five hospital trains and eight hospital ships with its outstanding effort.[33]

DOCTORS WINNING VICTORIA CROSSES DURING THE BOER WAR

The contributions by the doctors of the RAMC were well recognised and six doctors were awarded the Victoria Cross and are listed as follows:

- Major William Babtie: He was awarded this for his actions at Colenso on 15 December 1899. He rode across open ground to provide medical assistance and despite his horse sustaining three wounds he provided care for the wounded despite being under fire himself;
- Lieutenant W.H.S. Nikerson: This was awarded to him for his actions at Wakkerstroom, 22 April 1900. On the evening of this day, he went out in the face of heavy shell and rifle fire to attend a casualty. He provided immediate medical care and remained with him until the wounded man was evacuated from this exposed position;
- Lieutenant H.E.M. Douglas: On 11 December 1899, during the battle at Magersfontein, and in the face of severe fire and risk to himself he provided care to Captain Gordon and Major Robinson who had been wounded in addition to many other acts of bravery on the same day;
- Lieutenant E.T. Inkson: In Natal on 24 February 1900 he carried 2nd Lieutenant Devenish who was severely wounded for three or four hundred metres under heavy fire and over ground where he was completely exposed to enemy fire;

- Surgeon-Captain T.J. Crean: At Tygerkloof Spruit 18 December 1901, although he was himself wounded attended to the wounded whilst under fire and less than 150 yards from the Boers. He continued until he was stopped by being wounded on a second occasion, but survived to serve later in the Great War where he won the DSO;
- Surgeon Captain A. Martin-Leake: On 8 February 1902 at Vlakfontein he attended a wounded man despite being under heavy fire from a group of 40 Boers at about 100 yards distance from him. He then went to the assistance of a wounded officer and, while attending him was himself shot three times. Martin-Leake won a second Victoria Cross during the First battle of Ypres in 1914 during the Great War. By a curious coincidence, he attended the dying doctor Captain Noel Chavasse, awarded the VC and Bar in the Great War;
- Surgeon-Lieutenant N. R. Howse: at Vredefort on 24 July 1900. He was the first Australian ever to win the Victoria Cross when he rescued a wounded man under heavy fire.

HOSPITAL TRAINS AND SHIPS

Hospital trains

The British made full use of trains both for supplies and for evacuation of the wounded. It was better to transport wounded on comparatively well-equipped trains than on carts dragged over the land. There was uncertainty initially as to how far forwards the railway could go towards the front (e.g. short of Bloemfontein and Pretoria) and whether it would be feasible to keep replacing or repairing track damaged by the Boers.[34] However, the railway stopped short of the British front line and transport in wagons was necessary for the first part of the journey back to base.[35]

Any who had been wounded further forward than the railway could either be taken forward with the advancing army, or they could be sent overland to the rear and to the start of the active railway system (the railhead); if a hospital facility had been established between the railhead and the front, they could be sent there.[36]

The Princess Christian Hospital Train was the first of its kind and was capable of transporting 7,548 wounded soldiers. The number of hospital trains was increased to six. Four were based in Cape Town and two in Natal. The trains were relatively luxurious for their time and comprised ambulance vehicles of two types; those with a capacity for four officers and 12 men, or those for four officers and 20 men, and each train had a number of these vehicles. In addition, there was an ordinary salon for RAMC personnel, a pharmacy and a kitchen with refrigerated cupboards.

Two tiers of bunks ran along the length of the coach. Each bunk had its own locker and mattress made of horsehair covered by a waterproof canvas (which was used to make them cleanable). There was also a toilet and seats for the attendants and pigeon-holes for storage of dressings or other things which may have been needed during the journey. The carriage was well ventilated and lit by oil lamps.[37]

Hospital ships

The British made use of 15 specially fitted hospital ships which sailed from Durban to Cape Town or from Cape Town and Durban to England. Some of these ships were also used as temporary hospitals when in Durban harbour.

The *Illustrated London News* in 1989 (p.824) described the hospital ship *Princess of Wales* which had been converted from an ocean liner. There were specifically designed wards, with individual "wards" (single rooms) designated for officers, medically sick and convalescent cases. In addition there were operating theatres, a pharmacy and suitable accommodation for medical and nursing staff.

Another hospital ship, the *Nubia*, had initially brought the Scots Guards to the Cape but was then taken to Durban where it remained for the duration of the war. There was accommodation for 474 patients in seven wards. Cots were available for the wounded, while convalescent soldiers slept in hammocks. There was a well equipped operating theatre, dispensary and of course, a mortuary. There were six doctors, seven nursing sisters and 35 attendants and a small number of marines were billeted there to maintain discipline and act as guards.[38] The comforts of the soldiers were clearly considered and thought about and Ashton stated:

> The ladies of Durban came forward with their usual munificence and supplied numbers of deck chairs, small tables and screens, as well as many hanging ferns and palms; these enormously enhance the general comfort and cheerful aspect of the wards. Every day baskets of flowers and fruit, together with bundles of newspaper and illustrated periodicals, arrive. These contributions show that Tommy has won a large circle of sympathetic friends who are only too pleased to avail themselves of this opportunity to tender him a token of their appreciation.[39]

CONCENTRATION CAMPS AND MEDICAL CARE

The British under their commander Lord Roberts, established a system of 45 concentration camps for Boers, ostensibly to provide a home for civilian families who had lost their homes and lands during the fighting. Black Africans were interned in 64 camps, as they were a source of labour for the Boers, both in farming and mining. The reality was that by employing concentration camps, men would be forced to lay down their arms if they wanted to be reunited with their families who had been deprived of their freedom.

On 29 November 1900, Roberts was replaced by Lord Kitchener and Kitchener continued to use and to expand the concentration camp system. Tens of thousands of women and children were forcibly moved into them.

Conditions were appalling and shortages of food and water, inadequate standards of hygiene, poor accommodation and a lack of medical staff all led to malnutrition and rapid spread of infectious diseases such as typhoid and dysentery. There were lethal outbreaks of measles and pneumonia amongst the children. There was a shortage of doctors and nurses, who frequently resigned or left because of the conditions in the camps. Some nurses were provided by the British Colonial Association. Families of Boer men who continued to fight were actively discriminated against and were particularly badly treated. A total of 28,000 women and children and 20,000 Black Africans died in these camps, with a mortality rate of approximately 25%.[40] The high mortality rate was not intentional on the part of the British but happened because of poor administration, incompetence and the problems referred to above which led directly to these deaths.

A statement about the conditions in one of the camps, located at Brandfort, illustrates what was being experienced:

> Among us was a Mrs Coetzee; she had eight children, and four were already dead. One day I passed near her tent and saw three little boys lying on khaki blankets on the ground, and they were covered in ants. The mother, suffering from childbed fever – her newborn son was already dead – lay on a small bed. A girl of seven lay beside her also ill. To add to their misery, the tent was full of khaki lice. If it was necessary the poor boys had to stand up without assistance, although their little weak legs could barely carry them. (Neethling, E.m Mags Ons Vergeet? (Cape Town 1938), statement by Ms M Els (translation), p.34).

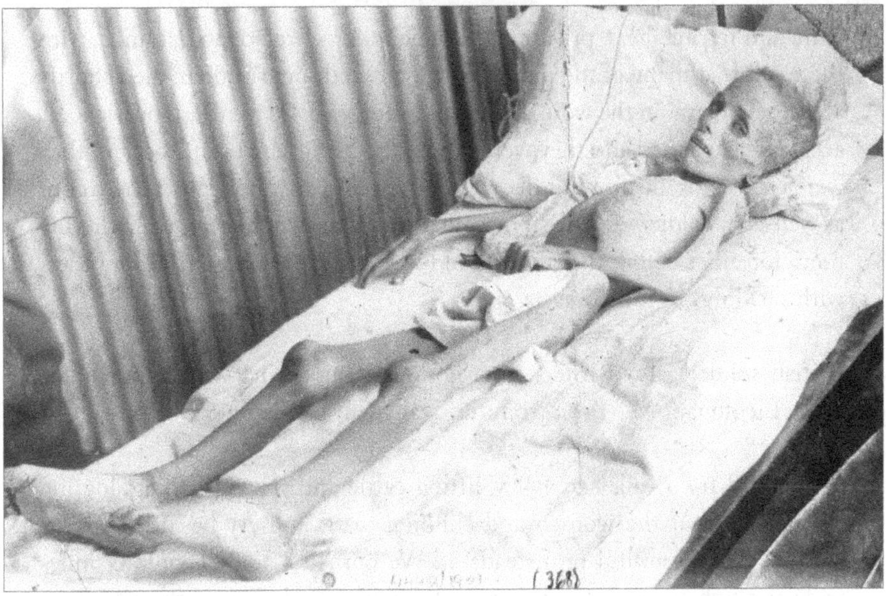

Figure 15.9. Lizzie van Zyl, who died in the Bloemfontein concentration camp. Her father neither surrendered, nor betrayed, his people, Lizzie was placed on the lowest rations and so perished with hunger. (http://www.boer.co.za/boerwar/hellkamp.htm)

There were difficulties in the camps inherent to the internees themselves. For example, the Boers believed in sweating out fevers by keeping the affected person sealed in a tent; they had remedies based on animal dung, animal body parts or animal blood. These of course contributed to the transmission of disease within the camp.

The Boers complained bitterly about the state of the camps and the worsening fates of the 120,000 internees. On 21 November 1901, Acting State President S.W. Burger and State Secretary F.W. Reitz sent a report to the British Prime Minister about a scorched earth raid which read:

> This removal took place in the most uncivilised and barbarous manner, while such action is ... in conflict with all the up to the present acknowledged rules of civilised warfare. The families were put out of their houses under compulsion, and in many instances by means of force ... (the houses) were destroyed and burnt with everything in them ... and these families among them were many aged ones, pregnant women, and children of very tender years, were removed in open trolleys (exposed) for weeks to rain, severe cold

> wind and terrible heat, privations to which they were not accustomed, with the result that many of them became very ill, and some of them died shortly after their arrival in the women's camps ... The vehicles were also overloaded, accidents happened and they were exposed to being caught in crossfire. They were exposed to insults and ill-treatment by Blacks in service of the troops as well as by soldiers ... British mounted troops have not hesitated in driving them for miles before their horses, old women, little children, and mothers with sucklings to their breasts ....[41]

British soldiers also wrote letters home detailing what was happening. For example, Lieutenant Morrison from the Transvaal stated:

> We moved from valley to valley, lifting cattle and sheep, burning, looting and turning out the women and children to sit and cry beside the ruins of their once beautiful farmsteads. ... We burned a track about six miles wide through these fertile valley, and completely destroyed the village of Wilpoort and the town of Dullstroom.[42]

Emily Hobhouse, who came from Cornwall, was the daughter of an Anglican rector and niece of Lord Hobhouse. She had carried out welfare work amongst Cornish miners working in Minnesota in the earlier part of her life but for various reasons had returned to England. She became involved with the South African Conciliation Committee where she heard about the high mortality in the concentration camps. She was the co-ordinator of the South African Women's and Children's Distress Fund.

In December 1900 she arrived in Cape Town and was authorised by Kitchener to visit the camp at Bloemfontein and others to the South but was denied permission to go north to the camps at Kroonberg, Winburg and Johannesburg.[43] She had heard that conditions in those camps were particularly poor. Hobhouse set out from Cape Town with several hundred pounds worth of food, clothing and hospital supplies and after a two day journey she reached the camp at Bloemfontein. She also visited camps at Cape Colony, Orange River Colony and Mafeking. On reaching Bloemfontein, she described the appalling conditions, with up to eight people living in a bell tent. There were shortages of food and water, of mattresses to sleep on, of fuel, and of soap for washing.[44]

She found similar conditions in other camps and described these in her report to the British government in 1901 entitled *Report of a visit to the camps of women and children in the Cape and Orange River colonies*. She stated that the camp system was "wholesale cruelty. It can never be wiped out of the memories of the people. It presses hardest on the children".[45]

This work was instrumental in establishing a Commission of Enquiry of four women led by Millicent Fawcett to report on the conditions in the camps. The Commission spent a total of five months visiting camps, taking statements from all concerned, including those who administered the camps, as well as the internees before publishing their report. Wholesale changes were made and as the condition improved in the camps the mortality dramatically fell.[46]

TYPHOID

Typhoid fever was the major cause of death during the Boer War. Of a total of 556,653 men who served in the British forces, 57,684 contacted typhoid fever and 8,255 died from the disease. This is in contrast to a slighter lower number of 7,582 men who were killed in action or who died of wounds.[47]

Contamination of water supplies inevitably led to outbreaks of typhoid. One of the biggest outbreaks occurred in Bloemfontein, which resulted in between 4,000 and 6,000 deaths from this disease.[48] A description of the conditions in which men fought and which predisposed to typhoid was given by an Irish surgeon, Sir William Thomson:

> ....Water is very scarce on the field, and when great masses of men and horses are moving through the streams they must soon become polluted; often the rivers are the receptacles of dead men and horses. Directions given to the average soldier as to the avoidance of such water are almost useless. After marching for hours in a broiling sun and going through the excitement of an engagement, little water remains in his bottle, and when a pool is reached men drink what they can get without considering the question of possible danger. A distinguished staff officer who was in the recent fighting which culminated at Paardeberg told me that he was glad to "drink his fill" of the Modder water and to replenish his bottle with it. True there were dead men and horses in it, and it was like the dirtiest puddle; but he must at any cost assuage his thirst, and enteric fever had no terrors for him at such a moment.[49]

Attempts to control the symptoms of typhoid were made but often with little effect:

> No special plan of treatment seems to be more favoured than another. Some use salol largely, others swear by Yeo's free chlorine and quinine mixture; others, again, use quinine simply. Apparently no difference in results is traceable to their divergences of treatment. At the Woodstock Hospital a trial has been made of the eliminative treatment on Woodbridge's or, rather, on Thistle's principle-powders of salol and calomel being administered at frequent intervals, in combination with small doses of magnesium sulphate. The medical officer in charge of the typhoid wards informs me, however, that, after a short trial he has definitively abandoned this line. He found it more or less unmanageable. A violent exacerbation of diarrhoea would sometimes set in quite suddenly and apparently without reason, and prove very difficult to check. At first he thought the treatment cleaned the tongue and relieved abdominal tenderness, but later he found that patients so dealt with seemed, independently of any complication, to take on a very asthenic aspect, and more or less to collapse. One point has been brought out clearly at both the Woodstock Hospital and No. 3-the great value of monsonia ovate in checking diarrhoea and haemorrhage in typhoid fever.[50]

Vaccination against typhoid fever had been developed prior to the start of the war by Sir Almroth Wright, Professor of Pathology at the Army Medical School in Netley. While a few soldiers had been vaccinated against typhoid the majority had not because of unfounded fears regarded the safety of vaccination. This has already been discussed in detail in Chapter 11.

SURGICAL MANAGEMENT OF DIFFERENT TYPES OF WOUNDS

Wounds of the limbs

Approximately 60% of wounds sustained during the Boer War were of the extremities. This is comparable to the numbers sustained in more modern conflicts. In World War 2 it was 65%; in the Korean War it was 67%; in Vietnam it was 66%.[51]

Wounds of the leg and thigh were commonly associated with fractures of the long bones. These were major wounds, often with comminution (extensive shattering of the bones) and sometimes involved bone loss over relatively large distances. There was always extensive associated soft tissue damage, particularly to muscles in cases of fractures of the femur, which made this one of the most severe wounds with a high mortality rate. There may also have been associated damage to major blood vessels and nerves which could threaten the viability of the limb as well as cause life-threatening haemorrhage.

In previous wars the usual treatment of these wounds would have been early amputation, because of the risk of infection and its complications. During the Boer War surgical practice was changing and fewer than 4% of all fractures of all long bones of limbs were treated by early amputation.[52] Stevenson noted that the mortality for this type of wound in the American Civil War was 50%. However, he also noted that the long time taken to transfer soldiers with such wounds to base hospitals for definitive treatment predisposed to infection.

Stevenson noted that when soldiers who had sustained compound fractures of the limbs were transferred all the way to base hospitals, they arrived in poor condition because of established sepsis which often resulted in amputation or death. In contrast, soldiers treated at a stationary hospital closer to the front for up to three weeks before being transferred to a base hospital, had a much greater chance of survival and without the need for an amputation.[53, 54] If urgent early transport to base hospitals had to be carried out for military reasons then there was a high risk of death but the mortality was less if a primary amputation had already been carried out before the journey to the next medical facility began.[55]

Penetrating wounds of the abdomen

There was little enthusiasm for operating on penetrating wounds of the abdomen during the Boer War and therefore surgery was not generally carried out for the following reasons.

1. There were many anecdotal reports of soldiers with gunshot wounds to the abdomen who had not had surgery and yet had survived. Treves described several cases after the Battle at Spion Kop where this had occurred:

> Point of entry near navel, and point of exit by side of second lumbar vertebra; entry directly over stomach, and exit by upper part of right loin; entry in anterior part-of one loin, and exit in other loin; entry at tip of eleventh rib, and escape through the opposite axilla.[56,57]

2. The perceived lack of damage from the Mauser bullet led to a mistaken belief that the damage caused was so limited, that any holes in the bowel could and would usually be sealed by nearby loops of small intestine sticking to and covering the hole.

The practical difficulties for abdominal surgery were very clear, the lack of clean water in particular (e.g. for hygiene, washing of towels) was cited as a reason why such surgery was difficult to undertake. There was a shortage of surgical instruments, and Treves stated that:

> The appliances I took with me for abdominal operations get over all difficulties as to really efficient and sterile sponges, sterile silk, etc., and a sterile instrument tray and sponge dish. They also provide a reliable means of making a carbolic solution. The whole tin is so small that three can be carried in a capacious coat pocket. They are, however, still far from perfect.[58]

3. Whilst it was possible for the surgeon undertake an abdominal operation and sometime to repair the damage, the supportive care that patients actually needed, e.g. blood transfusions, antibiotics, intensive supportive care etc, that we now have were simply not available at that time. The likely high mortality from abdominal wounds was a factor used in making a decision not to operate and a good illustration comes, again from Treves' experience.

> A man was knocked down by a Mauser in the engagement of Monday, February 5th. I witnessed the engagement, and saw the rifle fire and shell fire to which the men were exposed. He was hit at long range, and fell about 1 p.m. He was brought into hospital on a stretcher, having been carried by hand all the way. He came in at 5.30 p.m., having had to wait until the infantry and field artillery had retired. I saw him at once. He was blanched and somewhat collapsed. His pulse was small. He answered all questions promptly. He had had an injection of morphine when picked up, and had vomited twice. There was still much pain, but the abdomen was quite flat. There was evidence of considerable peritoneal haemorrhage. The wound was a Mauser wound, and was over the left tenth rib in the mid-axillary line. There was no point of exit, but a well-marked ecchymosis of the right parietes at the tip of the right twelfth rib suggested the position of the bullet. The case seemed favourable for operation, and I carried out a laparotomy by median incision at once. The following condition was found: fracture of the 10th rib, lacerated hole in the spleen, enormous quantity of blood in the peritoneal cavity and evidently from the spleen, a linear rent in the upper jejunum one inch long, four holes (entry and exit) in the jejunum at its very commencement, a hole in the lower part of the right lobe of the liver. All the five wounds in the bowel were carefully sutured, the smaller

> holes requiring in addition to a continuous suture of the mucous membrane - from 3 to 6 Lembert sutures. I found the bullet lying loose under the liver. The wounds in the solid organs had ceased to bleed, and were not touched. The whole peritoneal cavity was flushed out with hot water, which had been passed through a Berkefeld filter after having been boiled. The operation of necessity occupied a considerable time. The patient died shortly after.[59]

Interestingly there was an appreciation that a critical point was the time interval between the wound being sustained and when surgery was undertaken for a better chance of surviving.

> Everything depends, however, on the time that elapses between the infliction of the wound and the laparotomy. Hitherto, as far as I have been able to ascertain, the time that has elapsed has been so considerable that the chance of recovery was but remote. Very protracted operations are hardly feasible in a field hospital when there is any rush of wounded, and by the time that the patient has been transported to some place where there is opportunity for performing the exploration with due deliberation, the most favourable moment has passed are vastly increased. Moreover, as the above and other cases show, recovery may take place in cases in which if they were seen in civil hospitals soon after the injury, exploration would in most instances be advised.[60]

Some surgeons did undertake laparotomy and were of the opinion that some abdominal wounds could be dealt with in a straightforward way:

> The point of entry of the Mauser is very small-often, as Tommy says, like a bug bite; it is not difficult to overlook. The point of exit is also often very small, but is more apt to be slit-like. Several patients have been shot through the abdomen without inconvenience following. In some of these the bowel has been penetrated, as shown by blood in the motions. The hole made in the bowel by the Mauser is very small, and can be closed by from three to five Lembert's sutures. Several penetrating wounds of the liver and kidney have been followed by no symptoms. One distinguished officer had a shrapnel bullet pass through his liver and kidney. He had little collapse, and beyond some temporary tympanites and haematuria he had no trouble of any kind.[61]

However, the general consensus was that the results from operative treatment of abdominal wounds were disappointing and very little progress in the surgical management of abdominal wounds (other than the occasional laparotomy) was made during the Boer War. This was not helped by the opinion of the consulting surgeon to the British Army during the Boer War, Sir William MacCormac. He was firmly entrenched in his position when he stated:

> In this war a man wounded in the abdomen dies if he is operated upon and remains alive if he is left in peace.[62]

Penetrating wounds of the chest

If the casualty survived to reach hospital, the mortality from penetrating gunshot wounds of the chest was 27%, which was better than in previous wars. The bullets used were believed to be less damaging as already discussed and surgeons believed that the dry and clean air might also have contributed.[63] Surgery was never performed. It was not possible to operate inside the chest cavity although wounds of the chest wall were cleaned and debrided.

Gunshot wounds of the skull and head

There were some developments in neurosurgery during the late part of the 19th century and the early part of the 20th century. If patients with head wounds lived long enough to reach hospital almost one third of them survived.[64]

Soldiers who had sustained gunshot wounds of the head from close range (less than 150 yards) nearly all died, either immediately or within a few hours. As the distance between the casualty [65] and the point from which the bullet had been fired increased, the chances of survival increased and the wearing of helmets may have offered some protection at medium to long ranges. There were examples of soldiers who had been shot in the head and the bullet being retained within the helmet. There were some who survived where the bullet had lodged in the brain or had passed directly through and exited the skull.

The first category of wound was "guttering" of the skull.[66] This occurred when a bullet passed through the scalp and ran along the outer surface of the skull causing guttering as it passed by. Whilst there may have been extensive damage to the scalp and associated soft tissues the bone may not have been significantly damaged. However it was recommended that surgery should be performed to "trephine" the skull, even if the patient was well, on the basis that there might be extensive damage to bone on the inner aspect of the skull. Results were thought to be good and so surgeons commonly performed this procedure even if the casualty's clinical condition before surgery had appeared stable. While it is well recognised that deterioration in the clinical condition of a head-injured patient and death may occur due to blood clots developing and compressing the brain, it is quite conceivable that this group of patients would have done well without treatment.

Bullets which penetrated the skull caused much more damage and the amount of damage depended on the angle at which the bullet hit the skull. If the bullet hit at right angles, the outer and inner layers of the skull bone were usually perforated with a clean hole. If it struck at a more oblique angle then extensive damage would often be inflicted on the inner layer of skull and fragments of bone driven into the underlying brain. Victor Horsley was a pioneering surgeon with expertise in the treatment of wounds of the skull and brain who recommended that all cases of fractured skull associated with such depressed fragments should be treated by surgery. Wide access to the track of the wound was made and detached fragments of bone removed, suturing dura (a thick membrane surrounding the brain) and closing the wounds primarily.

Surgery was undertaken through a "trephine" and the wound was explored and underlying damaged bone removed, which could be at some distance from the original wound site.[67] There are reports of removal of extensively disrupted skulls and evacuation of large clots of blood from within the brain along with removal of damaged brain tissue and control of bleeding from the major venous sinuses within the skull. Sometimes such procedures were carried out successfully with good recoveries.[68] These are wounds that even today would challenge surgeons working under optimal conditions. Indeed, Surgeon-general Stevenson expressed the view:

> Even the most severe of gunshot fractures of the skull should be given the chance of recovery afforded by operative intervention.[69]

For those who survived such wounds the longer term effects depended on the anatomical site and the extent of damage caused. If the bullet had damaged the frontal lobe(s) then symptoms may have been minimal. If the motor cortex (that part of the brain exerting control over movement of arms and legs) had been damaged then hemiplegia or paralysis of certain muscles could occur.[70]

Wounds of the spinal cord

Wounds of the spinal cord were studied during the Boer War, and while the prognosis of cord injuries was very poor and most victims died, there was again little understanding about what happened after these wounds had been sustained in terms of effects on neurological function. It was recognised that a transverse wound might affect a very small area of the spinal cord and yet cause devastating paralysis. If a bullet had travelled longitudinally along the length of the spinal column (the vertebra surrounds the cord to offer some protection, with the cord running through the middle) then there might be more extensive cord destruction over a long distance. Bone fragments could be forced into the cord, or it could be damaged by bleeding causing its compression.

It was also documented that even if the soldier was initially paralysed, occasionally some recovery might occur at a later stage. Surgeons did not know why this occurred and wondered if it was caused by pressure on an otherwise intact cord by bleeding into the adjacent tissues or by stretching of tissues. The term "nerve shock" was coined to describe this clinical picture.[71]

Wounds of peripheral nerves

Wounds of the limbs were sometimes associated with peripheral nerve injuries and the large and complex nerve trunks which run into the arms and legs carrying the nerves to control the movement of muscles. Damage to these nerves results in loss of function of the muscle and loss of sensation since all these nerves are mixed nerves, which means they contain both sensory fibres which carry information from the skin, as well as motor fibres which innervate muscles. If the nerve is completely transected then loss of function is total and permanent.

During the Boer War it was noted that if the nerve was not transected but there was an adjacent soft tissue wound or fracture, then the nerve might stop functioning for a while before some or all function returned. There was no way of knowing how much function would return and surgeons recognised that all they could do was wait and see what happened to the wounded soldier subsequently. Typical examples of such cases were reported as follows:

> Thus in one case I saw the ulnar nerve carefully exposed in the lower part of the axilla in the hope of relieving symptoms of a similar nature to those described above. The cicatricial track of the missile was seen, but it did not affect the ulnar or any other of the nerve trunks, nor was the ulnar nerve

other than perfectly normal in appearance. In another case a large nerve trunk was involved in the cicatricial track of a Mauser bullet which had perforated the Ilium, and, judging by its direction, had injured the nerve a little below the sciatic notch. It may be observed incidentally that the almost undeviating-track of these bullets, whatever the tissues they meet with, renders the task of the surgeon to some extent easier. The patient suffered extremely from pain along the course and distribution of the sciatic nerve. The hyperaesthetic area was extensive and most marked. In this case, as in some others, the tenderness of the tibia was marked. There was foot drop. The diagnosis made was bruising of the sciatic nerve and involvement in cicatricial tissue. This diagnosis was borne out to the letter. Some two inches below the exit of the nerve trunk it was found caught in cicatricial tissue as tough and dry as that following a burn. This cicatricial tissue compressed the nerve and grooved it as a fibrous ring compresses a strangulated hernia. All this tough material was dissected off and the nerve set free. The immediate after-results as regards the pain were satisfactory, but the foot drop persisted, and the greatly wasted flexor muscles of the thigh acted only in the feeblest manner.[72]

SUMMARY

The Boer War marks the last major conflict to be discussed in this book. Many of the types of wounds that surgeons dealt with surgically during this conflict bore a close resemblance to the wounds that George James Guthrie and John Hennen were tackling during the Peninsular War ninety years before. Surgeons in the Boer War operated on wounds of the extremities, just as Guthrie and Hennen had done, although amputation was resorted to much less frequently than in the Crimean War or the Peninsular War. Thanks to microbiology surgeons understood about wound infections and anti-septic and aseptic surgery significantly reduced the risk of this happening. Instead of "inflammation" being regarded as part of the normal healing process, it was now perceived as a complication. Hospital gangrene, once the scourge of military hospitals during the nineteenth century was now an entity of the past.

Wounds of the skull and brain were treated more aggressively and surgery became the rule rather than the exception and became more widely applied and accepted compared with the more sporadic attempts at intervention in earlier conflicts. That much then denotes progress.

On the other hand, patients with penetrating chest wounds lived or died depending on whether or not there had been damage to vital structures. Likewise it was generally accepted that abdominal wounds should be left well alone, and Sir William MacCormac's stance did nothing to encourage surgical initiative in this field. Despite the fact that general anaesthesia had been available for more than half a century, very little progress had been made in military abdominal surgery.

ENDNOTES

1. James, T., "Gunshot Wounds of the South African War," *South African Medical Journal, 1971; 45: pp.1089-1095.*
2. Benton, E.H., "British surgery in the South African War: the work of Major Frederick Porter", *Medical History 1977; 21: pp.275-290.*
3. Stevenson, W.F., "Notes on surgical experiences of the Boer War", *Journal of the Royal Army Medical Corps* 1903: pp.91-94.
4. Benton, E.H., *op cit.*
5. Stevenson, W.F., *op. cit.*
6. de Villiers, J.C., "Hospitals in Cape Town during the Anglo-Boer War", *South African Medical Journal* 1999; 89: pp.75-82.
7. Benton, E.H., *op. cit.*
8. Treves, F., *Tales of a Field Hospital.* London: Cassell and Company Ltd, 1900, p.64.
9. Gubbins, W.L., "Field Medical Organisation – The lessons of the War." *Journal of the Royal Army Medical Corps* 1904; 2: pp.446-451.
10. "A South African Campaigner, the Medical aspects of the Boer War", *British Medical Journal* 1899; 2: pp.1485-7.
11. Pakenham, T., *The Boer War.* London: George Weidenfield and Nicolson Ltd, 1979.
12. Treves, F., *op. cit.*, p.14.
13. *Ibid*, p.20.
14. Treves, F., *Tales of a Field Hospital.* London: Cassell and Company Ltd, 1900.
15. *Ibid*, p.20.
16. *Ibid*, p.21.
17. Treves, F., *Tales of a Field Hospital.* London: Cassell and Company Ltd, 1900.
18. *Ibid*, p.15.

19. *Ibid*, p.15.
20. *Ibid*, p.16.
21. *Ibid*, p.21.
22. *Ibid*, p.69.
23. *Ibid*, p.44.
24. Gubbins, W.L., *op.cit.* pp.446-451.
25. Benton E.H., *op. cit.*, pp.275-290.
26. *Ibid.*
27. Scotland, T., S.D.Heys (eds.), *War Surgery 1914-1918*. Solihull: Helion & Company, 2012.
28. Gubbins, W.L., *op. cit.*, pp.446-451.
29. de Villiers, J.C., "Hospitals in Cape Town during the Anglo-Boer War "*South African Medical Journal* 1999; 89:pp.75-77.
30. Chamberlain M. Nurses in the Boer War. Available at: http://www.bwm.org.au/site/Nurses.asp. Accessed 07/14/2012.
31. Treves, F., *op. cit.*, p.35.
32. Scotland, T.R., S.D.Heys, *op. cit.*
33. The British Red Cross. The Second Boer War. Available at: http://www.redcross.org.uk/About-us/Who-we-are/Museum-and-archives/Historical-factsheets/Boer-wars. Accessed 05/05/2012.
34. "A South African Campaigner, The Medical aspects of the Boer War", *British Medical Journal* 1899; 2: pp.1485-87.
35. *Ibid.*
36. *Ibid.*
37. *Ibid.*
38. Ashton G. "The hospital ship *Nubia*", *British Medical Journal* 1900; pp.345-1.
39. *Ibid.*
40. Gellately R.K.B., *The Specter of Genocide: Mass Murder in Historical Perspective* Cambridge: Cambridge University Press; 2003. p.159.
41. Women and Children in White Concentration Camps during the Anglo-Boer War, 1900-1902 Available at: http://www.sahistory.org.za/topic/timeline-women-children-white-concentration-camps-during-anglo-boer-war-1900-1902. Accessed 04/30/2012.
42. Hobhouse, E., *The brunt of the war and where it fell.* London: Methuen and Co., 1902, p.41.
43. *Ibid*, p.115.
44. *Ibid*, p.117.

45. Hobhouse, E., *Report of a Visit to the Camps of Women and Children in the Cape and Orange River Colonies.* London: Friars Printing Association, Ltd., 1901.
46. Concentration Camps Commission. *Report on the Concentration Camps in South Africa, by the Committee of Ladies Appointed by the Secretary of State for War, containing Reports on the Camps in Natal, The Orange River Colony, and the Transvaal.* 1902. London: Printed for HMSO by Eyre and Spottiswoode, 1902.
47. de Villiers JC. The medical aspect of the Anglo-Boer War, 1899-1902 Part II. 1984; Available at: http://samilitaryhistory.org/vol063jc.html. Accessed 06/29/2012.
48. *Ibid.*
49. Thomson, W. "An advanced base hospital", *British Medical Journal* 1900; p.909-1.
50. Anonymous. "Notes on the base hospitals in Cape Colony", *British Medical Journal* 1900. pp.910-1.
51. Parker, P.J., "Surgical experiences from the Boer War", *Journal of the Royal Army Medical Corps* 2002; 148, pp.89-95.
52. Stevenson, W.F., *op. cit.* pp.91-4.
53. *Ibid.*
54. Stevenson, W.F., "Notes on surgical experiences of the Boer War", *Journal of the Royal Army Medical Corps* 1903. pp.91-4; discussion pp.89-90.
55. *Ibid.*
56. Treves, F. "The War in South Africa. After Spion Kop". *British Medical Journal* 1900; pp.599-607.
57. Dent, C.T., "Slighter bullet wounds", *British Medical Journal* 1900; p.662-1.
58. Treves, F. "The War in South Africa. After Spion Kop". *British Medical Journal* 1900; pp.599-607.
59. Treves, F. "The War in South Africa. After Spion Kop". *British Medical Journal* 1900; pp.599-607.
60. Dent, C.T., *op. cit.*
61. Treves, F., "The War in South Africa The battle of Tugela". *British Medical Journal* 1900; 1:pp.219-222.
62. Bennett, J.D., "Abdominal surgery in war-the early story" *Journal of the Royal Society of Medicine* 1991; 84(9): pp.554-557.
63. Parker, P.J., *op.cit.* pp.89-95.

64. Currie D., "Wounds of the skull and brain". In: Scotland T., S.D. Heys (eds.), *War Surgery 1914-1918*. Solihull: Helion & Company, 2012, pp.234-255.
65. Stevenson, W.F. *op. cit.*, pp.91-4.
66. Anonymous. "Bullet wounds of the head. A humane war", *British Medical Journal* 1900, pp.471-2.
67. Currie D., *op. cit.*
68. Anonymous. Bullet wounds of the head. A humane war," *British Medical Journal* 1900, pp.471-2.
69. Stevenson, W.F., *op. cit.*, pp.91-4.
70. *Ibid.*
71. Dent, C.T., "Bullet injuries of nerve trunks and of the spinal cord", *British Medical Journal*; 1900 pp.406-1.
72. *Ibid.*

16

The Russo-Japanese War

The Russo-Japanese War is often regarded as the first major war of the 20th century and as such is considered of particular interest. Both powers, with their expanding empires, had designs over Manchuria and Korea for a variety of reasons. Very important was the access to better sea-ports for both military and trading purposes. Whilst a discussion of the historical aspects of the war is beyond the subject matter of this book it is important to note that military attachés and observers from foreign powers had the opportunity to study how this war was conducted and to learn lessons from it for their own future use should they find themselves in further conflicts. They were particularly interested in the military tactics and the weapons used and also the medical care of the wounded. In terms of the human cost of the war, it has been estimated that the number of Japanese battle casualty deaths was approximately 47,000 and if non-battle casualties are included losses reached 80,000. Russian losses were between 40,000 and 70,000 men but it is not possible to know the exact figure.

JAPANESE ORGANISATION OF CARE FOR THE WOUNDED

The Japanese implemented a system which was designed to provide improved medical care for casualties.[1]

This was modelled on the Letterman plan which was introduced during the American Civil War (see Chapter 12) and which aimed to evacuate wounded rapidly to the rear. This was by a system where the initial step was to take the casualty to a first aid facility, then a field hospital where immediate and life saving care could be delivered, before finally reaching a hospital at the rear where definitive surgery would be undertaken.[2] The Japanese system was extremely well organised.

Battalion or regimental units

Battalion or regimental units provided immediate first aid including the application of field dressings and splints. If the fighting was very heavy this facility could also function as a minor temporary dressing station.

In terms of medical personnel, two medical officers were assigned to each battalion and they were equipped with four medical and surgical panniers. In addition a non-commissioned officer from the medical service was attached to each company. He was provided with a special "surgical" haversack with first aid equipment and he was accompanied by four stretcher bearers, with one stretcher for each company.

The stretcher bearer battalions

The first organised medical care was delivered by Stretcher Bearer Battalions and each division was provided with one such battalion. During peacetime, each infantry battalion contributed 16 men to help form a reserve battalion which was planned to be mobilised in the event of war. The main duty of the Stretcher Bearer Battalion was to form a Main Dressing Station (MDS) which was designed to provide first aid and to stabilise the wounded before they were transported to field hospitals. It was positioned approximately one kilometre behind the front line. However, if the military situation dictated, medical officers could set up temporary dressing stations closer to the front to carry out these functions until the MDS was established, at which time the personal manning the temporary stations were brought back to the MDS.[3]

The MDS itself comprised four departments:

1. Admission and Discharge Department (split into 2 sections, one for admitting the wounded and the other for evacuating them);
2. Department for serious cases;
3. Department for light cases;
4. Apothecaries department.

Stretcher bearers transported the wounded to the main dressing station where they were examined to assess the type of wound and its severity. Surgery was only undertaken if absolutely necessary as an immediate life saving measure. Otherwise the wounds of the casualties were dressed and fractures were splinted before they were taken by the stretcher bearer battalion to the field hospital.

There were approximately 160 stretcher bearers and the total number of stretchers was 40. The dressing station staff were all from the medical service and comprised:

- 8 medical officers;
- 2 apothecaries;
- 40 non-commissioned officers and men.

Their equipment was contained in 16 panniers and each man had a rucksack containing more medical equipment. The Japanese planned that dressing stations could be split into two identical sections so as to be flexible as circumstances demanded. Between engagements men carried out maintenance tasks and helped in the transport of casualties to the rear.

Field hospitals

Each Japanese army division was provided with six field hospitals which were numbered very simply 1 to 6. Each had 200 beds and was supplied with enough equipment to be able to provide medical care for 200 men for up to 2 weeks. It was staffed by:

- 6 medical officers;
- 2 apothecaries (or 1 apothecary and 1 compounder);
- 40 non-commissioned officers and men.

A field hospital could also be divided into two identically equipped hospitals to spread the medical care. There were no female nurses and the wounded were looked after by male sick attendants who were different from the male orderlies found in the British system.[4]

Reserve Medical Personnel

Each division had a medical reserve unit which gave the field hospital itself mobility. It moved in to replace the field hospital when the field hospital was required to move with the division to which it was attached. The hospital taken over by the reserve unit was designated a "stationary" field hospital with a staffing of:

- 14 medical officers;

- 3 apothecaries;
- 120 men.

Equipment and supplies were provided for up to 600 patients for one week. There were sufficient reserves of men to take over three field hospitals if these units had to move with their divisions.

The sick transport committees

The responsibility for the transport of the wounded along the established evacuation pathway lay with the sick transport committee, also known as the Sick and Wounded Transport Department, which was also responsible for procuring transport material and personnel from wherever it could. Each division had one of these committees with a medical officer and a combatant officer working together to supply the appropriate needs for the division.

The reserve medical store

Each division was provided with a single reserve medical store which followed wherever the reserve medical personnel went. It supplied and replenished field hospitals located in areas where fighting was taking place and also supplied regimental units, field hospitals, bearer battalions and the stationary hospitals formed by the reserve personnel.

Line of communication hospitals

Lines of communication hospitals may be regarded as the equivalent of what the British called stationary and general hospitals (see previous chapters). They varied in size and number and were usually an expansion of the stationary field hospitals which were staffed by the reserve personnel.[5]

Hospital ships

Hospitals ships were used to evacuate the wounded from Southern Manchuria to Japan. The number of ships varied according to demand and was generally around seven. Each ship could accommodate 200 wounded and two belonged to the Red Cross. They were all well equipped and catered for the most recent advances in medicine, e.g. X-rays and disinfecting facilities for surgical instruments. There were doctors, nurses (often female) and support staff. Wounded soldiers from both sides were often treated and convalesced together.

The Red Cross in Japan

The Red Cross had an extensive network in Japan with approximately one million members together with having the support of the Japanese Royal Family.[6]

It provided medical care for the wounded and often used hospitals in Japan when medical staff vacated them after they joined the military services. The Red Cross provided approximately 3,000 female and 2,000 male nurses and although the females were not sent to the front line they did provide care for the sick and wounded in hospitals in Japan.[7]

Sanitation

The Japanese paid very strict attention to hygiene with the germ theory of disease very much in mind. Strict measures were employed, including the sterilisation of water and provision of clean uniforms before battle, in case of wounding. Sterile dressings were routinely employed and wounds were disinfected. There were no cases of cholera or malaria amongst Japanese troops and the number of reported cases of typhus and dysentery was only one sixth that reported in the Russian troops.[8]

RUSSIAN MEDICAL ORGANISATION

Russian Army Medical Services were less well prepared than the Japanese although a great deal of assistance was provided by the Red Cross. The Adjutant-General of the Army was in overall command but the Chief Sanitary Inspector of the Manchurian Army, Lt-General Trepov, effectively ran the service. His authority extended to all hospitals, except mobile units positioned with the different divisions, which were under the jurisdiction of the divisional commander. [9]

Surgeon General Wreden worked directly under the Chief Sanitary Inspector and was responsible for medical care rather than for administration. His duties were:[10]

- Provision of sanitary and medical measures for the preservation of the health of the army;

- Treatment of the sick and wounded;
- Selection of men for evacuation;
- Preparation of lists of medical stores;
- General supervision of medical personnel in the army.

The importance of diseases and epidemics and their impact on the strength of the army were well known from previous conflicts. Working under the command of the Surgeon General were two military hygienists (one at a base and one working in the field with the divisions) who were both medical officers. They were tasked with reporting to the Surgeon General on issues relating to hygiene and took administrative control when there were outbreaks of disease. A civilian bacteriologist was appointed to provide additional support who was also under the orders of the Surgeon General.[11]

The role of the Red Cross was particularly important in the provision of care and the key figure in the Red Cross was the Plenipotentiary of the Red Cross Society who was in charge of all their resources.

The Red Cross was organised into five divisions located at Port Arthur, Vladivostok, Liao-yang, Chita, and Irkutsk. Care was delivered to the wounded by their "fling detachments" which comprised up to two surgeons, three or four medical students and a similar number of stretcher bearers.[12] They provided immediate treatment of the wounded although transport to the divisional hospitals was a regimental responsibility.

Organisation of services in each army corps

Reporting to the Surgeon General was a corps surgeon who was assisted by a corps sanitary officer. These posts carried the rank of Colonel and the incumbent officers supported each other; the surgeon was responsible for medical matters and the sanitary officer focussed mainly on administration. Falling into the surgeon's remit was the treatment of the wounded, the organisation of dressing stations before and during battles and command over the Red Cross resources attached to the corps. The sanitary officer provided support by taking responsibility for sanitation together with logistics such as the provision of food, horses and transport for the wounded.[13]

Organisation of Services in each army division

Within each army corps were army divisions, each with a chief surgeon who was responsible to the divisional commander in general but for medical matters was answerable to the corps surgeon. The chief surgeon also had the assistance of a sanitary inspector who was placed under his command.

Regimental Care

At the regimental level there was a hospital with 16 beds and with limited supplies of medicines and surgical instruments. There were up to five doctors supported by assistants and orderlies. Each soldier had a field dressing which he carried with him and if possible would apply to his wound should one be inflicted. If he was incapable of doing so, then staff from the regimental hospital would deal with him at the advanced dressing station.

TRANSPORT OF THE WOUNDED

Regimental transport for the wounded consisted of two-wheeled one-horse carts, but in addition, there were many Chinese country carts which were also utilised. The Red Cross provided chairs bound together and attached to pack animals. The Russians attempted to use four wheel ambulance wagons drawn by four horses but the condition of the roads were so bad that they frequently becoming "bogged down" in the mud.

Red Cross trains were employed in European Russia, bearing a small red cross painted on them and were used to evacuate the wounded. Trains reached as far forwards to the front as possible to locations such as Irkutsk. Usually these trains were deployed in readiness if a major battle was expected when an estimate was given to the Red Cross of the likely number of casualties. There were more than 75 trains and each usually had 16 coaches with a total of approximately 250 beds although after major battles up to 500 wounded could be accommodated. Even goods trains were prepared for use if needed. Each train was staffed by at least three appropriately trained doctors, up to 10 nursing sisters from the Red Cross Society and 40 hospital assistants.

The military also had hospital trains in eastern Russia which were kitted out in a similar fashion. They had medical supplies and instruments and the trains were prepared by the Red Cross although they were deployed by the military authorities.

These train carriages had stretchers to accommodate approximately 12 men but there were also carriages fitted out specifically for the seriously wounded, with 12 iron cots (each cot with its own linen), carriages for the staff, for supplies, kitchens and an operating theatre which was well-kitted out for surgery.[14]

The carriage containing the operating theatre was purpose built, in contrast to the other carriages which were converted from existing rolling stock. It consisted of a standard size railway carriage, constructed from steel, with a wooden interior and a zinc covered floor. It contained an operating table with other tables for instruments but nothing else. There was a further carriage which contained two compartments; the first was equipped as a pharmacy and the second was a small operating theatre specifically for cases requiring more minor surgery.

Considerable effort was made to ensure the best possible standard of hygiene. Each carriage had its own latrine (which emptied onto the track), fresh linen was provided in exchange for dirty linen at certain stops; the kitchen had a cold store for storage of food and there were boilers for its preparation. There were five sanitary detachments and ten disinfecting detachments which ensured the maintenance of hygiene and helped to prevent or minimise disease, and these were transported by the rail system to wherever outbreaks of disease occurred to deal with these outbreaks.[15]

WHAT WAS THE KEY LESSON TO EMERGE FROM THIS WAR?

High standards of sanitation and prevention of disease amongst the troops was very important, particularly in the Japanese army. Another extremely important ground-breaking piece of work in the Russo-Japanese War was the early surgical treatment of perforating abdominal wounds. At the outset, the standard management was to refrain from surgery and not to explore the abdomen to determine what damage had occurred (an operation called a laparotomy). The method of treatment used was the "expectant method." The wounded soldier was provided with pain relief and was fasted but nothing else that was effective was done for him.

"Expectant treatment "was standard practice in the Boer War and this British management policy for abdominal wounds influenced practice amongst both Russian and Japanese doctors. Surgeon General MacCormac, advocating this policy, personally influenced thinking and practice amongst Russian military surgeons through his membership of the Russian Imperial Military Academy of Medicine.

Not surprisingly when this expectant method of treatment was used for the management of perforating abdominal wounds, the results were extremely poor and the vast majority of casualties died. Fortunately for the wounded, one surgeon, called Vera Gedroits, was prepared to challenge this conventional approach and carried out early surgery in the treatment of abdominal wounds.

Vera Gedroits was born in Kiev in 1876 and was actually a Lithuanian princess. She was educated in Kiev and St Petersburg before studying medicine at the University of Lausanne in Switzerland. She was thought to have been involved in controversial political activities in pre-revolutionary Russia and had been sent back to her family's estate and told to remain there! However, this was not acceptable and she fled the country to Lausanne to study medicine. After graduating she initially practised in the clinic of Cesar Roux but due to her parents' deteriorating health and the death of her sister she returned to Russia in 1900.

After the outbreak of the war she led a Russian-supported Red Cross hospital train as chief surgeon. Gedroits' view, based on her experience of casualties in this conflict, was that hospitals which were capable of carrying out major surgical procedures, should be located as close as possible to the casualty if the best results were to be obtained from surgery. This was especially so for those with abdominal wounds. Her surgical teams operated on large numbers of casualties. For example, in one month there were 1,255 patients operated upon, many of whom had life-threatening abdominal wounds. She documented policies for treating abdominal wounds and advocated that these casualties should undergo early surgery. The results of her treatment were not reported by her in a formal way, but comments by her colleagues indicated that this was justifiable and correct. She presented the results of her work to the Russian Society of Military Doctors and her treatment regimes for perforating abdominal wounds were accepted as the new standard of care by Russian surgeons.

Her results were far better than those of any other surgeons. It is likely that this was because of the combination of a strict methodical approach to surgical care together with excellent technical skills. For example, one of the criteria she used was that the casualty should be operated upon within three hours of being wounded. When there was a delay in treatment the results of surgery were significantly poorer. This policy of early surgery complemented an observation made during the Boer War that the few soldiers with abdominal wounds who were successfully treated in that conflict had all undergone surgery within a short time of being wounded. This would become an extremely important surgical principle which was rediscovered and eventually applied during the Great War with even better results.

Following the Russo-Japanese War, Gedroits returned to civilian life but became involved again in military surgery during the Great War, working as a surgeon based with an army unit in Siberia.

She subsequently returned to civilian practice and decided to pursue an academic career, pushing forwards the frontiers of surgery just had she had done in her earlier work with abdominal wounds. The culmination of her academic achievements was her appointment as one of the first female Professors of Surgery in the world when she was appointed Professor of Surgery to the University of Kiev in 1929.

To the detriment of many soldiers in the Great War, the work of Vera Gedroits and her teams of surgeons was largely ignored in the West, despite the very good results they achieved. It is difficult to understand why this happened, because accepted practice in civilians with a penetrating abdominal injury at the commencement of the Great War was to undergo exploratory surgery. This principle was not applied to those wounded in battle.

Instead, British attention focused on the management of casualties in Japan. For example, in 1904 there were reports of the "high quality" of care provided to Japanese soldiers in their wars of the late 19th century from the British military attaché, Sir William Taylor, who later became Director-General of the Army Medical Department.

Sir Frederick Treves, an experienced surgeon from the Boer War, visited the Principal Medical Officer in the colony of Hong Kong where Russian casualties were treated. He also visited Tokyo and his comments perhaps reflect the attitude towards Japan:

> In Japan there is very little evidence that this wonderful nation is at war.[16]

He visited military hospitals in Japan with the support of Surgeon-General Koike, to understand how Japanese medical services had prepared themselves for war. As well as Treves, there was a British RAMC officer, Lt-Col Macpherson who had already been appointed specifically as the British medical attaché.

Further support for Japanese medical care came from the United States medical military observers who commented on the benefits of non-operative management of casualties of any sort and their transfer back to base hospitals for surgical treatment, including perforating abdominal wounds. In the *New York Times* a military visitor to Japan (Major Seaman) commented on the high quality of medical care given by the Japanese:[17]

> When I tell you that of more than 1,000 wounded received in Tokyo prior to July 1 not one had ended fatally, and that everyone remaining in the ward presented a favourable prognosis, you can appreciate the admirable work that is being accomplished there.

However, this article did comment on that fact that the Japanese surgeons did not operate on patients at the front unless there were cases of haemorrhage and so perhaps these patients were self-selected and the extent of their wounds was not sufficient to have been fatal and that is why they survived. The article went on to explain that:

> The Japanese soldier has been taught how to treat his intestines – and consequently his intestines are now treating him with equal consideration. His plain, rational diet is digested, metabolized and assimilated. It is not an irritating, indigestible, fermenting mess-acting as a dentist, enteritis, colitis, hepatitis and the long list of intestinal processes through which we were all so familiar in the hospital wards at Camp Alger, Chatanooga, Tampa, Cuba, Porto Rico, Montauk Point etc in 1898.

The same article denigrated the Russians and their medical systems stating that:

> Wine, women and song were certainly the undoing of Russia where a beauty and a bottle were the highest ambition of its officers – from general to corporal. This was Russia's preparation for war. But if the bloody conflict now waging serves to awaken her from her moral nightmare and brings about her moral regeneration, (and nothing less than such a catastrophe can do it) then civilisation will ultimately be promoted and the masses of suffering humanity in that grand old country will come in some measure by their own.

SUMMARY

The Russo-Japanese War was the first conflict during which abdominal wounds were treated effectively and aggressively by early surgery with good results. Despite the groundbreaking work of Vera Gedroits, British medical observers learned nothing of her work, or if they did, they ignored it. Perhaps the political backdrop adversely affected and clouded their judgement. Britain had been deeply suspicious of Russia throughout the nineteenth century and this persisted into the twentieth century, so much so that a military alliance was forged with Japan in 1902 to protect the mutual interests of the two countries in the Far East against Russian expansion.

There was therefore perhaps a pre-existing prejudice against all things Russian at the outbreak of the Russo-Japanese War. Whatever the reason for this medical ignorance, a great opportunity was lost because in the opening year of the Great War, many soldiers died from penetrating abdominal wounds before the lessons of the Russo Japanese War were re-learned by enterprising British surgeons and the prognosis of this most serious of wounds once again began to improve.

ENDNOTES

1. MacPherson, W.H., *The Russo-Japanese War. Medical and Sanitary Reports from Officers attached to the Japanese Forces in the Field.* London: His Majesty's Stationary Office, 1908, pp.142-2.
2. Tooker, J., "Antietam: Aspects of Medicine, Nursing and the Civil War", *Transactions of the American Clinical and Climatological Association* 2007; 118: pp.215-223.
3. MacPherson, W.H., *op. cit.*, p.22.
4. Treves, F., "Medical aspects of the Russo-Japanese War", *British Medical Journal* 1904; 1:pp.1395-1396.
5. MacPherson, W.H., *op. cit.*, pp.142-2.
6. The Red Cross in Japan. Available at: http://www.medicalmuseum.mil/index.cfm?p=exhibits.mcgee.page_01. Accessed 08/06/2012.
7. Treves, F., *op. cit.*, pp.1395-1396.
8. McCallum, J.E., "Russo-Japanese War" in: *Military Medicine: from ancient times to the 21st century.* Oxford: ABC-CLIO Ltd, 2008, p.282.
9. MacPherson, W.H., *op. cit.*, p.545.
10. *Ibid*, p.544.
11. *Ibid*, p.545.
12. *Ibid*, p.539.
13. *Ibid*, p.546.
14. *Ibid*, p.550.
15. *Ibid*, p.553.
16. Treves, F., *op. cit.*, pp.1395-1396.
17. Anonymous. Tribute to Japanese care for soldiers. *New York Times*, 1904.

17

Concluding Remarks

Military surgery throughout the nineteenth century was concerned mainly with operations on the arms and legs. It focussed on the treatment of bone and muscle wounds and did not progress much further than this. George James Guthrie and John Hennen operated almost exclusively on upper and lower limb wounds during the Peninsular War and at Waterloo. Soldiers who had sustained abdominal and chest wounds were not treated surgically and nearly always died; the same applied to wounds affecting the skull and brain. Surgical practice in the Crimean War was broadly similar.

During the Boer War, limb surgery was once again the main focus of activity. However, it is clear that fewer amputations were performed and surgeons were beginning to learn better ways of dealing with these wounds to avoid amputation. Whilst some surgeons did perform abdominal surgery it was generally believed that this type of surgery should be avoided and there was little enthusiasm to develop it. Chest wounds were treated conservatively and without surgical intervention. Interestingly, wounds to the head were treated more aggressively during the Boer War and were routinely dealt with surgically. This was a definite change in practice as it was believed that better outcomes for the casualty would be achieved if surgery was undertaken. Major progress in the management of abdominal wounds was only made in 1904-5 by Vera Gedroits during the Russo-Japanese War, but her observations passed unnoticed by surgeons in the West and would have to be re-learned during the Great War.

One might have anticipated that the advent of general anaesthesia in the middle of the nineteenth century would have acted as a catalyst for the development of surgery for abdominal and chest wounds, but this was not the case. Indeed, general anaesthesia was often regarded with suspicion and actually with good reason. When general anaesthetics were administered to severely shocked wounded soldiers, the pharmacological actions of various anaesthetic agents could cause sudden death and in the early days of anaesthesia it was not understood why this happened.

From the mid-nineteenth century, wars had cost a great many lives from a variety of wounds. The American Civil War and the Franco-Prussian War both resulted in very large numbers of casualties killed and wounded. Furthermore, the Russo-Japanese War provided ample evidence of the multiple, severe and contaminated wounds that shell splinters and machine gun bullets were capable of inflicting. Yet, apart from the work of Vera Gedroits, further surgical progress was not made until the Great War when massive numbers of casualties from the battlefields of France and Flanders would become the catalyst for significant surgical progress to be made. The reader is referred to *War Surgery 1914-1918* [1] for a detailed account of how this occurred and for the surgical developments made during the Great War and which were largely responsible for the emergence of surgical specialties.

Throughout the nineteenth century, diseases always caused more deaths than enemy action. James McGrigor made significant improvements in the health of Wellington's forces during the Peninsular War. However, the measures he put in place were forgotten by the time of the Crimean War when conditions for the soldiers were appalling and they suffered terrible hardships. Deaths from diseases in filthy and overcrowded hospitals led to urgent investigation by a Sanitary Commission in 1855 which made immediate recommendations to improve hospital hygiene in Scutari. After the Crimean War the Sanitary Commission of 1857 introduced further improvements for the benefit of soldiers in subsequent conflicts. The establishment of the Army Medical School in 1860 and the appointment of Chairs in Surgery, Medicine, Hygiene and Pathology put military medicine and surgery on a scientific footing.

These various changes resulted in significant and progressive reductions in deaths from disease during various conflicts in the latter half of the nineteenth century. Matters might have improved further if commanding officers always paid heed to the advice of their sanitary officers. The Franco-Prussian War in 1870-1 was the first conflict during which deaths from enemy action exceeded deaths from disease. Much to the shame of the British Army, the status quo was restored during the Second Boer War when twice as many died of disease as lost their lives as a result of enemy action, a sobering statistic attributable mainly to typhoid fever.

Almroth Wright, Professor of Pathology at the Army Medical School had developed a vaccine effective against typhoid fever which was available for use during the Boer War but fears about the safety of the vaccine meant that it failed to gain approval for use. Wright was so disgusted by the way in which his discovery was dealt with that he resigned from his position.

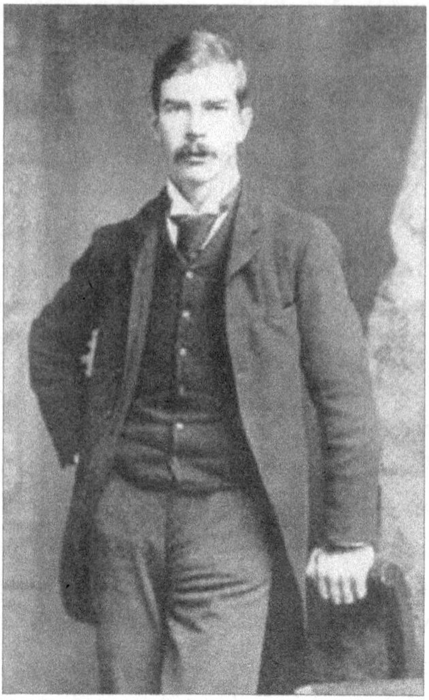

Figure 17.1. Sir Almroth Wright.
(Wikimedia Commons).

In 1906, the Secretary of State for War, Richard Haldane, and his very capable Director General of Army Medical Services, Sir Alfred Keogh, were very much aware that losses from disease were every bit as capable of depleting the strength of a fighting force as enemy action and anxious to minimise such losses, they improved the health of troops further by ensuring close cooperation between medical officers of the RAMC and combat officers.

Keogh drew on all the bitterly acquired experiences of the nineteenth century to ensure that soldiers in twentieth century warfare would be fitter and healthier than ever before. At the outbreak of the Great War in 1914, Secretary of State for War, Lord Kitchener, encouraged men to be inoculated against typhoid before being despatched to the front. As a result of this and all the other measures aimed at improving hygiene and troop welfare, the overwhelming majority of fatalities on the Western Front were the result of enemy action and only a small minority of deaths were caused by disease. Some lessons, at least, had been learned.

ENDNOTES

1. Scotland, T., S.D.Heys, (eds.), *War Surgery 1914-1918*. Solihull: Helion & Company, 2012.

Appendix I

Causes of Death in all Hospitals (Regimental & General) in Peninsular Campaign During Years 1812–1814

DISEASE	1812	1813	1814	TOTAL
Dysentery	2340	1629	748	4717
Febris Continua	2020	1598	387	4005
Vulnera (wounds)	905	1095	699	2699
Typhus	999	971	307	2277
Gangraena	35	446	122	603
Unknown	182	59	124	365
Febris Intermittens	148	139	4	291
Pneumonia	58	133	96	287
Phthisis Pulmonalis	49	158	72	279
Diarrhoea	79	106	34	219
Varii (various)	97	71	35	203
Morbi Chronici (chronic Morbidity)	102	58	15	175
Febris Remittens	67	65	18	150
Hydrops	26	72	21	119
Fractures		6	64	70
Apoplexia	19	21	16	56
Tetanus	4	23	24	51
Enteritis	4	32	7	43
Mortification		32	7	39
Febris Hectica		15	23	38
Hepatitis	5	23	8	36
Syphilis	19	11	5	35
Hydrothorax	5	13	15	33

Ulcus (ulcer)	5	20	6	31
Abscessus		8	8	16
Rheumatismus	2	11	2	15
Carditis	6	4	1	11
Epilepsia	3	6	1	10
Asthma		5	4	9
Paralysis		4	4	8
Gastritis		2	4	6
Variola (smallpox)	3	1	2	6
Icterus	1	3	2	6
Cynanche	1	3	1	5
Sphacelus		5		5
Haemorrhagica		2	2	4
Hydrocephalus		1	3	4
Peritonitis	1	1	2	4
Erysipelas	1	2	1	4
Phrenitis		1	2	3
Synochus			3	3
Haemoptysis	1	2		3
Cholera	2			2
Colica		2		2
Peri pneumonia		1		1
Cancer	1			1
Hernia	1			1
Empyema		1		1
Atrophia		1		1
Comata		1		1
Mania		1		1
Nostalgia		1		1
Anthrax		1		1
Ophthalmia		1		1

From: McGrigor, J., "Sketch of the Medical History of the British Armies in the Peninsula of Spain and Portugal during the late campaigns", *Medico Chirurgical Transactions* 1815; 6: pp.381-489

Appendix II

Nomenclature of Diseases in the Nineteenth Century

Abscessus (abscess)

This is a collection of pus under pressure and was most commonly secondary to a wound infection. The abscess itself might prove fatal, although its systemic effects after spreading to the bloodstream (septicaemia) would be a more likely cause of death in this group of patients. The organism *Staphylococcus pyogenes* was most commonly responsible.

Anthrax

Anthrax is a disease caused by the *Bacillus anthracis.* There may be a skin lesion, a so-called malignant pustule, with associated lymph node enlargement. Overwhelming spread of infection to the bloodstream proves fatal. Alternatively, anthrax spores may be inhaled (wool sorters' disease) causing a virulent haemorrhagic pneumonia which quickly causes death.

Apoplexia

Apoplexy is a descriptive term, and conveys nothing of any underlying pathology. From the late 14th to the late 19th century the word "apoplexy" was used to describe any sudden death that began with a sudden loss of consciousness, especially one in which the victim died within a matter of seconds after losing consciousness. Sudden cardiac deaths, ruptured cerebral aneurysms, certain ruptured aortic aneurysms and heart attacks may have been described as apoplexy in the past.

Asthma

This is a respiratory disorder associated with acute bronchospasm (constriction of the air passages). In severe cases, it may impossible for the patient to breathe in and out. Even today with broncho-dilating drugs and the facilities of an intensive therapy unit, an acute attack of asthma may prove fatal.

Atrophia

This means the decrease in size of a normally developed organ or tissue. This would never be cited as a cause of death today.

Carditis

Carditis is an inflammation of the heart and may be a complication of rheumatic fever (see below) with cardiac failure. Rheumatic fever also often affects the heart valves and may cause late cardiac failure. Cardio-myopathies which may cause sudden death in apparently fit and healthy individuals may also occur with fatal consequences.

Cholera

Cholera was not a cause of death during the Peninsular War but was a significant cause of morbidity and mortality during subsequent conflicts. It is an acute disease of the gastro-intestinal tract, caused by the bacterium *Vibrio cholerae*. Transmitted by contaminated food and drink, cholera vibrios multiply in the lumen of the small bowel and do not invade the bowel wall. They secrete a very powerful toxin which stimulates the bowel to produce massive amounts of fluid. Even although the absorptive ability of the bowel is unimpaired, there is so much fluid produced that severe dehydration quickly supervenes, with electrolyte loss and imbalance as a result of profuse diarrhoea. An untreated person with cholera may produce 10-20 litres of diarrhoea a day. Vomiting is also a clinical feature which further aggravates dehydration and electrolyte imbalance. Renal failure may quickly follow and death from circulatory failure may supervene within a few hours.

Whilst this is a description of the very worst type of case, in many instances the disease is less severe and the patient survives. There may even be asymptomatic carriers of the disease who can infect others who have less resistance.

Prevention of spread of cholera requires strict personal hygiene and water for drinking must come from a cleaned, piped supply, or else it must be boiled. Under no circumstances should flies be allowed anywhere near food, as they can carry the organisms on their legs.

Cynanche

Cynanche means inflammation of the throat region. Cynanche maligna was a putrid sore throat, with pus (presumably streptococcal) on the tonsils. Cynanche parotidaea was mumps; cynanche pharyngaea was inflammation of the pharynx (pharyngitis).

Quinsy is a complication of tonsillitis. It is a collection of pus (abscess) that develops between the back of one of the tonsils and the wall of the pharynx. The medical name for quinsy is peritonsillar abscess and it was a very dangerous condition before antibiotics became available.

Diarrhoea
This has been cited as the cause of death in a number of patients during various wars of the nineteenth century. It is descriptive, and conveys nothing of what caused the diarrhoea.

Dysentery
Dysentery may be viral, bacterial *(Shigella dysenteriae)* or parasitic (*amoebic*). It is characterised by damage to the intestinal lining, with blood and mucus passed in faeces. Water and mineral loss may occur rapidly leading to extreme dehydration and death.
Amoebic dysentery commonly infected troops stationed in tropical climates and was frequently associated with amoebic abscesses in the liver, with malaise, fever and weight loss. The abscess might rupture into the lung after penetrating the diaphragm, with the victim coughing up the contents of the abscess.

Empyema
This refers to a collection of pus between the chest wall and the underlying lung. It may occur as a complication of pneumonia (see below) or following a wound which penetrated the chest wall.

Enteritis
This is inflammation of the small bowel. There are specific inflammatory entities which may affect small bowel, such as Crohn's Disease (which was not described until 1932).

Epilepsia
Fits occurring in the age group of most soldiers would usually be associated with idiopathic (cause unknown) epilepsy and would be quite common. Death during fits no doubt occurred from time to time. It was a common late complication of penetrating head injury.

Erysipelas

This is an acute infection of the skin caused by *Streptococcus pyogenes*, with redness, swelling and induration of the skin and subcutaneous tissues. Nowadays, the condition can be cured using penicillin. In the pre-antibiotic era this was a very serious condition.

Febris continua (Continued fever)

This is a descriptive term of a pattern of fever, without any indication of the underlying cause of that fever. While it might have been an acceptable diagnosis in the early nineteenth century, it would not be regarded as so today. It may have been caused by a variety of conditions which include typhus, typhoid, smallpox, measles and scarlet fever.

Febris hectica (exhausting fever)

This type of fever is severe, persistent, exhausting and debilitating and is associated with wild swings in body temperature. It may be caused by tuberculosis or septic diseases e.g., where there may be deep seated collections of pus in a hidden location in the body. Nowadays, sophisticated investigations can help to establish the locations of such collections, but in the nineteenth century, if clinical examination was unhelpful there was nothing anyone could do to localise the source of hidden infection.

Febris Intermittens (Malaria)

Intermittent fever was Malaria. Only the descriptive nature of the fever was applied in the early 19th century. The fever was often attributed to the evil smells which emanated from stagnant water and swamps. Such regions of course were eminently suitable breeding grounds for the anopheles mosquito, the insect carrier of this disease.

Malaria is caused by infection with *Plasmodium Falciparum*, *P. Vivax*, *P. Ovale*, or *P. Malariae*. These are parasites carried by the anopheles mosquito and when they bite a human, they inject the parasites which then proliferate during the human phase of their life cycle. Malaria is widespread in tropical and subtropical regions, because of the significant amounts of rainfall and consistently high temperatures and humidity, along with stagnant pools of waters in which the larvae of mosquitoes mature. In the nineteenth century, malaria was found in Europe, for example during the Walcheren Expedition in 1809. Fever occurs when the red blood cells of the human host (within which the malaria parasite has been proliferating) rupture, releasing the parasites into the circulation. Typically, this occurs every two to three days, explaining the intermittent nature of the fever. Malaria caused by *P. Falciparum* is particularly dangerous and may be associated with sudden death due to cerebral involvement.

For once, treatment was effective in the early nineteenth century and involved giving Peruvian bark which contains quinine, a very effective agent for treating malaria.

Febris Remittens

This could also be malaria, but might also be in keeping with typhoid or dysentery. Once again, it is a descriptive term, and is not diagnostic of the underlying cause.

Gangraena

This is gangrene, which is derived from Latin, *gangraena,* and from Greek *gangraina*, an eating sore. In the nineteenth century there were frequently outbreaks of hospital gangrene, *gangraena nosocomialis,* where whole wards full of wounded soldiers developed hospital gangrene, which spread rapidly from one patient to the next. It was characterised, as the derivation of the name suggests, by "eating sores", and was graphically described by surgeon John Bell (1763-1820), who was a prominent Edinburgh trained surgeon.

We would now recognise the disease as allied to necrotising fasciitis, which is fortunately rare, as it still carries a high mortality. It is most often seen as a complication of intravenous drug abuse after addicts use contaminated, dirty needles. There is extensive and rapidly spreading infection within the skin and subcutaneous planes which quickly involves the deep fascia and sub-fascial plane, before it runs unchecked along and between muscle planes, culminating in the death (or necrosis) of the body tissues it affects. Septicaemia, circulatory collapse and death frequently occur. The causative organism is the *Streptococcus group A.* When it produces this type of clinical picture, the organism is referred to in lay terms as "a flesh-eating bug", a descriptive yet apt term, which fits closely with Bell's description of hospital gangrene.

Gas gangrene, which is different, is a condition we readily recognise today, and it occurs when a deep wound with much dead or necrotic muscle tissue becomes infected with *Clostridium perfringens.* This organism produces a toxin, which causes further destruction of muscle, and forms gas within the tissues, which is clinically apparent as crepitus within the deep muscle planes as the gas bubbles are compressed. The patient develops septicaemia and dies of multiple organ failure unless the condition is dealt with by radical surgery as soon as the diagnosis is suspected. By the time gas forms, it is often too late! Gas gangrene was very commonly associated with contaminated high-energy shell wounds during the Great War.

Gastritis

Inflammation of the stomach, or gastritis, is often seen today when patients swallow anti-inflammatory drugs to help reduce the pain of arthritis. There may be acute gastric erosions and bleeding. In the nineteenth century, alcohol abuse amongst soldiers would be a potent source of acute and chronic gastritis.

Haemorrhagica

It is not possible to deduce the source of haemorrhage in the cases enumerated in McGrigor's returns. He may have referred to bleeding from oesophageal varices, secondary to cirrhosis of the liver. Certainly gastro-intestinal haemorrhage secondary to alcohol abuse must have figured high on the list of possible causes of such a symptom in the nineteenth century.

Hepatitis

This is inflammation of the liver. Hepatitis may be caused most often by viruses producing Hepatitis A, Hepatitis B and Hepatitis C. Hepatitis A would certainly have occurred in the nineteenth century. Although hepatitis B and C are regarded as "modern" diseases having their origins in blood transfusion and intravenous drug abuse, hepatitis B was described as serum hepatitis in 1885. Hepatitis may also be caused by alcohol abuse, an all too common condition in the British Army of the early nineteenth century. All forms of hepatitis may be associated with jaundice. Some of the fevers (e.g. yellow fever) which killed so many soldiers in the nineteenth century caused severe liver damage.

Hydrocephalus

"Water on the brain" or excessive production or blocked resorption (e.g. after meningitis) of cerebro-spinal fluid gives rise to this condition. It is commoner in infants and young children, whose unfused skull bones expand away from each other, and the head gets bigger and bigger as a result of the excessive production of CSF. In adults, the bones of the skull have fused, and there is no opportunity for expansion. There is therefore a rapid rise in intracranial pressure with headaches, visual disturbance and progressive neurological impairment. This would be an unusual condition for an adult, and perhaps physicians mistook the diagnosis for a chronic subdural haematoma occurring as a complication of a head wound.

Hernia

This must have been a strangulated hernia in McGrigor's series, where the hernia becomes trapped and the bowel within it becomes gangrenous resulting in septicaemia and death. It is surprising that there was only one such case in McGrigor's figures from the Peninsula. One might well have expected to see more.

Hydrops

Hydrops is what we now call oedema. It was also called dropsy. Hydrops Universalis was extreme, widespread oedema. Oedema is often more prominent in the lower legs and feet toward the end of the day as a result of pooling of fluid from the upright position usually maintained during the day.

In itself, it would no longer be regarded as a cause of death, but rather as a demonstrable physical sign associated with an underlying disorder, such as renal or cardiac failure secondary to some specific cause. Use of the term "hydrops" as a cause of death reflects the lack of medical knowledge in the nineteenth century.

Hydrothorax

A hydrothorax (a pleural effusion, either transudate e.g. cardiac failure or exudate, e.g. due to pleurisy, underlying pneumonia, TB, etc) is a condition that results from an accumulation of serous fluid in the pleural cavity. It is often associated with liver cirrhosis and ascites (free fluid in abdominal cavity) in which ascitic fluid leaks into the pleural cavity. Hepatic hydrothorax is often difficult to manage in end-stage liver failure. Given that alcohol abuse was endemic, this probably explains the prevalence of this condition in soldiers during the nineteenth century.

Icterus

This means jaundice, and may be caused by a variety of conditions affecting the liver, gall bladder or bile ducts. It may be infective, or it may have its origins in a mechanical obstruction to the flow of bile from the liver and gall bladder to the duodenum in the common bile duct. The term jaundice is descriptive (the yellow discolouration of the skin), and does not give any clue as to the underlying pathology. Yellow fever was the commonest cause of jaundice in the nineteenth century.

Mania

A manic episode is not a disorder in itself, but rather is a part of a bipolar disorder associated with extremes of mood ranging from complete elation to terrible depression. Suicide during a trough of depression is not uncommon.

Mortificatio

This means the death of tissues which turn black and are clearly dead. Mortification could affect either the legs or hands. It was often the result of arterial damage to the limb and Guthrie talked about mortification in his book, citing the example of a wound around the elbow resulting in the fingers of the hand turning progressively black and of the thigh, where transaction of the femoral artery resulted in a cold limb, with marbling of the skin, followed by progressive discolouration and obvious death of the blackened limb. He distinguished mortification resulting from this local cause, from progressive blackening of the extremities associated with pre-existing systemic disease, such as typhus fever. Patients suffering from typhus fever often displayed peripheral mortification of fingers or toes secondary to extreme peripheral vasoconstriction.

Nostalgia

The term was coined in 1688 by Johannes Hofer (1669–1752). Hofer introduced the term nostalgia or mal du pays ("homesickness") for the condition also known as mal du Suisse "Swiss illness" or Schweizerheimweh ("Swiss homesickness") because of its frequent occurrence in Swiss mercenaries who were pining for their native mountain landscapes while fighting in the plains of lowlands of France or Italy. In English, homesickness is a loose translation of nostalgia. Nostalgia would not cause death, although perhaps the individual who succumbed in McGrigor's series took his own life, or "turned his face to the wall", and stopped eating and drinking till he died.

Ophthalmia

Ophthalmia affected the armies of Egypt in 1801, in what was described as "malignant ophthalmia" by James McGrigor. In Egypt it resulted in many cases of total blindness. It was characterised by purulent conjunctivitis, leading to suppuration of the globe and destruction of the eye. It was easily spread by contagion from one to another. Egyptian ophthalmia was associated with a granular condition of the inner lining of the eyelids (trachoma).

It was treated by the usual methods of blistering and bleeding, needless to say without any benefit. Mercury was administered orally and aggressive surgery was employed to remove congested conjunctiva and to scarify conjunctival vessels. French troops too, suffered from ophthalmia, but Larrey did not interfere surgically and the prognosis was better, suggesting that it was the treatment administered by the British which caused blindness, rather than the disease itself.

After the British Army returned to Europe, ophthalmia persisted and continued to cause blindness. There was a theory that in some cases at least, it was self-inflicted. "Ophthalmia conspiracy" was regarded as a means to escape floggings and the terrible monotony of army barrack life. Men were allegedly egged on by womenfolk to persist with the dangerous practice of aggravating their symptoms in order to obtain a discharge from the army with a pension.

In fact, Egyptian Ophthalmia (trachoma) is caused by *Chlamydia trachomatis* and it is spread by direct contact with eye, nose, and throat secretions from affected individuals, or contact with fomites (inanimate objects that carry infectious agents), such as towels and/or wash cloths, that have had similar contact with these secretions. Flies can also be a route of mechanical transmission. Untreated, repeated trachoma infections result in entropion—a painful form of permanent blindness when the eyelids turn inward, causing the eyelashes to scratch the cornea and cause abrasions.

Ophthalmia caused significant problems in the army for many years after its introduction to Europe from Egypt. A civilian oculist, Dr William Adams, claimed surgical success in treating ophthalmia and his appointment brought him into direct conflict with James McGrigor, who was of the opinion that there was no need for a civilian to become involved with military matters.

Paralysis

This would most likely be due to wounding following injury of the spine, when the outcome was invariably fatal. In non-traumatic cases, paralysis might be secondary to a stroke or some progressive neurological disorder.

Peritonitis

Peritonitis is an inflammation of the membrane which lines the inner aspect of the abdominal and pelvic cavities and also envelops the viscera. It might result from the perforation of a hollow abdominal organ following a wound, or occur after appendicitis, or perforated gall bladder as a result of infection, or be associated with a perforated gastric or duodenal ulcer, often secondary to alcohol abuse. Occasionally there might be a large bowel perforation as a result of a condition known as diverticulitis. All these conditions require urgent surgery, which was not an available option for most of the nineteenth century, and consequently most of these men would have died.

Peri-pneumonia
This is a rather meaningless term, and is not used at all today. It refers to a particularly severe pneumonia when there is a sense of suffocation, loss of speech and breathing, culminating in a speedy death.

Phrenitis (encephalitis)
This is inflammation of the brain and is usually caused by a virus; symptoms include headache and neck pain and drowsiness and nausea and may lead to unconsciousness and death.

Phthisis Pulmonalis
This is pulmonary tuberculosis, a common condition in the nineteenth and early twentieth century. It is caused by the organism *Mycobacterium tuberculosis*, which was first described by Robert Koch in 1882, who subsequently received the Nobel Prize in Medicine for his discovery in 1905. The organism has also been known as the *Tubercle bacillus*, or "*Koch's bacillus*"

The disease is spread directly from one individual to another by droplet inhalation associated with coughing. Overcrowded conditions associated with poor housing accommodation in a malnourished population of poor general health predisposes to the spread of tuberculosis. Treated nowadays with antibiotics, tuberculosis is "enjoying" resurgence in immunologically compromised individuals suffering from AIDS.

Plague
Bubonic plague is an infection of the lymphatic system usually resulting from the bite of an infected flea, Xenopsylla cheopis (the rat flea). The fleas are often found on rodents such as rats and mice, and seek out other prey when their rodent hosts die. The bacteria form aggregates in the gut of infected fleas and this results in the flea regurgitating ingested blood, which is now infected, into the bite site of a rodent or human host. Once established, bacteria rapidly spread to the lymph nodes and multiply. *Yersinia Pestis* (formerly known as *Pasteurella Pestis*) bacilli can resist phagocytosis (the engulfing, ingestion and destruction of bacteria by the body's white blood cells, the defence mechanism against invading bacteria) and even reproduce inside phagocytes (white cells). As the disease progresses, the infected lymph nodes can bleed and become swollen and necrotic. Bubonic plague can progress to lethal septicaemic plague in some cases, meaning that it spreads through the blood stream. The bacteria may spread to the lungs, when they cause the disease known as the pneumonic plague. This form of the disease is

highly communicable as the bacteria can be transmitted in droplets emitted when coughing or sneezing.

The nursery rhyme

A ring a ring o' roses, a pocket full o' posies:
Atishoo! Atishoo! We all fall down!

refers to transmission of and death from pneumonic plague.

Bubonic plague is generally believed to be the cause of the Black Death that swept through Europe in the 14th century and killed an estimated 75 million people, or 30-60% of the European population.

Pneumonia

Pneumonia is an infection of the lungs, which may be a primary infection occurring in previously fit individuals, and is caused by the *Pneumococcus*. It may also be caused by a variety of different organisms as a terminal event following a pre-existing debilitating condition such as a severe wound, where prolonged morbidity and immobilisation results in pulmonary stasis, with a resultant broncho-pneumonia which carries the victim off.

Rheumatismus

This refers to diseases producing painful joints, and is a descriptive term giving little understanding of the underlying disease process. It might include rheumatoid arthritis, which results in painful swollen joints, although death would be unlikely in this condition. It might also include an acute septic arthritis of a joint, (hip or knee, for example) and without antibiotic treatment, this would be a very serious condition and be frequently associated with overwhelming sepsis and death. Rheumatic fever, while usually affecting children and adolescents, may also affect young adults and be associated with cardiac involvement, as well as affecting multiple joints.

Scurvy

Scurvy is caused by a deficiency of Vitamin C, which results in defective formation of collagen, the building block of connective tissue in the body. It was prevalent amongst sailors who spent very long periods at sea and who existed on a poor diet deficient in Vitamin C. Dr James Lind (1716-1794), a Scot who was born in Edinburgh in 1716, discovered that scurvy could be cured by giving oranges and lemons to sailors affected by the condition. Scurvy affected troops in the Crimea, and can only have been due to an appalling diet deficient in fresh fruit and vegetables. It was not described by McGrigor in the Peninsular War, and thus provides evidence for the particularly bad conditions in the Crimea.

Scurvy is characterised by painful swollen and bleeding gums. Teeth become loose and in severe cases may fall out. There is bleeding in the subcutaneous tissue with bruising almost anywhere on the body surface. Haemorrhage may occur into joints, into the gastro-intestinal tract and the patient may suffer severe nose bleeds. Wounds fail to heal, a clinical feature of importance to surgeons. Death from cardiac failure is not infrequently the eventual outcome in untreated individuals.

Sphacelus

This is gangrene, or a gangrenous mass. McGrigor classified it in a different category from *Gangraena nosocomialis* or hospital gangrene. This may be what we recognise today as gas gangrene, although despite there being contaminated wounds which in many cases must have been dealt with inadequately, there were surprisingly few cases described.

Synochus

This was a form of continuous fever. Why it was classified separately in Appendix I is not clear.

Syphilis

Syphilis is a sexually transmitted disease and is caused by the organism *Treponema Pallidum*. It was prevalent throughout the nineteenth century. Primary syphilis presents with a sore (chancre) at the site of infection after an incubation period of 9 to 90 days, often with regional lymph node enlargement; secondary syphilis is associated with general infection with malaise, fever and a widespread rash in most patients. Condylomata lata are flat papules in moist areas and are full of treponemes. There is widespread lymph node enlargement. Mucous patches may occur in the mouth, throat and genitalia. Tertiary syphilis takes many years to develop and mainly affects the skin and long bones. The classic lesion is a lesion called a gumma. Quaternary syphilis occurs many years after primary infection and affects the central nervous system, when it presents as General Paralysis of the Insane (GPI) when the cerebral cortex is affected or as Tabes Dorsalis when the spinal cord is targeted. Syphilis may mimic any neurological disease. Cardiovascular syphilis may result in syphilitic aortitis, when the main artery from the heart (the aorta) is affected by an aneurysmal dilatation of the vessel which may rupture causing immediate death.

The admission rate for all venereal diseases, including syphilis, in 1860 was so great, at 309 per 1,000 ration strength that in 1864 the Contagious Diseases Act was made law. Any woman charged by a man of having given him syphilis, was compulsorily examined medically and if found diseased, was retained for treatment. Inspection of registered prostitutes was carried out every fourteen days. The act only applied to the military setting to begin with, but was extended to include the civilian population in 1871. The Act resulted in a dramatic fall in numbers of admissions. Objections to the Act on moral grounds, however, particularly relating to the compulsory examination of women, resulted in it being abolished in 1887.

Treatment of syphilis from the early nineteenth century was mercury, which continued to be the mainstay of treatment throughout the nineteenth century. The first effective treatment (Salvarsan) was developed in 1910 by Paul Ehrlich. Salvarsan was used until penicillin became available. Clinical trials confirmed the effectiveness of penicillin in 1943. Before the advent of effective treatment, mercury and isolation were commonly used, when treatment was often worse than the disease.

Tetanus

Tetanus is caused by the bacterium *Clostridium Tetani*, which lives in richly manured soil. If conditions are favourable, particularly in devitalised tissue following a wound, when there is an absence of oxygen, then the organism proliferates and produces a potent neurotoxin (toxic to nerve tissue) resulting in unrelenting spasm of skeletal muscle, frequently culminating in death. It is characterised by an uncontrollable hyperextension of the spine, with arching of the back and a spasm of the masseter muscle in the jaw resulting in an apparent grin, the "risus sardonicus". Well recognised and described, it was almost invariably fatal.

Typhus Fever

Typhus fever is transmitted by body lice, which become contagious by feeding on the blood of infected humans. The lice then defecate while feeding on another person and the faeces, (which contain the typhus fever bacteria, *Rickettsia Prowazekii*) can get rubbed into small wounds such as those caused by scratching lice-infected areas. It is the faeces, not the bite of the louse that transmits the illness to humans. It is also possible to become infected through contact with the mucous membranes of the mouth and eyes or by inhaling the dust of dried lice faeces. Typhus fever is not spread directly from person-to-person. Typhus Fever is most likely to occur among people living in overcrowded, dirty conditions, with few opportunities to wash themselves or their clothing. As a result typhus fever often occurs when cold weather, poverty, war and other disasters result in people living in squalid and crowded conditions, where body lice can thrive and spread.

The illness usually starts suddenly with a headache, chills, prostration, fever, and generalized body aches. A rash appears in four to seven days, initially on the upper trunk, followed by spread to the entire body, but usually not to the face, palms, or soles. The rash starts as maculopapular, becomes petechial or hemorrhagic and then develops into brownish-pigmented areas. The rash may be more concentrated in the axillae (armpits). Changes in mental status are common with delirium or coma. Toxaemia is usually pronounced. Heart and kidney failure can occur when the disease is severe and this is usually followed fairly closely by death.

Circulatory failure often resulted in gangrene of the extremities due to circulatory shutdown.

Nowadays, prompt treatment with antibiotics can cure most cases, but antibiotics were of course not available in McGrigor's day, and there was no effective treatment.

Ulcus (Ulcer)

Leg ulcers were a common disability and were caused by the tight gaiters worn by the soldiers. Sometimes they were aggravated by the men themselves as a means of malingering. Occasionally as a result of chronic infection and venous stasis, such ulcers caused death. Perhaps they did so by increasing the risk of thrombi-embolic disease (deep vein thrombosis, with dislodgement of clot from leg and fatal outcome when the clot travelled to the heart and from there caused obstruction of the pulmonary artery).

Variola

Smallpox was a disease caused by either of two viruses –*Variola major* and *Variola minor*. It has now been eradicated from the whole world. During the nineteenth century, it was a significant cause of death.

Smallpox virus preferentially attacked skin cells, causing the characteristic pimples (called macules) associated with the disease. A rash developed on the skin 24 to 48 hours after lesions on the mucous membranes appeared. Typically the macules first appeared on the forehead, then rapidly spread to the whole face, proximal portions of extremities, the trunk and lastly to distal portions of extremities. The process took no more than 24 to 36 hours, after which no new lesions appeared.

The disease progressed in four different ways. Ordinary smallpox produced a discrete rash, which sometimes became confluent and carried a mortality of around

60%; modified smallpox occurred in those who had been previously vaccinated and was never fatal; malignant smallpox, which usually affected children, was almost invariably fatal; haemorrhagic smallpox was associated with bleeding under the skin rather than pustules and was nearly always fatal. Death resulted from multi organ failure.

Vaccination against smallpox was introduced to the British Army in 1800, Jenner having introduced vaccination in 1796. Two British units, the Coldstream Guards and 85th Foot were vaccinated. In 1801, two civilian doctors, Walker and Marshall, went to Egypt to vaccinate all the troops in Abercromby's army.

Yellow Fever

Yellow fever is caused by a virus, and is transmitted by the bite of female mosquitoes, Aedes Aegyptii. In 1881, a Cuban by the name of Carlos Finlay, (who was actually of French and Scottish descent), showed that the disease is carried by mosquitoes. It is found in tropical and subtropical areas. It may be transferred from monkeys to man by the bite of the mosquito. The disease probably originated in Africa, and was introduced to the Caribbean and South America through the slave trade. In the nineteenth century, yellow fever was one of the most lethal of the infectious diseases.

It presents with fever, nausea and joint pains, and subsides after a few days. In some patients, a toxic phase ensues, with multiple haemorrhages making it one of the groups of conditions known as "haemorrhagic fevers". Hepatic damage may occur, giving rise to jaundice. The liver may become greatly enlarged, as jaundice becomes more pronounced. There is profuse bleeding from gums, nose, stomach, intestine and urinary tract. Petechial haemorrhages occur in the skin and conjunctivae. Renal failure may also occur. Death is preceded by coma.

Index